Introduction to
Medical Terminology

Pam Besser, PhD

Professor
Business Division
Jefferson Community College
Louisville, Kentucky

J. Patrick Fisher

Retired Instructor
Medical Secretary Program
Elkhart Area Career Center
Elkhart, Indiana

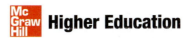 **Higher Education**

Boston   Burr Ridge, IL   Dubuque, IA   Madison, WI   New York   San Francisco   St. Louis
Bangkok   Bogotá   Caracas   Kuala Lumpur   Lisbon   London   Madrid   Mexico City
Milan   Montreal   New Delhi   Santiago   Seoul   Singapore   Sydney   Taipei   Toronto

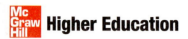

Higher Education

INTRODUCTION TO MEDICAL TERMINOLOGY

Published by McGraw-Hill, a business unit of The McGraw-Hill Companies, Inc., 1221 Avenue of the Americas, New York, NY 10020.

Some ancillaries, including electronic and print components, may not be available to customers outside the United States.

This book is printed on acid-free paper.

10 11 12 DOW/DOW 1 0 9 8 7 6

ISBN 978-0-07-301310-7
MHID 0-07-301310-2

Publisher, Career Education: *David T. Culverwell*
Senior Sponsoring Editor: *Roxan Kinsey*
Managing Developmental Editor: *Patricia Hesse*
Editorial Coordinator: *Connie Kuhl*
Senior Marketing Manager: *James F. Connely*
Lead Project Manager: *Joyce Berendes*
Senior Production Supervisor: *Sherry L. Kane*
Lead Media Project Manager: *Audrey A. Reiter*
Media Technology Producer: *Janna Martin*
Designer: *Laurie B. Janssen*
Cover Design and Illustration: *Lisa Gravunder*
Senior Photo Research Coordinator: *Lori Hancock*
Supplement Producer: *Tracy L. Konrardy*
Compositor: *Electronic Publishing Services Inc., NYC*
Typeface: *11/13 Minion*
Printer: *R. R. Donnelley Willard, OH*

Formerly titled *Basic Medical Terminology* by Patrick Fisher

All pronunciations and definitions presented in this textbook appear in Dorland's *Illustrated Medical Dictionary*, 30th ed.

Chapter Openers:
1: © Corbis Royalty Free; **2:** © Vol. 43/PhotoDisc; **3:** © Corbis Royalty Free; **4:** © Vol. 46/PhotoDisc; **5:** © PhotoDisc; **6:** © Vol. 113/PhotoDisc; **7:** © PhotoDisc; **8:** © Vol. 59/PhotoDisc; **9:** © Vol. 110/PhotoDisc; **10:** © Corbis Royalty Free; **11:** © Vol. 40/PhotoDisc; **12:** © Vol. 37SS/PhotoDisc; **13:** © Vol. 18/PhotoDisc; **14:** © Vol. 67/PhotoDisc; **15:** © Corbis Royalty Free; **16:** © Corbis Royalty Free; **17:** © Vol. 154/Corbis.

www.mhhe.com

Brief Table of Contents

Contents

PART 3   MEDICAL SPECIALTIES   451

Appendices

About the Authors

Pam Besser, Ph.D.

Pam Besser, author of the Mayfield/McGraw-Hill textbook *A Basic Handbook of Writing Skills*, has a varied academic background that spans 34 years. She has a Ph.D. in rhetoric and composition and currently is a Professor of Rhetoric at Jefferson Community College in Louisville, Kentucky, where she teaches courses in medical terminology (online and on campus) as well as classes in business writing (online and on campus). Her administrative positions at Jefferson Community College include, but are not limited to, the following: Business Division Chair, Acting Dean of Academic Affairs, Acting Allied Health Division Chair, Acting Respiratory Care Program Coordinator, and Acting Human Resources Director. She has published numerous articles in such journals as *Teaching English in the Two-Year College* and *Exercise Exchange*. In addition, she teaches regular medical terminology classes for two of the major hospital complexes in Louisville.

Dr. Besser has taught at the University of Louisville, where she was Assistant Director of Composition, and the University of Southern Illinois–Carbondale. Prior to teaching in university, she taught introductory courses in algebra, trigonometry, and biology to advanced junior high school students.

J. Patrick Fisher

This edition was co-authored by J. Patrick Fisher, former teacher (now retired) at the Elkhart Area Career Center, Elkhart, Indiana. Mr. Fisher hold a bachelor's degree in business education from Ball State University, Muncie, Indiana. He has also done extensive graduate work at Indiana/Purdue University. Mr. Fisher graduated from the U.S. Army Court Reporters School at Fort Benjamin Harrison, Indianapolis, and served as a court reporter.

Before joining the staff at the Career Center, Mr. Fisher was Dean of Education at the Elkhart Institute of Technology, and he taught courses such as medical shorthand, medical terminology, and medical transcription. He helped develop the curriculum for the medical secretary, medical transcription and secretarial programs at the Institute and the Career Center.

Dedication

For Rita, Tom, Tony, Alicia, Tighe, Lisa, Molly, Sarah, and Bennett
Castigat Ridendo Mores and *Veritas Vos Liberabit*

For Joel and Hannah

Preface

Getting the Most Out of Your Textbook

McGraw-Hill and the authors of this book, Pam Besser and Patrick Fisher, have invested their time, research, and talent to help you succeed. Our goal is to make learning easier. Throughout the textbook, you will find sketches and a variety of artwork that will enhance the study of medical terminology.

Introduction to Medical Terminology has 17 chapters and is divided into 3 parts:

Part 1 Learning About Medical Words has 3 chapters that focus on suffixes, prefixes, numbers, amounts, colors, and positions. These chapters provide the foundation for the terms presented throughout the textbook.

Part 2 Systems of the Body has 12 chapters that focus on separate systems of the body. These chapters provide common terms associated with the following body systems:

Integumentary system	Male reproductive system
Respiratory system	Female reproductive system
Digestive system	Nervous system
Cardiovascular system	Endocrine system
Hematic and lymphatic systems	Musculoskeletal system
Urinary system	Special senses

Part 3 Medical Specialties and Psychiatric Terminology has 2 chapters. The first provides terms for a variety of medical specialties and medical specialists, and the second provides psychiatric terms.

The Learning System

Students differ in how they learn and how they respond to various learning situations. Effective instruction and lasting retention don't just happen; they result from materials that are carefully planned and organized in a logical sequence so that learning will occur.

Introduction to Medical Terminology has the following learning system features:

- **Objectives**—guide you with the key points of the chapter
- **Orientation**—educates you with relevant background information for the chapter
- **Terminology Presentation**—informs you with words and word parts that are the basis of medical language
- **Terminology Application**—motivates you with a chance to review the terms and their definitions
- **Drug Terminology** (in the body system and psychiatric terminology chapters)— provides you with common categories of drugs appropriate to the specific system of the body that you are studying. Generic and brand-name drugs for each category are included.
- **Terminology Review for Tests**—challenges you with practice in identifying the words and word parts that you have learned
- **Word Element Review**—allows you with the opportunity for further practice identifying words and definitions
- **Case Studies** (in the body system chapters)—stimulate you with practice using medical terms in appropriate and real-life contexts

Special Features

Chapters have been organized to make learning medical terminology easier for your students. *Introduction to Medical Terminology* has the following features:

- Part 1 Learning About Medical Words
- Part 2 Systems of the Body
- Part 3 Medical Specialties
- More than 1000 medical terms and definitions
- Drug Terminology sections added to the body systems and psychiatric terminology chapters
- 52 Case Studies
- List of endocrine glands and hormones (Chapter 13)
- Information regarding the axial and appendicular skeletal structures (Chapter 14)
- End-of-chapter labeling exercise
- CD-ROM audio presentations
- Perforated Flashcards
- Six appendices, listing medical and chemical abbreviations; pharmaceutical abbreviations; common Latin and Greek singular and plural endings; common prefixes; common suffixes; and common STDs for Male and Female

This textbook is supplemented with a CD-ROM audio presentation to help you learn how to pronounce medical terms. Within each chapter you will find four or five separate lessons. For each lesson, follow these simple steps:

- At the beginning of each lesson's Terminology Presentation, look for . Start the CD, read the words, and pay attention to the pronunciations.
- Look for which means pause the CD. Practice the words and word parts until you feel that you know and understand them.
- Look for and start the CD again. As each word is pronounced again, write it in the appropriate space provided in your textbook. Then check your work for accuracy.

Once you complete these steps, you should be ready to complete the Terminology Application section for that lesson. Simply follow the directions in your textbook. After completing each lesson, you will be ready to begin the Terminology Review for the chapter test. Again, follow the directions in your textbook.

Teaching and Learning Supplements

For the Instructor

Instructor's Manual

The Instructor's Manual includes the following information to aid the instructor:

- A sample test for each chapter
- A sample 16-week syllabus
- Complete orientation per chapter
- Answers to all lessons in the textbook
- Two generic answer sheets
- Answers to the testing CDs per chapter

All of this information is presented in a clear and easy-to-use format.

Instructor Productivity Center (IPC CD-Rom)

This CD-ROM provides instructors with *PowerPoint* presentations for each chapter in the textbook. Each presentation includes a list of objectives, chapter topics, and drugs (as appropriate). Easy Test questions for each chapter in the book.

Online Learning Center—www.mhhe.com/besser

Instructors who adopt *Introduction to Medical Terminology* have access to an online course for their students. This OLC includes a variety of activities and exercises for students such as the following:

- Audio flashcards
- Concentration games
- Crossword puzzles
- Case studies
- Labeling exercises
- Chapter objectives

All of these exercises are designed to enhance student learning.

Instructor Lab Audio CDs

The Audio CD is designed to be used in conjunction with the textbook. Students have the opportunity to listen to, and to practice, the pronunciations of all of the terms presented in the textbook.

Instructor Testing Audio CDs

This CD provides 20 words per chapter to use with the answer sheets provided in the Instructor's Manual. This CD is designed for individual testing or a group setting. Students will be tested on the spelling of each word and the definition for that word.

For the Student

Student Audio CD-ROM

Your textbook also includes a CD-ROM for you to use for practicing the words and word parts presented in your textbook. Use this CD-ROM at home, in the car, or wherever you are comfortable listening to the terminology that you are learning.

Online Learning Center—www.mhhe.com/besser

The on-line learning center of this course provides you with the following supplementary exercises to further enhance and reinforce your learning of medical terminology:

- Animations
- Audio flashcards
- Case studies
- Concentration games
- Crossword puzzles
- Labeling exercises

These various exercises are designed to help you enjoy studying medical terminology.

Student Flashcards

Flashcards included with the textbook will help you practice key words and definitions presented in your textbook. Use these flashcards to study the terminology you are learning.

Acknowledgements

This textbook is the result of the hard work and the insights of many individuals. Thanks go to Todd Turner who insisted that I be considered as the lead author for this textbook. In addition, I appreciate the support of each of the following members of the incredible team that has worked on this textbook:

David Culverwell, Publisher

Roxan Kinsey, Senior Sponsoring Editor

Patricia Hesse, Managing Developmental Editor

Connie Kuhl, Editorial Coordinator

James F. Connely, Senior Marketing Manager

Joyce Berendes, Lead Project Manager

Faye Schilling, Managing Editor

Sherry Kane, Production Supervisor

Laurie Janssen, Designer

Tracy Konrardy, Supplement Producer

Janna Martin, Media Producer

Audrey Reiter, Media Project Manager

Wendy Nelson, Manuscript Editor

Jody McAdam, PowerPoint Presentations

The insight and dedication of each of these team members helped me through the initial stages of this project. Accolades go to Connie Kuhl, Editorial Coordinator, whose wisdom, honesty, instinct, patience, good humor, and friendship motivated me and sustained me throughout the various drafts. Her ideas and suggestions permeate the text. The incredible expertise and sense of humor of all of these team members have provided me with the impetus to refine the manuscript and to enjoy learning from them.

REVIEWERS

I wish to thank the following reviewers for their perceptive comments and suggestions:

Kay Aloi, MSN, RN, C, CNS
*Florida State University School of Nursing–
    Tallahassee, FL 32312*

Vickie Barth, EdD, RN
Florida State University–Tallahassee, FL

Holly A. Barton, CMA, MSM, PhD
Glen Oaks Community College–Centreville, MI

Paula Bostwick, RN, MSN
Ivy Tech State College-Northeast–Fort Wayne, IN

Mary L. Brown
Arapahoe Community College–Englewood, CO

Jean M. Chenu
Genesee Community College–Batavia, NY

Karen Cheung
Mission College–Santa Clara, CA

Stephanie Cox
York Technical Institute–Lancaster, PA

Nancy J. Fieldhouse
Ivy Tech State College–Fort Wayne, IN

Tammy T. Gant, RHIT, MA
Surry Community College–Dobson, NC

Kathaleen M. Gilliam RN, MSN, Assistant Professor
*Brevard Community College, Health Science Campus Associate
    Degree Nursing Program–Cocoa, FL*

Elaine Gillingham
Gateway Community College–Phoenix, AZ

Dawn Jackson
Eastern Kentucky University–Richmond, KY

JoAnna Jensen, ARNP, MS
Brevard Community College–Cocoa, FL

Elizabeth P. Keene, BSN, RN
Lansdale School of Business–North Wales, PA

Vicki L Khouli
Ivy Tech State College–Fort Wayne, IN

Sandy Ludwig, RN, MSN, NNP
Eastern Arizona College–Thatcher, AZ

Ann M Lunde
Waubonsee Community College–Sugar Grove, IL

Suzanne LyBarger, RRT
Hawaii Business College–Honolulu, HI

Gloria Madison, MS, RHIA
Moraine Park Technical College–West Bend, WI

Mary Jane McClain
Fresno City College–Fresno, CA

Janet McBride, BSN, RN
Mission College–Santa Clara, CA

Patti McCormick, RN, PhD.
Institute of Holistic Leadership–Beavercreek, OH

Linda Miedema
Brevard Community College–Cocoa, FL

Nancy Moorhead, CMA, CPC
Eastern New Mexico University, Roswell–Roswell, NM

Roxann Moran, RN, BSN, M.Ed.
*St. Paul College of Customized Training & Consulting–
St. Paul, MN*

Patricia C. Moyer, CMA
Berks Technical Institute–Wyomissing, PA

Susan Pazynski
Glen Oaks Community College–Centreville, MI

James H. Phillips, BS, CMA, RMA, CT
Central Florida College–Winter Park, FL

Donna Jeanne Pugh, RN, BSN
Florida Metropolitan University–Jacksonville, FL

Lael J. Richards
Aakers Business College–Fargo, ND

Renee Roach, Director of Education
Andover College–Portland, ME

Candace S. Schladenhauffen
Ivy Tech State College–Fort Wayne, IN

Michael Eric Seeherman
Harrisburg, PA

Timothy J. Skaife, RT(R), MA
National Park Community College–Hot Springs, AR

Ellen Marie Smith, NRCMA-A
Berks Technical Institute–Wyomissing, PA

Patricia A. Stich
Waubonsee Community College–Sugar Grove, IL

Barbara Stoner
Arapahoe Community College–Littleton, CO

Deborah Tchorz
Brevard Community College–Cocoa, FL

Marilyn Fuqua Thompson
Lakeland College–Mattoon, IL

Linda A Walter
Northwestern Michigan College–Traverse City, MI

Jay W. Wilborn, M.Ed.
National Park Community College–Hot Springs, AR

Jackie Whipple, R.T., (R)
Carl Sandburg College–Galesburg, IL

Peggy A Wolff, MBA, RHIA
Western Nebraska Community College–Scottsbluff, NE

Terri D. Wyman, CMRS
Sanford Brown Institute–Springfield, MA

Content and Art Organization

Two opening chapters introduce suffixes and prefixes with a focus on how to learn medical words.

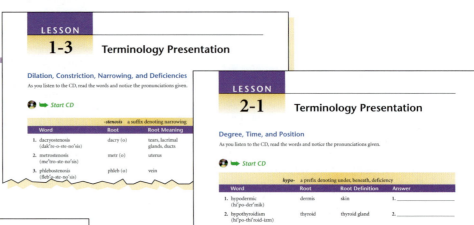

LESSON 1-3 — Terminology Presentation

Dilation, Constriction, Narrowing, and Deficiencies
As you listen to the CD, read the words and notice the pronunciations given.

➡ *Start CD*

		-stenosis	a suffix denoting narrowing
	Word	**Root**	**Root Meaning**
1.	dacryostenosis (dak′re-o-ste-no′sis)	dacry (o)	tears, lacrimal glands, ducts
2.	metrostenosis (me′tro-ste-no′sis)	metr (o)	uterus
3.	phlebostenosis (fleb′o-ste-no′sis)	phleb (o)	vein

LESSON 2-1 — Terminology Presentation

Degree, Time, and Position
As you listen to the CD, read the words and notice the pronunciations given.

➡ *Start CD*

		hypo-	a prefix denoting under, beneath, deficiency
	Word	**Root**	**Root Definition**	**Answer**
1.	hypodermic (hi′po-der′mik)	dermis	skin	1. _____
2.	hypothyroidism (hi′po-thi′roid-izm)	thyroid	thyroid gland	2. _____

LESSON 10-2 — Terminology Presentation

Glans Penis and Terms Indicating the Male Gender
As you listen to the CD, read the words and notice the pronunciations given.

➡ *Start CD*

Look at Figure 10-1 on page 269.

		balan(o)	a combining form indicating relationship to the glans penis
	Word	**Word Part**	**Definition**	**Answer**
1.	balanoplasty (bal′ah-no-plas′te)	-plasty	plastic surgery	1. _____
2.	balanitis (bal′ah-ni′tis)	-itis	inflammation	2. _____
3.	balanorrhagia (bal′ah-no-ra′je-ah)	-rrhagia	excessive flow, bleeding	

andr(o)

		gyn(o), gynec(o)	word elements denoting women or the female gender
	Word	**Word Part**	**Definition**	**Answer**
9.	gynecology (gi′ne-kol′o-je)	-logy	study of, science of	9. _____
10.	gynecologist (gi′ne-kol′o-jist)	-logist	specialist	10. _____
11.	gynecopathy (jin′e-kop′ah-the)	-pathy	disease	11. _____
12.	gynoplasty (ji′no-plas′te)	-plasty	plastic surgery	12. _____

⏹ *Stop CD*
After practicing each word several times, use a sheet of paper to cover all columns except the Answer column. As each word is pronounced again on the CD, write it in the space provided.

➡ *Start CD*
Check the words you have written against the words in the left-hand column. If you have misspelled any words, practice writing them correctly.

Practice
_____
_____

Color coded icons to show the use of lab CDs

Space to practice hard to spell words

Separate chapters for the male and female reproductive systems give extra detail.

This textbook includes all the learning processes: visual, audio, kinesthetic, and vocal.

Mary Jane McClain, Fresno City College

Each body system chapter displays a new labeling exercise. The four color image offers practice identifying various areas of that system.

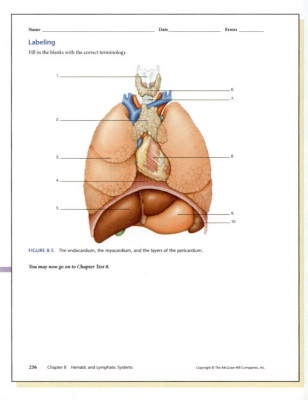

Name _____ Date _____ Errors _____

Labeling
Fill in the blanks with the correct terminology.

FIGURE 8-5 The endocardium, the myocardium, and the layers of the pericardium.

You may now go on to Chapter Test 8.

Real-Life Connection

52 Cases Studies facilitate practice using medical terms in appropriate and real-life contexts.

The Case Studies are wonderful. They are great for a variety of classes.

Suzanne Lybarger, Hawaii Business College

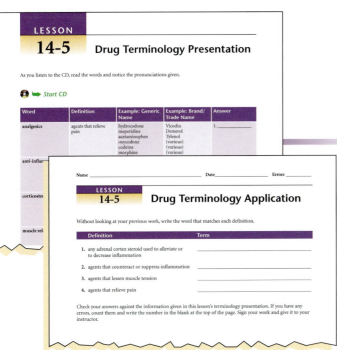

Drug Terminology Presentation and **Application** focus on common categories of drugs appropriate to specific systems of the body. Both generic and brand-name drugs are included.

Chapter 13, The Endocrine System includes **Hormone Presentation** and **Application** sections.

Name _____ Date _____ Errors _____

CHAPTER 7 **Terminology Review**

Case Studies

Read the following brief case studies. In each case study, some terms are followed by a superscript letter. Write a brief definition for each of those terms on the corresponding lines below.

1. M.K. is an elderly patient with cardiomyopathy[a] that has caused considerable endocarditis[b]. His arterial[c] flow is not good, and he has had two angioplasty[d] procedures within the past year. Since his last angioplasty, he has been on an antianginal[e], a thrombolytic[f], and an antilipidemic[g].

   a. _____
   b. _____
   c. _____
   d. _____
   e. _____
   f. _____
   g. _____

2. V. has had carditis[a] for several years and has recently experienced severe pain. She has recently met with her cardiologist[b], who first diagnosed her with this problem. The doctor has scheduled her for a battery of cardiac tests, and she will need to be hospitalized for a few days.

   a. _____
   b. _____

3. After suffering a stab wound to the chest, this ER patient underwent arteriorrhaphy[a] and phleborrhaphy[b] to repair damage. During the surgery, the patient suffered severe arterial[c] bleeding, after which the blood began to coagulate too quickly. Rather than have this patient risk thrombosis[d], the doctor put the patient on an IV (intravenous) blood thinner.

   a. _____
   b. _____
   c. _____
   d. _____

Chapter 7   Terminology Review   **205**

LESSON 14-5 **Drug Terminology Presentation**

As you listen to the CD, read the words and notice the pronunciations given.

🔊 ➡ *Start CD*

Word	Definition	Example: Generic Name	Example: Brand/Trade Name	Answer
analgesics	agents that relieve pain	hydrocodone meperidine acetaminophen oxycodone codeine morphine	Vicodin Demerol Tylenol (various) (various)	1. _____
anti-inflam				
corticoster				
muscle rel				

Name _____ Date _____ Errors _____

LESSON 14-5 **Drug Terminology Application**

Without looking at your previous work, write the word that matches each definition.

Definition	Term
1. any adrenal cortex steroid used to alleviate or to decrease inflammation	_____
2. agents that counteract or suppress inflammation	_____
3. agents that lessen muscle tension	_____
4. agents that relieve pain	_____

Check your answers against the information given in this lesson's terminology presentation. If you have any errors, count them and write the number in the blank at the top of the page. Sign your work and give it to your instructor.

LESSON 13-5 **Terminology Presentation**

As you listen to the CD, read the words and notice the pronunciations given.

🔊 ➡ *Start CD*

Gland	Hormone	Purpose	Answer
1. adenohypophysis cerebri (ad'e-no-hi-pof'i-sis) (se-re'bree)			1. _____

Name _____ Date _____ Errors _____

LESSON 13-5 **Hormone Terminology Application**

Without looking at your previous work, write the name of the gland that matches each definition.

Definition	Term
1. produces estrogen and progesterone	_____
2. produces calcitonin	_____
3. produces steroid hormones	_____

PART
1

Learning About Medical Words

1

Suffixes

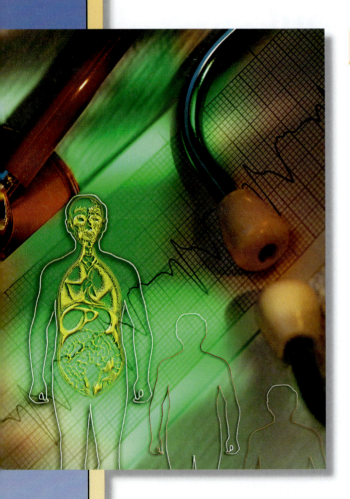

Objectives

After completing Chapter 1, you should be able to do the following:

1. identify common suffixes;

2. categorize common suffixes as noun spellings, verbs, and adjectives;

3. recognize plural forms of terms;

4. understand that suffixes can denote a process: an incision, a visual examination, a surgery, an excision, the process of recording, a surgical reattachment, or a surgical puncture;

5. understand that suffixes can denote pain, excessive bleeding, a disease, a prolapse, an inflammation, an abnormal condition, a fungal condition, a tumor, an enlargement, or an abnormal softening; and

6. recognize that suffixes can denote narrowing, expansion, and deficiency; identify suffixes that denote paralysis, dissolution, a flow, a formation, a fracture, and the study of an area.

Orientation to Suffixes

To completely understand a medical term, you need to learn ways to look at the various parts of the term. For example, the word *splenectomy* has a suffix *(-ectomy)*, an ending that changes the meaning of the word, and a root *(splen-)*, which is the main part of the word. The suffix *(-ectomy)* tells you that the word refers to a process (the process of removing something) and the root *(splen-)* tells you that the spleen is the part being removed.

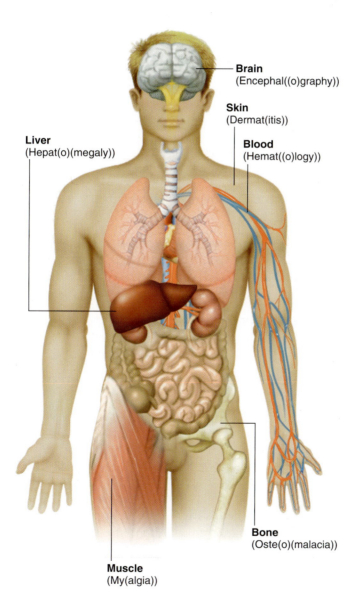

Brain
(Encephal((o)graphy))

Skin
(Dermat(itis))

Liver
(Hepat(o)(megaly))

Blood
(Hemat((o)logy))

Bone
(Oste(o)(malacia))

Muscle
(My(algia))

Learning About Medical Words

Medical words consist of a root (the main part of the word), a suffix (an ending used to alter the meaning of the root), and sometimes a prefix (a qualifying word part placed at the beginning of the root). When a suffix is added to a root (also called a "word root" or "root word"), a vowel (called a "combining vowel") is sometimes used to facilitate pronunciation. This vowel changes the root into a combining form to which a suffix can easily be added. The following examples indicate the use of combining vowels when adding a suffix that begins with a consonant.

Word Root	Combining Vowel	Combining Form	Suffix	Word	Meaning
gastr (stomach)	o	gastro	-scope	gastroscope	instrument used to view inside of stomach
hyster (uterus)	o	hystero	-ptosis	hysteroptosis	prolapse of the uterus
hepat (liver)	o	hepato	-megaly	hepatomegaly	abnormally enlarged liver
rhin (nose)	o	rhino	-plasty	rhinoplasty	surgical repair of the nose
dermat (skin)	o	derma	-itis	dermatitis	inflammation of the dermis/skin
quadr (four)	i	quadri	-plegia	quadriplegia	paralysis in four limbs

Note that combining vowels may not be necessary when a suffix beginning with a vowel is added to a root.

Word Root	Combining Vowel	Combining Form	Suffix	Word	Meaning
arthr (joint)	none	arthr	-algia	arthralgia	pain in a joint
bronch (bronchus)	none	bronch	-itis	bronchitis	inflammation of the bronchus
hyster (uterus)	none	hyster	-ectomy	hysterectomy	excision/removal of the uterus
dermat (skin)	none	dermat	-osis	dermatosis	abnormal condition of the skin

Suffix

A suffix is a word part that is added to the end of a word root (unit of meaning) to change its meaning. For example: in English, suffixes are often used to change verb tenses (*sigh, sighed; talk, talked*); to indicate progression of action (*ride, riding; think, thinking*); to change nouns from singular to plural (*arm, arms; bench, benches*); to change verbs to nouns (*expectorate, expectorant; intoxicate, intoxicant*); to indicate comparatives and superlatives (*happy, happier, happiest; tall, taller, tallest*); and to change word meanings (*admire, admirer, sad, sadly*).

Many of the suffixes used in medical language originated from Greek and Latin words—often prepositions. These suffixes now, when added to word roots or to combining forms, indicate diagnoses, symptoms, procedures, and disorders or diseases. Examples are provided in the lessons in this chapter.

Some suffixes, when added to word roots, indicate noun, adjective, or plural spellings. Review the following examples.

-ion, -ant, -logy		suffixes denoting noun spellings	
Word	**Root**	**Root Meaning**	**Definition**
1. transfusion	transfuse	to pour from one vessel to another	the transfer of blood or blood components from a donor to a receptor
2. auscultation	auscultate	to perform auscultation	listening to sounds made by body structures
3. intubation	intubate	to insert a tube	the process of inserting a tube for anesthesia or for pulmonary assistance
4. expectorant	expectorate	to expel from the chest	any agent that promotes the expelling of bronchial secretions
5. etiology	eti (o)	cause	the study of the cause of a disease
6. pathology	path (o)	feeling, disease	the study of diseases

-ate, -tripsy, -plasty, -pexy, -lysis		suffixes denoting processes	
Word	**Root**	**Root Meaning**	**Definition**
7. dehydrate	hydrate	to add water	to remove water from a substance, such as the body
8. lithotripsy	lith (o)	stone	the operation of crushing a stone
9. blepharoplasty	blephar (o)	eyelid	plastic surgery on the eyelid
10. cheiroplasty	cheir (o)	hand	plastic surgery on the hand
11. hysteropexy	hyster (o)	uterus	surgical fixation or fastening of the uterus
12. hemolysis	hem (o)	blood	breaking down or destroying blood cells

-ic, -al, -ac, -ar, -ary, -al, -eal, -ous		suffixes denoting adjective spellings	
Word	**Root**	**Root Meaning**	**Definition**
13. septic	sepsis	the presence of pathogenic organisms	pertaining to the presence of pathogenic organisms
14. thoracic	thorac(o)	chest	pertaining to the chest
15. arterial	arteri(o)	artery	pertaining to an artery
16. cardiac	card(i)	heart	pertaining to the heart
17. celiac	celi(o)	abdomen	pertaining to the abdomen
18. muscular	muscul(o)	muscle	pertaining to a muscle
19. vascular	vascul(o)	blood vessel	pertaining to a blood vessel
20. pulmonary	pulmon(o)	lung	pertaining to a lung
21. neural	neur(o)	nerve	pertaining to a nerve

continued

Word	Root	Root Meaning	Definition
22. bronchial	bronch(i)	bronchus	pertaining to a bronchus
23. laryngeal	laryng(o)	larynx	pertaining to the larynx
24. esophageal	esophag(o)	esophagus	pertaining to the esophagus
25. venous	ven(o)	vein	pertaining to a vein

-es, -ices, -i, -ae, -nges, -a, -mata suffixes denoting plurals			
Word	**Root**	**Root Meaning**	**Definition**
26. diagnoses	diagnosis	a determination of the nature of a disease	more than one determination of the nature of a disease
27. appendices	appendix	the appendix	more than one appendix
28. bronchi	bronchus	the bronchus	more than one bronchus
29. pleurae	pleura	the pleura	more than one pleura
30. meninges	meninx	a membrane surrounding the brain or spinal cord	membranes surrounding the brain and spinal cord
31. ova	ovum	an ovum(egg)	more than one ovum
32. ganglia	ganglion	a knotlike mass of nerve fibers	more than one ganglion
33. carcinomata	carcinoma	cancer	more than one cancer

LESSON

1-1

Terminology Presentation

Diagnoses, Symptoms, and Procedures

As you listen to the CD, read the words and notice the pronunciations given.

  Start CD

-algia	a suffix denoting pain		
Word	**Root**	**Root Meaning**	**Answer**
1. myalgia (mi-al'je-ah)	my (o)	muscle	1. *Muscle pain*
2. arthralgia (ar-thral'je-ah)	arthr (o)	joint	2. *Joint pain*

-tomy	a suffix denoting an incision		
Word	**Root**	**Root Meaning**	**Answer**
3. thoracotomy (tho'rah-kot'o-me)	thorac (o)	chest	3. *Chest incision*
4. tracheotomy (tra'ke-ot'o-me)	trache (o)	trachea, windpipe	4. *trachea incision*

-scopy	a suffix denoting a visual examination		
Word	**Root**	**Root Meaning**	**Answer**
5. gastroscopy (gas-tros'ko-pe)	gastr (o)	stomach	5. *visual exam in stomach*
6. colonoscopy (ko'lon-os'ko-pe)	col (o)	large intestine, colon	6. *visual exam in colon*

-plasty	a suffix denoting plastic surgery or a surgical repair		
Word	**Root**	**Root Meaning**	**Answer**
7. stomatoplasty (sto'mah-to-plas'te)	stomat (o)	mouth	7. *Mouth repair surgery*
8. mastoplasty (mas'to-plas'te)	mast (o)	breast	8. *Breast repair surgery*

continued

-ectomy   a suffix denoting an excision or removal

Word	Root	Root Meaning	Answer
9. hysterectomy (his′te-rek′to-me)	hyster (o)	uterus	9. _____
10. thrombectomy (throm-bek′to-me)	thromb (o)	blood clot or thrombus	10. _____

-graphy   a suffix denoting the process of recording

Word	Root	Root Meaning	Answer
11. encephalography (en-sef′ah-log′rah-fe)	encephal (o)	brain	11. _____
12. cardiography (kar′de-og′rah-fe)	cardi (o)	heart	12. _____

-pexy   a suffix denoting a surgical reattachment; to fix, or to fasten

Word	Root	Root Meaning	Answer
13. syndesmopexy (sin-des′mo-pek′se)	syndesm (o)	ligament	13. _____
14. nephropexy (nef′ro-pek′se)	nephr (o)	kidney	14. _____

-centesis   a suffix denoting a surgical puncture to remove fluid or tissue

Word	Root	Root Meaning	Answer
15. amniocentesis (am′ne-o-sen-te′sis)	amni (o)	fluid-filled sac containing fetus	15. _____
16. cephalocentesis (sef′ah-lo-sen-te′sis)	cephal (o)	head	16. _____

-pathy   a suffix denoting disease

Word	Root	Root Meaning	Answer
17. arteriopathy (ar′te-re-op′ah-the)	arteri (o)	artery	17. _____
18. lymphopathy (lim-fop′ah-the)	lymph (o)	lymph, or lymph glands or vessels	18. _____

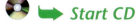

Pause CD

After practicing each suffix and word several times, use a sheet of paper to cover all columns except the Answer column. As each word is pronounced again on the CD, write it in the space provided.

Start CD

Check the words you have written against the words in the left-hand column. If you have misspelled any words, practice writing them correctly.

Practice

Practice

LESSON 1-1

Terminology Application

Without looking at your previous work, write the word that matches each definition.

Definition	Term
1. visual examination of the inside of the stomach	-scopy & gastroscopy
2. incision into the chest	-tomy & thoracotomy
3. removal of a blood clot	-ectomy & thrombectomy
4. any disease of the arteries	-pathy & Arteriopathy
5. reattachment of a kidney	-pexy & Nephropexy
6. recording of heart activity	-graphy & cardiography
7. surgical puncture of the head to remove fluid	-centesis & cephalocentesis
8. reattachment of a ligament	-pexy & syndesmopexy
9. surgical repair of the breast	-plasty & mastoplasty
10. joint pain	-algia & Artralgia
11. removal of the uterus	-ectomy & Hysterectomy
12. recording of brain activity	-graphy & Encephalography
13. visual examination of the inside of the colon	-scopy & colonoscopy
14. incision into the trachea	-tomy & tracheatomy
15. any disease of the lymphatic system	-pathy & lymphopathy
16. muscle pain	-algia & Myalgia
17. surgical puncture of the amnion to remove fluid	-centesis & Amniocentesis
18. surgical repair of the mouth	-plasty & stomatoplasty

Check your answers against the information given in this lesson's terminology presentation. If you have any errors, count them and write the number in the blank at the top of the page. Sign your work and give it to your instructor.

Practice

Terminology Presentation

Diseases and Abnormal Conditions

As you listen to the CD, read the words and notice the pronunciations given.

🔘 ➡️ **Start CD**

-ptosis   a suffix denoting falling, downward displacement, prolapse

Word	Root	Root Meaning	Answer
1. nephroptosis (nef'rop-to'sis)	nephr(o)	kidney	1. *falling kidney*
2. cystoptosis (sis'top-to'sis)	cyst(o)	sac or bladder	2. *falling bladder*

-itis   a suffix denoting an inflammation—note that a combining vowel is not used

Word	Root	Root Meaning	Answer
3. dermatitis (der'mah-ti'tis)	dermat	skin	3. _____
4. pharyngitis (far'in-ji'tis)	pharyng	throat, pharynx	4. _____

-osis   a suffix denoting an abnormal condition—note that a combining vowel is not used

Word	Root	Root Meaning	Answer
5. pyosis (pi-o'sis)	py	pus	5. _____
6. onychosis (on'i-ko'sis)	onych	nails	6. _____

-mycosis   a suffix denoting an abnormal condition of fungus

Word	Root	Root Meaning	Answer
7. rhinomycosis (ri'no-mi-ko'sis)	rhin (o)	nose	7. _____
8. otomycosis (o'to-mi-ko'sis)	ot (o)	ear	8. _____

continued

-cele	a suffix denoting a tumor, swelling, or hernia		
Word	**Root**	**Root Meaning**	**Answer**
9. ovariocele (o-va′re-o-sel′)	ovari (o)	ovary	9. _____
10. thyrocele (thi′ro-sel)	thyr (o)	thyroid gland	10. _____

-megaly	a suffix denoting an abnormal enlargement		
Word	**Root**	**Root Meaning**	**Answer**
11. hepatomegaly (hep′ah-to-meg′ah-le)	hepat (o)	liver	11. _____
12. splenomegaly (sple′no-meg′ah-le)	splen(o)	spleen	12. _____

-malacia	a suffix denoting abnormal softening		
Word	**Root**	**Root Meaning**	**Answer**
13. osteomalacia (os′te-o-mah-la′she-ah)	oste (o)	bone	13. _____
14. onychomalacia (on′i-ko-mah-la′she-ah)	onych (o)	nails	14. _____

-rrhagia	a suffix denoting excessive flow, bleeding		
Word	**Root**	**Root Meaning**	**Answer**
15. metrorrhagia (me′tro-ra′je-ah)	metr (o)	uterus	15. _____
16. rhinorrhagia (ri′no-ra′je-ah)	rhin (o)	nose	16. _____

  Pause CD

After practicing each word several times, use a sheet of paper to cover all columns except the Answer column. As each word is pronounced again on the CD, write it in the space provided.

  Start CD

Check the words you have written against the words in the left-hand column. If you have misspelled any words, practice writing them correctly.

Practice

_____

_____

LESSON 1-2

Terminology Application

Without looking at your previous work, write the word that matches each definition.

Definition	Term
1. inflammation of the throat/pharynx	_____
2. hernia of an ovary	_____
3. abnormal condition of pus	_____
4. falling kidney	_____
5. abnormally soft bone	_____
6. abnormal nasal hemorrhage	_____
7. abnormal condition of fungus in the nose	_____
8. tumor of the thyroid gland	_____
9. falling urinary bladder	_____
10. abnormal bleeding from uterus	_____
11. abnormally large liver	_____
12. abnormal condition of the nails	_____
13. abnormal condition of fungus in the ear	_____
14. abnormally large spleen	_____
15. abnormally soft nails	_____
16. inflammation of the skin	_____

Check your answers against the information given in this lesson's terminology presentation. If you have any errors, count them and write the number in the blank at the top of the page. Sign your work and give it to your instructor.

Practice

Terminology Presentation

Dilation, Constriction, Narrowing, and Deficiencies

As you listen to the CD, read the words and notice the pronunciations given.

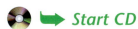 **Start CD**

		-stenosis a suffix denoting narrowing		
Word	**Root**	**Root Meaning**	**Answer**	
1. dacryostenosis (dak're-o-ste-no'sis)	dacry (o)	tears, lacrimal glands, ducts	1. _____	
2. metrostenosis (me'tro-ste-no'sis)	metr (o)	uterus	2. _____	
3. phlebostenosis (fleb'o-ste-no'sis)	phleb (o)	vein	3. _____	
4. esophagostenosis (e-sof'ah-go-ste-no'sis)	esophag (o)	esophagus	4. _____	

		-ectasis a suffix denoting expansion, dilation—note that the first example includes the use of a combining vowel		
Word	**Root**	**Root Meaning**	**Answer**	
5. bronchiectasis (brong'ke-ek'tah-sis)	bronch (i)	bronchus	5. _____	
6. arteriectasis (ar'te-re-ek'tah-sis)	arteri	artery	6. _____	
7. iridectasis (ir'i-dek'tah-sis)	irid	iris	7. _____	
8. pyelectasis (pi'e-lek'tah-sis)	pyel	pelvis of the kidney	8. _____	

continued

	-penia	a suffix denoting a deficiency, a decreased amount	

	WordRoot	Root Meaning	Answer
9.	leukopenia (loo′ko-pe′ne-ah)	leuk (o)	white blood cell	9. _____
10.	lymphopenia (lim′fo-pe′ne-ah)	lymph (o)	lymph cell	10. _____
11.	erythropenia (e-rith′ro-pe′ne-ah)	erythr (o)	red blood cell	11. _____
12.	glycopenia (gli′ko-pe′ne-ah)	glyc (o)	glucose, sugar	12. _____

➡ *Pause CD*

After practicing each word several times, use a sheet of paper to cover all columns except the Answer column. As each word is pronounced again on the CD, write it in the space provided.

➡ *Start CD*

Check the words you have written against the words in the left-hand column. If you have misspelled any words, practice writing them correctly.

Practice

_____

_____

_____

_____

_____

_____

_____

_____

_____

_____

_____

_____

_____

LESSON
1-3
Terminology Application

Without looking at your previous work, write the word that matches each definition.

Definition	Term
1. dilation of an artery	_____
2. deficiency of white blood cells	_____
3. narrowing of lacrimal ducts	_____
4. expansion of the bronchus	_____
5. deficiency of lymph cells	_____
6. deficiency of glucose in tissues	_____
7. narrowing of uterus	_____
8. dilation of an iris	_____
9. narrowing of a vein	_____
10. deficiency of red blood cells	_____
11. dilation of the pelvis of the kidney	_____
12. narrowing of the esophagus	_____

Check your answers against the information given in this lesson's terminology presentation. If you have any errors, count them and write the number in the blank at the top of the page. Sign your work and give it to your instructor.

Practice

Terminology Presentation

Miscellaneous Suffixes

As you listen to the CD, read the words and notice the pronunciations given.

 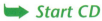 **Start CD**

	-plegia a suffix denoting paralysis		
Word	**Root**	**Root Meaning**	**Answer**
1. bronchoplegia (brong′ko-ple′je-ah)	bronch (o)	bronchus	1. _____
2. quadriplegia (kwod′ri-ple′je-ah)	quadr (i)	referring to four	2. _____

	-lysis a suffix meaning to dissolve, to break down		
Word	**Root**	**Root Meaning**	**Answer**
3. pancreolysis (pan′kre-ol′i-sis)	pancreat (o)	pancreas	3. _____
4. osteolysis (os′te-ol′i-sis)	oste (o)	bone	4. _____

	-rrhea a suffix denoting a flow		
Word	**Root**	**Root Meaning**	**Answer**
5. dacryorrhea (dak′re-o-re′ah)	dacry (o)	tears, lacrimal glands or ducts	5. _____
6. proctorrhea (prok′to-re′ah)	proct (o)	rectum, anus	6. _____

	-logy a suffix denoting the study of		
Word	**Root**	**Root Meaning**	**Answer**
7. hematology (hem′ah-tol′o-je)	hemat (o)	blood	7. _____
8. nephrology (ne-frol′o-je)	nephr (o)	kidney	8. _____

continued

-*poiesis* a suffix denoting form, formation			
Word	**Root**	**Root Meaning**	**Answer**
9. leukopoiesis (loo′ko-poi-e′sis)	leuk (o)	white blood cell	**9.** _____
10. erythropoiesis (e-rith′ro-poi-e′sis)	erythr (o)	red blood cell	**10.** _____

-*clasis* a suffix denoting break, fracture			
Word	**Root**	**Root Meaning**	**Answer**
11. thromboclasis (throm-bok′lah-sis)	thromb (o)	blood clot or thrombus	**11.** _____
12. osteoclasis (os-te-ok′lah-sis)	oste (o)	bone	**12.** _____

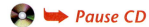 ➡ *Pause CD*

After practicing each word several times, use a sheet of paper to cover all columns except the Answer column. As each word is pronounced again on the CD, write it in the space provided.

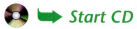 ➡ *Start CD*

Check the words you have written against the words in the left-hand column. If you have misspelled any words, practice writing them correctly.

Practice

_____

_____

_____

_____

_____

_____

_____

_____

_____

_____

_____

LESSON 1-4

Terminology Application

Without looking at your previous work, write the word that matches each definition.

Definition	Term
1. study of blood	_____
2. breaking down the pancreas	_____
3. paralysis in four limbs	_____
4. breaking a blood clot	_____
5. study of the kidney	_____
6. flow from the rectum or anus	_____
7. paralysis of the bronchus	_____
8. formation of white blood cells	_____
9. breaking or fracturing a bone	_____
10. flowing of tears, usually excessive	_____
11. formation of red blood cells	_____
12. breaking down bone	_____

Check your answers against the information given in this lesson's terminology presentation. If you have any errors, count them and write the number in the blank at the top of the page. Sign your work and give it to your instructor.

Practice

CHAPTER 1

Terminology Review

This is a review of the suffixes and words you have learned in the preceding lessons. Some of the medical terms listed below may be new, but they are composed of the suffixes and word roots that you have already learned. Read the words below as they are pronounced on the CD.

  Start CD

Word Element Review

Word	Word Part	Meaning of Word Part
1. nephrectomy	nephr (o)	_____
nephrectomy	-ectomy	_____
(ne-frek'-to-me)	Meaning of Word	_____
2. myalgia	my (o)	_____
myalgia	-algia	_____
(my-al'-je-a)	Meaning of Word	_____
3. thoracentesis	thora	_____
thoracentesis	-centesis	_____
(tho'rah-sen-te'sis)	Meaning of Word	_____
4. phlebitis	phleb (o)	_____
phlebitis	-itis	_____
(fle-bi'tis)	Meaning of Word	_____
5. hysteroptosis	hyster (o)	_____
hysteroptosis	-ptosis	_____
(his'ter-op-to'sis)	Meaning of Word	_____
6. tracheotomy	trache (o)	_____
tracheotomy	-tomy	_____
(tra'ke-ot'o-me)	Meaning of Word	_____
7. metrorrhagia	metr (o)	_____
metrorrhagia	-rrhagia	_____
(me'tro-ra'je-ah)	Meaning of Word	_____

Word	Word Part	Meaning of Word Part
8. glycopenia	glyc (o)	_____
glycopenia	-penia	_____
(gli′ko-pe′ne-ah)	Meaning of Word	_____
9. gastroscopy	gastr (o)	_____
gastroscopy	-scopy	_____
(gas-tros′ko-pe)	Meaning of Word	_____
10. myocele	my (o)	_____
myocele	-cele	_____
(mi′o-sel)	Meaning of Word	_____
11. bronchiectasis	bronch (i)	_____
bronchiectasis	-ectasis	_____
(brong′ke-ek′tah-sis)	Meaning of Word	_____
12. pyosis	py	_____
pyosis	-osis	_____
(pi′o-sis′)	Meaning of Word	_____
13. cystopexy	cyst (o)	_____
cystopexy	-pexy	_____
(sis′to-pek′se)	Meaning of Word	_____
14. esophagostenosis	esophag (o)	_____
esophagostenosis	-stenosis	_____
(e-sof′ah-go-ste-no′sis)	Meaning of Word	_____
15. osteolysis	oste (o)	_____
osteolysis	-lysis	_____
(os′te-ol′i-sis)	Meaning of Word	_____

 ➡ *Stop CD*

On the lines provided, write in the meanings of as many suffixes, roots, and words as you can from memory. Check your definitions in the glossary or a medical dictionary, and make any needed corrections.

CHAPTER 1
Terminology Review

Complete this review, and turn it in to your instructor when you are finished.

Definition

Each phrase below defines one of the words you have just studied. Without looking at your previous work, write in the word that matches each definition.

Definition	Term
1. recording of brain activity	_____
2. surgical puncture of the amnion to remove fluid	_____
3. any disease of the lymphatic system	_____
4. reattachment of a kidney	_____
5. visual examination of the inside of the stomach	_____
6. inflammation of the throat/pharynx	_____
7. falling urinary bladder	_____
8. abnormal bleeding from the uterus	_____
9. dilation of the pelvis of the kidney	_____
10. deficiency of glucose in tissues	_____
11. narrowing of the esophagus	_____
12. removal of a blood clot	_____
13. surgical repair of the mouth	_____
14. reattachment of a ligament	_____
15. determination of the nature of a disease	_____

continued

CHAPTER 1

Terminology Review

Matching

Match the following terms with the definitions given. Write the letter of the correct term to the left of the definition.

	Definition	Term
_____	16. pertaining to blueness of extremities due to lack of oxygenation	**a.** erythropenia
_____	17. visual examination of the inside of the colon	**b.** bronchoplegia
_____	18. abnormal nasal hemorrhage	**c.** iridectasis
_____	19. abnormally large spleen	**d.** ovariocele
_____	20. hernia of an ovary	**e.** splenomegaly
_____	21. deficiency of red blood cells	**f.** rhinorrhagia
_____	22. dilation of an iris	**g.** cyanotic
_____	23. formation of white blood cells	**h.** leukopoiesis
_____	24. flowing of tears, usually excessive	**i.** colonoscopy
_____	25. paralysis of the bronchus	**j.** dacryorrhea

You may now go on to Chapter Test 1.

2

Prefixes

Objectives

After completing Chapter 2, you should be able to do the following:

1. identify common prefixes;

2. categorize common prefixes as denoting degree, time, and position;

3. understand prefixes used to indicate direction;

4. recognize prefixes that indicate negation, number, and color; and

5. identify miscellaneous prefixes.

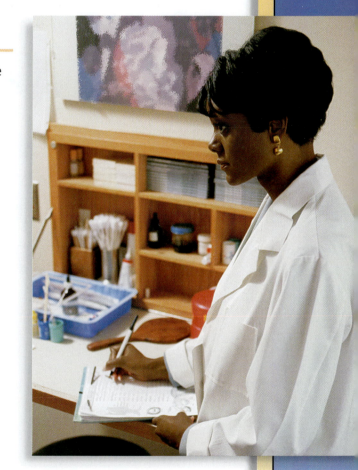

Orientation to Prefixes

A prefix is a word part that is added to the beginning of a word root (unit of meaning) to change the meaning of the word. For example: in English, prefixes are often used to qualify the meaning of a word (intelligent, superintelligent); to indicate number (angle, triangle); to indicate time (view, preview); or to change meaning (scope, microscope).

Many of the prefixes used in medical terminology originated from Greek and Latin words for such things as prepositions, numbers, and colors. When added to word roots, these prefixes indicate degree, time, and position; direction; and negation, number, and color. Examples are provided in the lessons in this chapter.

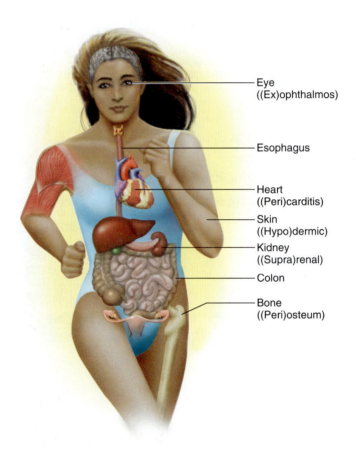

Eye
((Ex)ophthalmos)

Esophagus

Heart
((Peri)carditis)

Skin
((Hypo)dermic)

Kidney
((Supra)renal)

Colon

Bone
((Peri)osteum)

Terminology Presentation

Degree, Time, and Position

As you listen to the CD, read the words and notice the pronunciations given.

  Start CD

hypo- a prefix denoting under, beneath, deficiency

Word	Root	Root Definition	Answer
1. hypodermic (hi′po-der′mik)	dermis	skin	1. _____
2. hypothyroidism (hi′po-thi′roid-izm)	thyroid	thyroid gland	2. _____

hyper- a prefix denoting an excessive amount

Word	Root	Root Definition	Answer
3. hyperalgesia (hi′per-al-je′ze-ah)	algesia	pain or ache	3. _____
4. hyperpnea (hi′perp-ne′ah)	pnea	breathing, or air	4. _____

peri- a prefix denoting around

Word	Root	Root Definition	Answer
5. pericarditis (per′i-kar-di′tis)	cardi (o)	the heart	5. _____
6. periosteum (per′e-os′te-um)	osteum	bone	6. _____

anti- a prefix denoting against

Word	Root	Root Definition	Answer
7. antiemetic (an′ti-e-met′ik)	emesis	vomit	7. _____
8. anticoagulant (an′ti-ko-ag′u-lant)	coagulate	to clot	8. _____

continued

	inter-	a prefix denoting between		
	Word	**Root**	**Root Definition**	**Answer**
9.	intercostal (in′ter-kos′tal)	cost (o) -al	rib pertaining to	**9.** _____
10.	interdigital (in′ter-dij′i-tal)	digit -al	fingers, toes pertaining to	**10.** _____

	pre-	a prefix denoting before		
	Word	**Root**	**Root Definition**	**Answer**
11.	prenatal (pre-na′tal)	natus -al	birth pertaining to	**11.** _____ _____
12.	premenstrual (pre-men′stroo-al)	menses -al	menstruation pertaining to	**12.** _____ _____

	supra-	a prefix denoting above		
	Word	**Root**	**Root Definition**	**Answer**
13.	suprarenal (soo′prah-re′nal)	renal	kidney	**13.** _____
14.	supratympanic (soo′prah-tim-pan′ik)	tympanum	eardrum	**14.** _____

	intra-	a prefix denoting within		
	Word	**Root**	**Root Definition**	**Answer**
15.	intrabuccal (in′trah-buk′al)	buccal	pertaining to the cheek	**15.** _____
16.	intravenous (in′trah-ve′nus)	vena -ous	vein pertaining to	**16.** _____ _____

	epi-	a prefix denoting above		
	Word	**Root**	**Root Definition**	**Answer**
17.	epiglottis (ep′i-glot′is)	glottis	vocal apparatus of the larynx	17. _____
18.	epidermis (ep′i-der′mis)	dermis	skin	18. _____

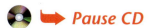 *Pause CD*

After practicing each word several times, use a sheet of paper to cover all columns except the Answer column. As each word is pronounced again on the CD, write it in the space provided.

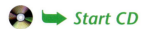 *Start CD*

Check the words you have written against the words in the left-hand column. If you have misspelled any words, practice writing them correctly.

Practice

_____

_____

_____

_____

_____

_____

Some examples of common prefixes are listed below.

Prefix	Meaning	Root Word and Prefix	Meaning
re-	again, backward	rename	to name again
		regurgitate	to flow backward; to vomit
de-	away from	decapitate	to remove the head
multi-	much, many	multipolar	having more than two poles
pre-	before	preoperative	occurring before an operation
ab-	away from	abnormal	not normal
anti-	against	antibacterial	agent that counters (goes against) bacteria
trans-	through, across	transdermal	through the skin
im-	not	impossible	not possible
tri-	three	triceps	three-headed muscles
dia-	across, through	diameter	straight line going through the center point and connecting two opposite points on a circle

Practice

LESSON 2-1

Terminology Application

Without looking at your previous work, write the word that matches each definition.

Definition	Term
1. increased sensitivity to pain	_____
2. an agent that prevents or alleviates nausea and vomiting	_____
3. before the onset of menses	_____
4. situated above or upon the skin	_____
5. deficiency of thyroid secretion	_____
6. within the cheek or mouth	_____
7. connective tissue covering the bone	_____
8. situated above the kidney (adrenal gland)	_____
9. increase in the depth and rate of breathing	_____
10. situated between the ribs	_____
11. administered beneath the skin	_____
12. situated above the tympanum	_____
13. before childbirth	_____
14. the lidlike structure that covers the larynx to prevent food from entering the trachea	_____
15. within a vein	_____
16. situated between the fingers or toes	_____
17. an agent that prevents blood clotting	_____
18. inflammation of the membrane surrounding the heart	_____

Check your answers against the information given in this lesson's terminology presentation. If you have any errors, count them and write the number in the blank at the top of the page. Sign your work and give it to your instructor.

Practice

Direction

As you listen to the CD, read the words and notice the pronunciations given.

 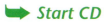 **Start CD**

de- a prefix denoting away from			
Word	**Root**	**Root Definition**	**Answer**
1. dehydrate (de-hi′drat)	hydr(o)	water	1. _____
2. detoxify (de-tok′si-fi)	toxic	poison	2. _____

ex- a prefix denoting away from			
Word	**Root**	**Root Definition**	**Answer**
3. expectorant (ek-spek′to-rant)	pectoral	chest	3. _____
4. exophthalmos (eks′sof-thal′mos)	ophthalmos	eye	4. _____

ab- a prefix denoting away from			
Word	**Root**	**Root Definition**	**Answer**
5. abnormal (ab-nor′mal)	normal	agreeing with the regular and the established	5. _____
6. aboral (ab-o′ral)	oral	mouth	6. _____

ad- a prefix denoting toward			
Word	**Root**	**Root Definition**	**Answer**
7. adrenal (ah-dre′nal)	renal	kidney	7. _____
8. adduct (ah-dukt′)	duct(o)	to draw	8. _____

dextro-	a prefix denoting to the right		
Word	**Root**	**Root Definition**	**Answer**
9. dextral (deks′tral)	dexter	right	9. _____
10. dextrogastria (deks′tro-gas′tre-ah)	gastr(o)	stomach	10. _____

sinistro-	a prefix denoting to the left		
Word	**Root**	**Root Definition**	**Answer**
11. sinistral (sin′is-tral)	sinister	left	11. _____
12. sinistrocardia (sin′is-tro-kar′de-ah)	cardi(o)	heart	12. _____

trans-	a prefix denoting through		
Word	**Root**	**Root Definition**	**Answer**
13. transdermal (trans-der′mal)	dermis	skin	13. _____
14. transabdominal (trans′ab-dom′i-nal)	abdominal	pertaining to the abdomen	14. _____

dia-	a prefix denoting through		
Word	**Root**	**Root Definition**	**Answer**
15. diarrhea (di′ah-re′ah)	-rrhea	a flowing	15. _____
16. dialysis (di-al′i-sis)	-lysis	dissolution	16. _____

➡ *Pause CD*

After practicing each word several times, use a sheet of paper to cover all columns except the Answer column. As each word is pronounced again on the CD, write it in the space provided.

➡ *Start CD*

Check the words you have written against the words in the left-hand column. If you have misspelled any words, practice writing them correctly.

Practice

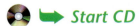

_____

_____

LESSON 2-2

Terminology Application

Without looking at your previous work, write the word that matches each definition.

Definition	Term
1. displacement of the stomach to the right	_____
2. situated away or remote from the mouth	_____
3. an agent that promotes the ejection of mucus from the lungs	_____
4. process of separating elements in a solution through a semipermeable membrane	_____
5. entering through the dermis or skin	_____
6. to remove water from a substance, such as the body	_____
7. situated near the kidney	_____
8. abnormal frequency and liquidity of fecal discharges	_____
9. location of the heart in the left side of the thorax	_____
10. pertaining to the right	_____
11. through the abdominal wall	_____
12. not normal	_____
13. pertaining to the left	_____
14. to draw toward	_____
15. abnormal protrusion of the eyeball	_____
16. to remove the toxic quality of a substance	_____

Check your answers against the information given in this lesson's terminology presentation. If you have any errors, count them and write the number in the blank at the top of the page. Sign your work and give it to your instructor.

Practice

Terminology Presentation

Negation, Number, and Color

As you listen to the CD, read the words and notice the pronunciations given.

 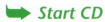 **Start CD**

im-, in-	prefixes denoting not		
Word	**Root**	**Root Definition**	**Answer**
1. immature (im′ah-tur)	mature	adult, fully developed	1. _____
2. insomnia (in-som′ne-ah)	somni	sleep	2. _____

a-, an-	prefixes denoting not, without		
Word	**Root**	**Root Definition**	**Answer**
3. apnea (ap-ne′ah)	pnea	breathing, air, or gas	3. _____
4. analgesic (an′al-je′zik)	algesia	pain or ache	4. _____

non-	a prefix denoting not		
Word	**Root**	**Root Definition**	**Answer**
5. nonviable (non-vi′ah-b′l)	viable	capable of living	5. _____
6. nonspecific (non-spe-sif′ik)	specific	pertaining to a species	6. _____

primi-, mono-	prefixes denoting one		
Word	**Root**	**Root Definition**	**Answer**
7. primipara (pri-mip′ah-rah)	-para	to bring forth, produce	7. _____
8. monochromatic (mon′o-kro-mat′ik)	chromatic	pertaining to color	8. _____

continued

bi-, di-, diplo-   prefixes denoting two, double, both

	Word	Root	Root Definition	Answer
9.	biceps (bi′seps)	ceps	head	9. _____
10.	diplophonia (dip′lo-fo′ne-ah)	phonia	voice, sound	10. _____

tri-   a prefix denoting three

	Word	Root	Root Definition	Answer
11.	triorchidism (tri-or′ki-dizm)	orchidism	condition of the testes	11. _____

quadri-   a prefix denoting four

	Word	Root	Root Definition	Answer
12.	quadruped (kwod′roo-ped)	ped(o)	foot, feet	12. _____

multi-   a prefix denoting much or many

	Word	Root	Root Definition	Answer
13.	multicellular (mul′ti-sel′u-lar)	cell	fundamental, structural and functional unit of living organisms	13. _____

pan-   a prefix denoting all

	Word	Root	Root Definition	Answer
14.	panhysterectomy (pan′his-ter-ek′to-me)	hyster(o)	uterus	14. _____

hemi-   a prefix denoting half

	Word	Root	Root Definition	Answer
15.	hemianesthesia (hem′e-an′es-the′ze-ah)	anesthesia	lack of perception	15. _____

alb-, leuko-   prefixes denoting white

	Word	Root	Root Definition	Answer
16.	albuminuria (al′bu-mi-nu′re-ah)	-uria	urine condition	16. _____
17.	leukemia (loo-ke′me-ah)	-emia	blood condition	17. _____

erythro-	a prefix denoting red		
Word	**Root**	**Root Definition**	**Answer**
18. erythrocyte (e-rith′ro-sit)	-cyte	cell	**18.** _____

cyano-	a prefix denoting blue		
Word	**Root**	**Root Definition**	**Answer**
19. cyanemia (si′ah-ne′me-ah)	-emia	pertaining to blood	**19.** _____

xantho-	a prefix denoting yellow		
Word	**Root**	**Root Definition**	**Answer**
20. xanthochromic (zan′tho-kro′mik)	chromic	pertaining to color	**20.** _____

melano-	a prefix denoting black		
Word	**Root**	**Root Definition**	**Answer**
21. melanuria (mel′an-u′re-ah)	-uria	urine	**21.** _____

➡️ *Pause CD*

After practicing each word several times, use a sheet of paper to cover all columns except the Answer column. As each word is pronounced again on the CD, write it in the space provided.

➡️ *Start CD*

Check the words you have written against the words in the left-hand column. If you have misspelled any words, practice writing them correctly.

Practice

_____

_____

_____

_____

_____

_____

_____

Practice

LESSON 2-3

Terminology Application

Without looking at your previous work, write the word that matches each definition.

Definition	Term
1. the production of double vocal sounds	_____
2. not due to any single known cause, such as a particular pathogen	_____
3. a red blood cell	_____
4. composed of many cells	_____
5. denoting a yellow discoloration of the skin or spinal fluid	_____
6. not fully developed	_____
7. black or dark discoloration of the urine	_____
8. excessive number of white blood cells	_____
9. bluishness of the blood	_____
10. not capable of living	_____
11. total removal of the uterus and cervix (total hysterectomy)	_____
12. having only one color	_____
13. presence of serum albumin in the urine	_____
14. the condition of having three testes	_____
15. pertaining to the giving of a medicine to relieve or remove pain	_____
16. condition denoting anesthesia (lack of feeling) on one side of the body	_____
17. a woman who has had one pregnancy with a viable offspring	_____
18. four-footed, such as many animals	_____

Definition	Term
19. inability to sleep	_____
20. a muscle having two heads	_____
21. temporary absence of breathing	_____

Check your answers against the information given in this lesson's terminology presentation. If you have any errors, count them and write the number in the blank at the top of the page. Sign your work and give it to your instructor.

Terminology Presentation

Miscellaneous Prefixes

As you listen to the CD, read the words and notice the pronunciations given.

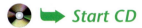 **Start CD**

nocti-	a prefix denoting night		
Word	**Root**	**Root Definition**	**Answer**
1. noctiphobia (nok′te-fo′be-ah)	phobia	fear	1. _____
2. nocturia (nok-tu′re-ah)	-uria	urine	2. _____

post-	a prefix denoting after (time), behind (position, location)		
Word	**Root**	**Root Definition**	**Answer**
3. postmortem (post-mor′tem)	mortis	death	3. _____
4. postnasal (post-na′zal)	nasal	pertaining to the nose	4. _____

brady-	a prefix denoting slowness		
Word	**Root**	**Root Definition**	**Answer**
5. bradycardia (brad′e-kar′de-ah)	cardi(o)	heart	5. _____
6. bradypnea (brad′e-ne′ah)	pnea	breathing, air, or gas	6. _____

auto-	a prefix denoting self		
Word	**Root**	**Root Definition**	**Answer**
7. autopsy (aw′top-se)	-opsy	view	7. _____
8. autograft (aw′to-graft)	graft	tissue for transplant	8. _____

cryo-	a prefix denoting cold		
Word	**Root**	**Root Definition**	**Answer**
9. cryotherapy (kri′o-ther′ah-pe)	therapy	treatment of disease	9. _____
10. cryosurgery (kri′o-sur′jer-e)	surgery	treatment of diseases, injuries, and deformities by manual or operative methods	10. _____

neo-	a prefix denoting new		
Word	**Root**	**Root Definition**	**Answer**
11. neonatal (ne′o-na′tal)	natal	childbirth	11. _____
12. neoplasm (ne′o-plazm)	-plasm	formation, growth	12. _____

ortho-	a prefix denoting straight		
Word	**Root**	**Root Definition**	**Answer**
13. orthodontics (or′tho-don′tiks)	odont(o)	tooth, teeth	13. _____
14. orthopnea (or′thop-ne′ah)	pnea	breathing, air, or gas	14. _____

 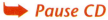 *Pause CD*

After practicing each word several times, use a sheet of paper to cover all columns except the Answer column. As each word is pronounced again on the CD, write it in the space provided.

 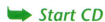 *Start CD*

Check the words you have written against the words in the left-hand column. If you have misspelled any words, practice writing them correctly.

Practice

_____

_____

_____

_____

_____

_____

LESSON 2-4

Terminology Application

Without looking at your previous work, write the word that matches each definition.

Definition	Term
1. abnormally slow heartbeat	_____
2. the therapeutic use of cold	_____
3. inability to breathe unless one is in an upright position	_____
4. a graft of tissue derived from the patient's body	_____
5. the branch of dentistry that deals with the prevention and correction of irregularities of the teeth and malocclusion	_____
6. occurring or performed after death	_____
7. pertaining to the first 4 weeks after birth	_____
8. irrational fear of night and darkness	_____
9. abnormally slow breathing	_____
10. any new or abnormal growth	_____
11. situated or occurring behind the nose	_____
12. destruction of tissue by the application of extreme cold	_____
13. excessive urination at night	_____
14. postmortem examination of a body	_____

Check your answers against the information given in this lesson's terminology presentation. If you have any errors, count them and write the number in the blank at the top of the page. Sign your work and give it to your instructor.

Practice

CHAPTER 2

Terminology Review

This is a review of the prefixes and words you have learned in the preceding lessons. Some of the medical terms listed below may be new, but they are composed of the prefixes and word roots that you have already learned. Read the words below as they are pronounced on the CD.

  Start CD

Word Element Review

Word	Word Part	Meaning of Word Part
1. orthopnea	orth(o)	_____
orthopnea	pnea	_____
(or'thop-ne'ah)	Meaning of Word	_____
2. detoxify	de-	_____
detoxify	toxify	_____
(de-tok'si-fi)	Meaning of Word	_____
3. hemianesthesia	hemi-	_____
hemianesthesia	anesthesia	_____
(hem'e-an'es-the'ze-ah)	Meaning of Word	_____
4. analgesic	an-	_____
analgesic	algesia	_____
(an'al-je'zik)	Meaning of Word	_____
5. monochromatic	mono-	_____
monochromatic	chromatic	_____
(mon'o-kro-mat'ik)	Meaning of Word	_____
6. aboral	ab-	_____
aboral	oral	_____
(ab-o'ral)	Meaning of Word	_____
7. antiemetic	anti-	_____
antiemetic	emetic	_____
(an'ti-e-met'ik)	Meaning of Word	_____

Word	Word Part	Meaning of Word Part
8. dialysis	dia-	_____
dialysis	-lysis	_____
(di-al′i-sis)	Meaning of Word	_____
9. primipara	primi-	_____
primipara	-para	_____
(pri-mip′ah-rah)	Meaning of Word	_____
10. hypothyroidism	hypo-	_____
hypothyroidism	thyroidism	_____
(hi′po-thi′roid-izm)	Meaning of Word	_____
11. cyanosis	cyan(o)	_____
cyanosis	-osis	_____
(si′ah-no′sis)	Meaning of Word	_____
12. intrauterine	intra-	_____
intrauterine	uterine	_____
(in′trah-u′ter-in)	Meaning of Word	_____
13. adduct	ad-	_____
adduct	duct	_____
(ah-dukt′)	Meaning of Word	_____
14. diplopia	dipl-	_____
diplopia	-opia	_____
(di-plo′pe-ah)	Meaning of Word	_____
15. epiglottis	epi-	_____
epiglottis	glottis	_____
(ep′i-glot′is)	Meaning of Word	_____

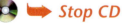 *Stop CD*

On the lines provided, write in the meanings of as many prefixes, roots, and words as you can from memory. Check your definitions in the glossary or a medical dictionary, and make any needed corrections.

CHAPTER 2
Terminology Review

Complete this review, and turn it in to your instructor when you are finished.

Definition

Each phrase below defines one of the words you have just studied. Without looking at your previous work, write in the word that matches each definition.

Definition	Term
1. connective tissue covering the bone	_____
2. temporary absence of breathing	_____
3. administered beneath the skin	_____
4. having only one color	_____
5. condition denoting anesthesia (lack of feeling) on one side of the body	_____
6. an agent that prevents blood clotting	_____
7. abnormally slow heartbeat	_____
8. a woman who has had one pregnancy with a viable offspring	_____
9. displacement of the stomach to the right	_____
10. excessive urination at night	_____
11. situated above or upon the skin	_____
12. entering through the dermis or skin	_____
13. presence of serum albumin in the urine	_____
14. inability to sleep	_____
15. a yellow discoloration of the skin or the spinal fluid	_____

continued

Matching

Match the following terms with the definitions given. Write the letter of the correct term to the left of the definition.

Definition	Term
_____ 16. before childbirth	a. postmortem
_____ 17. a graft of tissue derived from the patient's body	b. neoplasm
_____ 18. any new or abnormal growth	c. intrabuccal
_____ 19. irrational fear of night and darkness	d. prenatal
_____ 20. situated between the fingers or toes	e. cryosurgery
_____ 21. occurring or performed after death	f. interdigital
_____ 22. the branch of dentistry that deals with the prevention and correction of irregularities of the teeth and malocclusion	g. pericarditis
	h. orthodontics
_____ 23. destruction of tissue by the application of extreme cold	i. noctiphobia
_____ 24. within the cheek or mouth	j. autograft
_____ 25. inflammation of the membrane surrounding the heart	

You may now go on to Chapter Test 2.

3

Numbers, Amounts, Colors, and Positions

Objectives

After completing Chapter 3, you should be able to do the following:

1. identify word parts that indicate numbers;

2. recognize word parts that indicate amounts and positions; and

3. understand word parts that indicate colors.

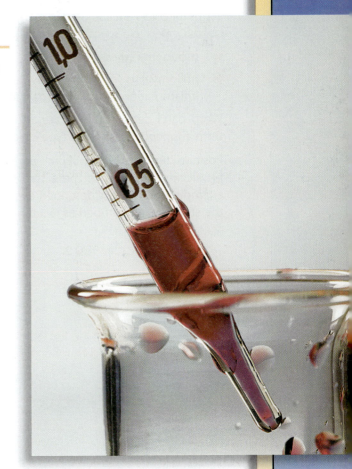

Orientation to Numbers, Amounts, Colors, and Positions

This section involves numbers, amounts, colors, and positions. Numbers and amounts are quite important for anyone working in the medical field because they are commonly used in lab reports and in many physicians' reports to denote weights and measurements. The following examples illustrate the ways in which numbers are used to describe the shapes of various parts of the body:

▶ *biceps* (two-headed muscle),

▶ *bicuspid* (a heart valve with two leaflets),

▶ *triceps* (a three-headed muscle),

▶ *tricuspid* (a heart valve with three leaflets).

Health-care professionals use amounts such as metric measurements (millimeters, centimeters) when determining the length, width, and depth of incisions, fractures, tumors, etc. They also will use milliliters and liters to measure liquids and grams to measure liquids and solids.

Terms for colors are also used in many types of medical reports. For example, the term *erythrocyte* (*erythr(o)* = red) refers to a specific type of cell—a red blood cell. Many disease symptoms are identified by color:

▶ melanoma (*melan(o)* = black + *-oma* = tumor): a black tumor

▶ poliomyelitis (*poli(o)* = gray + *myel(o)* = spinal cord + *-itis* = inflammation): an inflammation of the gray matter of the spinal cord.

Word parts denoting color are also widely used in reporting laboratory findings. For example, the term *eosinophil*, refers to a type of leukocyte that readily accepts an *eosin* (rose-colored) stain.

Position terms such as *supra*, *infra*, etc., are commonly used in anatomical descriptions. Many physicians' reports use these terms to indicate the site of a symptom or injury to the body. For example, the heart is described as *superior* to the intestine (i.e., located above the intestine), just as the stomach is described as located *inferior* to (i.e., located below) the oral cavity.

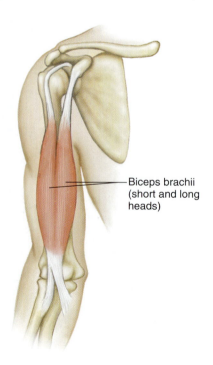

Biceps brachii (short and long heads)

LESSON

3-1

Terminology Presentation

Numbers

As you listen to the CD, read the words and notice the pronunciations given.

  Start CD

Word	Word Part	Definition	Answer
1. monorchism (mon′or-kizm)	mono- orchis	one testicle	**1.** _____
2. centimeter (sen′ti-me′ter)	centi- meter	100 or 1/100 measure (1 meter = 39.37 inches)	**2.** _____
3. hectogram (hek′to-gram)	hect(o) gram	100 weight (1 gram = 0.035 oz.)	**3.** _____
4. kilounit (kil′o-u′nit)	kilo- unit	1000 unit	**4.** _____
5. pentad (pen′tad)	pent- -ad	five (5) pertaining to	**5.** _____
6. millivolt (mil′i-volt)	milli- volt	1/1000 volt (electric force)	**6.** _____
7. decagram (dek′ah-gram)	deca- gram	10 weight (1 gram = 0.035 oz.)	**7.** _____
8. deciliter (des′i-le′ter)	deci- liter	1/10 measure (1 liter = 1.0567 quarts)	**8.** _____
9. tetradactyly (tet′rah-dak′ti-le)	tetra- dactyl(o)	four (4) finger, toe, digit	**9.** _____
10. diplopia (di-plo′pe-ah)	dipl(o) -opia	double eye, vision	**10.** _____
11. triorchidism (tri-or′ki-dizm)	tri- orchid(o) -ism	three (3) testes, testicle condition	**11.** _____

continued

Word	Word Part	Definition	Answer
12. hemianesthesia (hem′e-an′es-the′ze-ah)	hemi- an- esthesia	half (1/2) without, lack of perception, sense	12. _____
13. semilunar (sem′e-lu′nar)	semi- lun(a) -ar	half (1/2) moon pertaining to	13. _____

 ➡ *Pause CD*

After practicing each word several times, use a sheet of paper to cover all columns except the Answer column. As each word is pronounced again on the CD, write it in the space provided.

 ➡ *Start CD*

Check the words you have written against the words in the left-hand column. If you have misspelled any words, practice writing them correctly.

Practice

_____

_____

_____

_____

_____

_____

_____

_____

_____

_____

_____

_____

_____

_____

LESSON
3-1

Terminology Application

Without looking at your previous work, write the word that matches each definition.

Definition	Term
1. resembling a crescent or half-moon	Semilunar
2. a unit of mass being 100 grams	Hectogram
3. the condition of having four digits on the hands or feet	tetradactyl
4. one-tenth of a liter	Deciliter
5. the condition of having three testes	triorchidism
6. a unit of the metric system being 1/100 meter	centimeter
7. 1/1000 volt	millivolt
8. any group of five	pentad
9. a quantity equaling 1000 units	kilounit
10. condition denoting anesthesia (lack of feeling) on one side of the body	Hemianesthesia
11. ten grams	Decagram
12. double vision	Diplopia
13. having only one descended testicle in the scrotum	monorchidism

Check your answers against the information given in this lesson's terminology presentation. If you have any errors, count them and write the number in the blank at the top of the page. Sign your work and give it to your instructor.

Practice

Terminology Presentation

Amounts and Positions, Part 1

As you listen to the CD, read the words and notice the pronunciations given.

 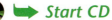 **Start CD**

Word	Word Part	Definition	Answer
1. anterosuperior (an'ter-o-su-per'e-or)	anter(o) super(ior)	before above	1. _____
2. hypogastric (hi'po-gas'trik)	hypo- gaster -ic	under stomach of, pertaining to	2. _____
3. anastomosis (ah-nas'to-mo'sis)	ana- stom(a) -osis	up mouth, opening abnormal condition	3. _____
4. sublingual (sub-ling'gwal)	sub- lingu(a) -al	under tongue pertaining to	4. _____
5. hyperglycemia (hi'per-gli-se'me-ah)	hyper- glyc(o) -emia	excessive sugar, glucose pertaining to blood	5. _____
6. inframammary (in'frah-mam'ah-re)	infra- mammary	below, beneath breast	6. _____
7. semicoma (sem'e-ko'mah)	semi- coma	half (1/2) stupor, unconscious	7. _____
8. contraindication (kon'trah-in'di-ka'shun)	contr(a) indicati(o) -ion	against indicate, point to denotes noun	8. _____
9. supratympanic (soo'prah-tim-pan'ik)	supra- tympan(o) -ic	above tympanum, eardrum pertaining to	9. _____
10. infratracheal (in'frah-tra'ke-al)	infra- trache(a) -al	beneath trachea pertaining to	10. _____
11. tertian (ter'shun)	ter(ti)- -an	three (3) pertaining to	11. _____

continued

Word	Word Part	Definition	Answer
12. ultrasonic (ul'trah-son'ik)	ultra- son(o) -ic	above, excess sound pertaining to	12. _____
13. unilateral (u'ni-lat'er-al)	uni- lateral	one side	13. _____

 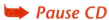 *Pause CD*

After practicing each word several times, use a sheet of paper to cover all columns except the Answer column. As each word is pronounced again on the CD, write it in the space provided.

 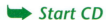 *Start CD*

Check the words you have written against the words in the left-hand column. If you have misspelled any words, practice writing them correctly.

Practice

_____

_____

_____

_____

_____

_____

_____

_____

_____

_____

_____

_____

_____

_____

_____

_____

_____

_____

LESSON
3-2

Terminology Application

Without looking at your previous work, write the word that matches each definition.

Definition	Term
1. situated below the stomach	_____
2. situated beneath the tongue	_____
3. recurring every third day	_____
4. situated in front and above something	_____
5. situated beneath the trachea	_____
6. an opening or connection between two vessels or organs	_____
7. having a frequency above sound	_____
8. any condition which renders a certain treatment undesirable or not indicated	_____
9. a stupor from which the patient may be aroused	_____
10. situated above the tympanum	_____
11. abnormally high level of sugar in the blood	_____
12. situated beneath the breast	_____
13. pertaining to or affecting only one side	_____

Check your answers against the information given in this lesson's terminology presentation. If you have any errors, count them and write the number in the blank at the top of the page. Sign your work and give it to your instructor.

Practice

Amounts and Positions, Part 2

As you listen to the CD, read the words and notice the pronunciations given.

  Start CD

Word	Word Part	Definition	Answer
1. bifurcate (bi-fur′kat)	bi- furcate	two forked	1. _____
2. ectoderm (ek′to-derm)	ect(o) derm	outside skin	2. _____
3. intercostal (in′ter-kos′tal)	inter- cost(o) -al	between rib of, pertaining to	3. _____
4. intrabuccal (in′trah-buk′al)	intra- bucc(o) -al	within cheek, mouth of, pertaining to	4. _____
5. epiotic (ep′e-ot′ik)	epi- otic	above, upon pertaining to the ear	5. _____
6. monochromatic (mon′o-kro-mat′ik)	mon(o) chromat(o) -ic	one (1) color pertaining to	6. _____
7. panhysterectomy (pan′his-ter-ek′to-me)	pan- hyster(o) -ectomy	all uterus excision	7. _____
8. pericardium (per′i-kar′de-um)	peri- cardi(o)	around heart	8. _____
9. polydipsia (pol′e-dip′se-ah)	poly- -dipsia	many, much thirst	9. _____
10. polyphagia (pol′e-fa′je-ah)	poly- phagia	many, much to eat	10. _____
11. protoplasia (pro-to-pla′se-ah)	prot(o) -plasia	first formation	11. _____
12. postmortem (post-mor′tem)	post- mortem	after death	12. _____

continued

Word	Word Part	Definition	Answer
13. retractor (re-trak′tor)	re- tract(or)	back to draw or pull, to hold	**13.** _____
14. retroflexed (ret′ro-flekst)	retr(o) flexed	backward bent	**14.** _____

  Pause CD

After practicing each word several times, use a sheet of paper to cover all columns except the Answer column. As each word is pronounced again on the CD, write it in the space provided.

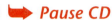 *Start CD*

Check the words you have written against the words in the left-hand column. If you have misspelled any words, practice writing them correctly.

Practice

_____

_____

_____

_____

_____

_____

_____

_____

_____

_____

_____

_____

_____

_____

_____

LESSON 3-3

Terminology Application

Without looking at your previous work, write the word that matches each definition.

Definition	Term
1. the outermost of the layers of skin	_____
2. divide into two branches	_____
3. excessive thirst	_____
4. the fibroserous sac surrounding the heart	_____
5. situated between the ribs	_____
6. the primary formation of tissue	_____
7. occurring or performed after death	_____
8. bent backward	_____
9. within the cheek or mouth	_____
10. an instrument to draw back and hold the edges of a wound	_____
11. having only one color	_____
12. situated above or upon the ear	_____
13. total removal of the uterus and cervix (total hysterectomy)	_____
14. excessive eating, overeating (bulimia)	_____

Check your answers against the information given in this lesson's terminology presentation. If you have any errors, count them and write the number in the blank at the top of the page. Sign your work and give it to your instructor.

Practice

3-4 Terminology Presentation

Colors and Positions

As you listen to the CD, read the words and notice the pronunciations given.

 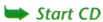 **Start CD**

Word	Word Part	Definition	Answer
1. aberrant (ab-er'ant)	ab- errant	away from wander	1. _____
2. adduct (ah-dukt')	ad- duct(o)	toward to draw	2. _____
3. melena (me-le'nah)	melan(o)	black	3. _____
4. biceps (bi'seps)	bi- ceps	two, double head	4. _____
5. dorsal (dor'sal)	dors(o)- -al	back (of the body) of, pertaining to	5. _____
6. dehydrate (de-hi'drat)	de- hydr(o)	from, not, down water	6. _____
7. chlorophyll (klo'ro-fil)	chlor(o) -phyll(o)	green leaf	7. _____
8. cirrhosis (sir-ro'sis)	cirrh(o) -osis	yellow abnormal condition	8. _____
9. erythrocyte (e-rith'ro-sit)	erythr(o) -cyte	red cell	9. _____
10. leukocyte (loo'ko-sit)	leuk(o) -cyte	white cell	10. _____
11. rubeosis (roo'be-o'sis)	rub(e) -osis	red abnormal condition	11. _____
12. xanthoderma (zan'tho-der-mah)	xanth(o) derma	yellow skin	12. _____

continued

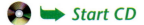

Pause CD

After practicing each word several times, use a sheet of paper to cover all columns except the Answer column. As each word is pronounced again on the CD, write it in the space provided.

Start CD

Check the words you have written against the words in the left-hand column. If you have misspelled any words, practice writing them correctly.

Practice

_____

_____

_____

_____

_____

_____

_____

_____

_____

_____

_____

_____

_____

_____

_____

_____

_____

_____

_____

_____

_____

LESSON
3-4

Terminology Application

Without looking at your previous work, write the word that matches each definition.

Definition	Term
1. the green coloring matter of plants	_____
2. dark or black feces containing blood	_____
3. a liver disorder in which a primary symptom is jaundice (yellow skin)	_____
4. deviating from the norm	_____
5. redness of an area	_____
6. white blood cell	_____
7. to draw toward	_____
8. any yellow discoloration of the skin	_____
9. red blood cell	_____
10. to remove water from a substance, such as the body	_____
11. pertaining to the back of the body	_____
12. a muscle having two heads	_____

Check your answers against the information given in this lesson's terminology presentation. If you have any errors, count them and write the number in the blank at the top of the page. Sign your work and give it to your instructor.

Practice

CHAPTER 3

Terminology Review

This is a review of the word parts and words you have learned in the preceding lessons. Some of the medical terms listed below may be new, but they are composed of the word parts and word roots that you have already learned. Read the words below as they are pronounced on the CD.

  Start CD

Word Element Review

Word	Word Part	Meaning of Word Part
1. hemianesthesia	hemi-	_____
hemianesthesia	an-	_____
hemianesthesia	esthesia	_____
(hem′e-an′es-the′ze-ah)	Meaning of Word	_____
2. tertian	ter(ti)-	_____
tertian	-an	_____
(ter′shun)	Meaning of Word	_____
3. protoplasia	prot(o)	_____
protoplasia	-plasia	_____
(pro-to-pla′ze-ah)	Meaning of Word	_____
4. biceps	bi-	_____
biceps	ceps	_____
(bi′seps)	Meaning of Word	_____
5. rubeosis	rub(e)	_____
rubeosis	-osis	_____
(roo′be-o′sis)	Meaning of Word	_____
6. polyphagia	poly-	_____
polyphagia	phagia	_____
(pol′e-fa′je-ah)	Meaning of Word	_____
7. aberrant	ab-	_____
aberrant	errant	_____
(ab-er′ant)	Meaning of Word	_____

Word	Word Part	Meaning of Word Part

8. infra costal — infra- — _____

infra cost al — cost(o) — _____

infracost al — -al — _____

(in′frah-kos′tal) — Meaning of Word — _____

9. centi meter — centi- — _____

centi meter — meter — _____

(sen′ti-me′ter) — Meaning of Word — _____

10. ana stomosis — ana- — _____

ana stom osis — stoma — _____

anastom osis — -osis — _____

(ah-nas′to-mo′sis) — Meaning of Word — _____

11. hypo gastric — hypo- — _____

hypo gastric — -gastric — _____

(hi′po-gas′trik) — Meaning of Word — _____

12. post mortem — post- — _____

post mortem — mortem — _____

(post-mor′tem) — Meaning of Word — _____

13. chloro phyll — chlor(o) — _____

chloro phyll — -phyll(o) — _____

(klo′ro-fil) — Meaning of Word — _____

14. xantho derma — xanth(o) — _____

xantho derma — -derma — _____

(zan′tho-der-mah) — Meaning of Word — _____

15. pent ad — penta — _____

pent ad — -ad — _____

(pen′tad) — Meaning of Word — _____

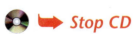 ➡ *Stop CD*

On the lines provided, write in the meanings of as many suffixes, prefixes, roots, and words as you can from memory. Check your definitions in the glossary or a medical dictionary, and make any needed corrections.

CHAPTER 3

Terminology Review

Complete this review, and turn it in to your instructor when you are finished.

Definition

Each phrase below defines one of the words you have just studied. Without looking at your previous work, write in the word that matches each definition.

Definition	Term
1. abnormally high level of sugar in the blood	_____
2. redness of an area	_____
3. situated below a rib	_____
4. dark, black feces containing blood	_____
5. anesthesia (lack of feeling) on one side of the body	_____
6. an opening or connection between two vessels or organs	_____
7. overeating	_____
8. the green-coloring substance in plants	_____
9. recurring every third day	_____
10. the primary formation of tissue	_____
11. excessive thirst	_____
12. a muscle having two heads	_____
13. a unit of the metric system being 1/100 meter	_____
14. occurring or performed after death	_____
15. divide into two branches	_____

continued

Matching

Match the following terms with the definitions given. Write the letter of the correct term to the left of the definition.

Definition	Term
_____ **16.** any group of five	**a.** intrabuccal
_____ **17.** the primary formation of tissue	**b.** epiotic
_____ **18.** red blood cell	**c.** millivolt
_____ **19.** situated above or upon the ear	**d.** pentad
_____ **20.** within the cheek or mouth	**e.** leukocyte
_____ **21.** situated beneath the breast	**f.** cirrhosis
_____ **22.** white blood cell	**g.** protoplasia
_____ **23.** a liver disorder in which the primary symptom is jaundice	**h.** erythrocyte
_____ **24.** being 1/1000 of a volt	**i.** supratympanic
_____ **25.** situated above the tympanum	**j.** inframammary

You may now go on to Chapter Test 3.

PART
2

Systems of the Body

4

Integumentary System

Objectives

After completing Chapter 4, you should be able to do the following:

1. identify word roots pertaining to the skin;
2. know the three layers of the skin—the epidermis, the dermis, and the subcutaneous layers;
3. identify the terms for hair and the nails;
4. name and identify glands in the skin; and
5. identify several types of drugs associated with skin conditions and treatments.

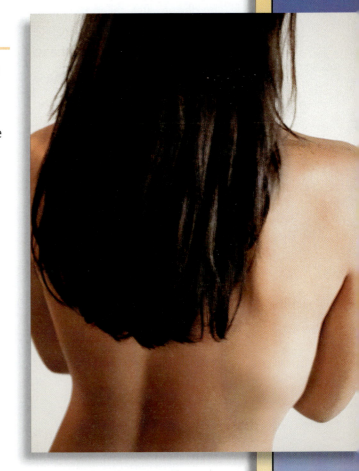

Orientation to the Integumentary System

The integumentary system consists of the skin, nails, hair, and glands embedded in the skin. The skin (*integument*—"a covering") has been called the largest organ of the body because of its great surface area. The skin provides a protective covering, acts as a sensing unit to note changes in the environment, and helps regulate body temperature.

The skin consists of three layers: the epidermis (the outer layer), the dermis (the middle layer), and the subcutaneous layer (the innermost layer of tissue). The epidermis is a protective covering of scale-like cells made up of the protein keratin. Color in the epidermis results from pigment granules called melanin, which occur in various amounts in each person. This pigment protects the body from excess ultraviolet light rays.

The dermis, also called the corium, contains hair follicles (roots), sebaceous (oil) glands, sudoriferous (sweat) glands, and sensory receptors that transmit pain, heat, cold, or pressure to the brain.

The subcutaneous layer of the skin is a combination of fibrous and fatty (adipose) tissues.

Hair and nails are forms of skin cells in which keratin is the major structure of the tissue.

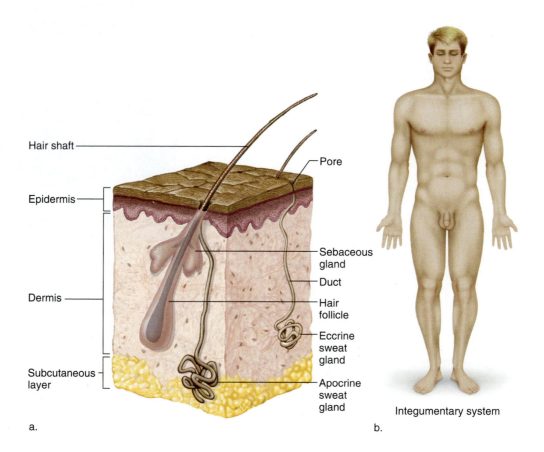

a.

b. Integumentary system

4-1 Terminology Presentation

Skin

As you listen to the CD, read the words and notice the pronunciations given.

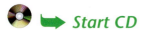 **Start CD**

Look at Figure 4-1

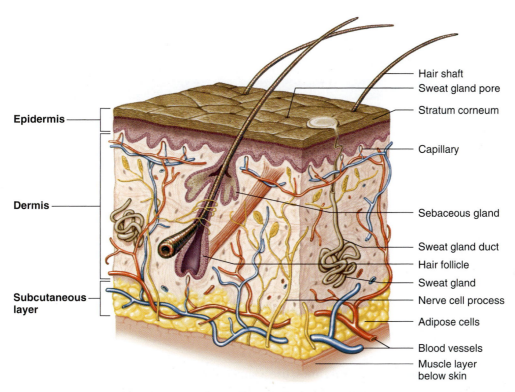

FIGURE 4-1   Structure of skin: epidermis, dermis, subcutaneous layer, sebaceous gland, sudoriferous (sweat) gland, nerve endings, blood vessels, hair, and adipose tissue.

derm(o), *derm(a), dermat(o)* combining forms denoting the skin			
Word	**Word Part**	**Definition**	**Answer**
1. dermatologist (der′mah-tol′o-jist)	-(o)logist	specialist	1. _____
2. dermatoautoplasty (der′mah-to-aw′to-plas′te)	auto -plasty	self plastic surgery	2. _____

continued

Word	Word Part	Definition	Answer
3. dermatitis (der′mah-ti′tis)	-itis	inflammation	3. _____
4. dermal (der′mal)	-al	of, pertaining to	4. _____
5. dermatophobia (der′mah-to-fo′be-ah)	-phobia	fear	5. _____
6. dermatosis (der′mah-to′sis)	-osis	abnormal condition	6. _____
7. dermatome (der′mah-tom)	-tome	an instrument for cutting	7. _____
8. dermomycosis (der′mo-mi-ko′sis)	myc(o) -osis	fungus abnormal condition	8. _____

kerat(o)	a combining form denoting horny tissue or the cornea of the eye

Word	Word Part	Definition	Answer
9. keratiasis (ker′ah-ti′ah-sis)	-iasis	diseased condition	9. _____
10. keratoderma (ker′ah-to-der′mah)	derm(a)	skin	10. _____
11. keratoid (ker′ah-toid)	-oid	like, resembling	11. _____
12. keratogenous (ker′ah-toj′e-nus)	-genous	to produce	12. _____
13. keratoma (ker′ah-to′mah)	-oma	tumor	13. _____

  ➡ *Pause CD*

> After practicing each word several times, use a sheet of paper to cover all columns except the Answer column. As each word is pronounced again on the CD, write it in the space provided.

  ➡ *Start CD*

> Check the words you have written against the words in the left-hand column. If you have misspelled any words, practice writing them correctly.

LESSON
4-1   Terminology Application

Without looking at your previous work, write the word that matches each definition.

Definition	Term
1. of or pertaining to the skin	_____
2. autografting of skin taken from another part of the patient's own body	_____
3. a horny skin or covering	_____
4. the presence of horny warts on the skin	_____
5. an instrument for cutting the skin or cutting thin transplants	_____
6. specialist in the diagnosis and treatment of skin diseases	_____
7. any fungus disease of the skin	_____
8. a morbid fear of acquiring a skin disease	_____
9. a tumor or growth of horny tissue	_____
10. producing cells that result in the formation of horny tissue such as fingernails	_____
11. any generalized skin disease	_____
12. inflammation of the skin	_____
13. like or resembling a horny skin	_____

Check your answers against the information given in this lesson's terminology presentation. If you have any errors, count them and write the number in the blank at the top of the page. Sign your work and give it to your instructor.

Practice

4-2 Terminology Presentation

Hair and Nails

As you listen to the CD, read the words and notice the pronunciations given.

  Start CD

Look at Figure 4-1 on page 81

trich, trich(o)	combining forms denoting hair or capillary (hairlike) vessels		
Word	**Word Part**	**Definition**	**Answer**
1. trichoglossia (trik′o-glos′e-ah)	-gloss	pertaining to the tongue	1. _____
2. trichalgia (trik-al′je-ah)	-algia	pain	2. _____
3. trichology (tri-kol′o-je)	-ology	the study of	3. _____
4. trichoschisis (trik-os′ki-sis)	-schisis	splitting	4. _____
5. trichopathy (tri-kop′ah-the)	-pathy	disease	5. _____
6. trichomycosis (trik′o-mi-ko′sis)	-myc(o) -osis	fungus abnormal condition	6. _____
7. trichogenous (tri-koj′e-nus)	-genous	to produce	7. _____

Look at Figure 4-2 below

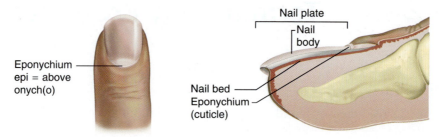

FIGURE 4-2 Structure of a nail.

	onych(o) a combining form denoting the nails		
Word	**Word Part**	**Definition**	**Answer**
8. onychomalacia (on'i-ko-mah-la'she-ah)	-malacia	softening	8. _____
9. onychophagia (on'i-ko-fa'je-ah)	-phagia	to eat	9. _____
10. onychorrhexis (on'i-ko-rek'sis)	-rrhexis	rupture	10. _____
11. onychoma (on'i-ko'mah)	-oma	tumor	11. _____
12. onychomycosis (on'i-ko-mi-ko'sis)	-myc(o) -osis	fungus abnormal condition	12. _____
13. onychosis (on'i-ko'sis)	-osis	abnormal condition	13. _____
14. onychoptosis (on'i-kop-to'sis)	-ptosis	falling	14. _____
15. onychogenic (on'i-ko-jen'ik)	-genic	produce	15. _____

  ➡ *Pause CD*

After practicing each word several times, use a sheet of paper to cover all columns except the Answer column. As each word is pronounced again on the CD, write it in the space provided.

  ➡ *Start CD*

Check the words you have written against the words in the left-hand column. If you have misspelled any words, practice writing them correctly.

Practice

_____

_____

LESSON 4-2

Terminology Application

Without looking at your previous work, write the word that matches by each definition.

Definition	Term
1. softening of the fingernail	_____
2. a hairy condition of the tongue	_____
3. falling off of the nail	_____
4. habitual biting of the nails	_____
5. pain when the hair is touched	_____
6. a tumor of the nail or nail bed	_____
7. promoting growth of hair	_____
8. splitting or rupture of the nails	_____
9. the study of the hair	_____
10. a disease of the hair	_____
11. fungus condition of the nails	_____
12. fungus infection of the hair	_____
13. producing nail substance	_____
14. splitting of the hair	_____
15. a disease of the nails	_____

Check your answers against the information given in this lesson's terminology presentation. If you have any errors, count them and write the number in the blank at the top of the page. Sign your work and give it to your instructor.

Practice

4-3 Terminology Presentation

Tissues

As you listen to the CD, read the words and notice the pronunciations given.

 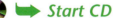 **Start CD**

Look at Figure 4-1 on page 81

hist(o), histi(o) combining forms denoting relationship to tissue			
Word	**Word Part**	**Definition**	**Answer**
1. histology (his-tol'o-je)	-(o)logy	study of, science of	1. _____
2. histoneurology (his'to-nu-rol'o-je)	neur(o) -(o)logy	nerves study of, science of	2. _____
3. histokinesis (his'to-ki-ne'sis)	-kinesis	movement	3. _____
4. histocyte (his'to-sit)	-cyte	cell	4. _____
5. histotoxic (his'to-tok'sik)	tox -ic	poison pertaining to	5. _____
6. historrhexis (his'to-rek'sis)	-rrhexis	rupture	6. _____

sarc(o) a combining form denoting flesh or connective tissue			
Word	**Word Part**	**Definition**	**Answer**
7. sarcopoietic (sar'ko-poi-et'ik)	-poiesis -ic	formation pertaining to	7. _____
8. sarcoid (sar'koid)	-oid	like, resembling	8. _____
9. sarcolysis (sar-kol'i-sis)	-lysis	dissolve, break down	9. _____
10. sarcogenic (sar'ko-jen'ik)	genic	to produce	10. _____
11. sarcoma (sar-ko'mah)	-oma	tumor	11. _____

continued

Word	Word Part	Definition	Answer
12. sarcosis (sar-ko′sis)	-osis	abnormal condition	12. _____
13. sarcoblast (sar′ko-blast)	-blast	immature cell	13. _____

  Pause CD

After practicing each word several times, use a sheet of paper to cover all columns except the Answer column. As each word is pronounced again on the CD, write it in the space provided.

 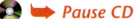 *Start CD*

Check the words you have written against the words in the left-hand column. If you have misspelled any words, practice writing them correctly.

Practice

_____

_____

_____

_____

_____

_____

_____

_____

_____

_____

_____

_____

_____

_____

_____

_____

LESSON 4-3

Terminology Application

Without looking at your previous work, write the word that matches each definition.

Definition	Term
1. the histology of the nervous system	_____
2. tumor of fleshy or connective tissue	_____
3. destruction or dissolution of flesh	_____
4. forming flesh	_____
5. the study of tissue	_____
6. producing flesh or muscle	_____
7. breaking up of tissue	_____
8. movement in the tissues of the body	_____
9. like or resembling flesh	_____
10. a tissue cell	_____
11. primitive or immature cell that develops into connective tissue	_____
12. abnormal increase in flesh	_____
13. being poisonous to tissue or tissues	_____

Check your answers against the information given in this lesson's terminology presentation. If you have any errors, count them and write the number in the blank at the top of the page. Sign your work and give it to your instructor.

Practice

4-4

Terminology Presentation

Fat and Sweat

As you listen to the CD, read the words and notice the pronunciations given.

⬤ ➡ *Start CD*

Look at Figure 4-1 on page 81

	adip(o)	a combining form denoting a relationship to fat, adipose tissue		
Word	**Word Part**	**Definition**	**Answer**	
1. adipoid (ad′i-poid)	-oid	resembling	1. _____	
2. adiposis (ad′i-po′sis)	-osis	abnormal condition	2. _____	
3. adiposuria (ad′i-po-su′re-ah)	-uria	condition of the urine	3. _____	
4. adipoma (ad′i-po-mah)	-oma	tumor	4. _____	

	lip(o)	a combining form denoting relationship to fat or to lipids		
Word	**Word Part**	**Definition**	**Answer**	
5. lipemia (li-pe′-me-ah)	-emia	condition of the blood	5. _____	
6. lipopenia (lip′o-pe′ne-ah)	-penia	deficiency	6. _____	
7. lipedema (lip′e-de′mah)	-edema	swelling	7. _____	

	steat(o)	a combining form denoting relationship to fat		
Word	**Word Part**	**Definition**	**Answer**	
8. steatorrhea (ste′ah-to-re′ah)	-rrhea	a flow	8. _____	

continued

	hidr(o)	a combining form denoting relationship to sweat or to a sweat gland	
Word	**Word Part**	**Definition**	**Answer**
9. hidropoiesis (hid'ro-poi-e'sis)	-poiesis	formation	9. _____
10. hidradenitis (hi'drad-e-ni'tis)	-aden(o) -itis	gland inflammation	10. _____

➡ Pause CD

After practicing each word several times, use a sheet of paper to cover all columns except the Answer column. As each word is pronounced again on the CD, write it in the space provided.

➡ Start CD

Check the words you have written against the words in the left-hand column. If you have misspelled any words, practice writing them correctly.

Practice

_____

_____

_____

_____

_____

_____

_____

_____

_____

_____

_____

_____

_____

_____

_____

_____

LESSON
4-4
Terminology Application

Without looking at your previous work, write the word that matches each definition.

Definition	Term
1. a fatty tumor; lipoma	_____
2. deficiency of lipids in the body	_____
3. excessive amounts of fats in the feces	_____
4. obesity or corpulence; excessive accumulation of fat in the body	_____
5. inflammation of a sweat gland	_____
6. resembling fat; lipoid	_____
7. excess fat or lipids in the blood	_____
8. the formation and secretion of sweat	_____
9. accumulation of excess fat and fluid in subcutaneous tissue	_____
10. presence of fat in the urine; lipuria	_____

Check your answers against the information given in this lesson's terminology presentation. If you have any errors, count them and write the number in the blank at the top of the page. Sign your work and give it to your instructor.

Practice

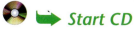
Drug Terminology Presentation

As you listen to the CD, read the words, and notice the pronunciations given.

 Start CD

Word	Definition Name	Example: Generic Name	Example: Brand/ Trade Name	Answer
anti-infectives	agents that can kill infectious agents or prevent them from spreading	azithromycin moxifloxacin amoxicillin/ clavulanate potassium cephalexin cefaclor	Zithromax Avalox Augmentin Keflex Ceclor (various)	1. _____
anti-inflammatories	agents that counteract or suppress inflammation	celecoxib	Celebrex	2. _____
antifungals	agents that destroy fungus or suppress its growth	itraconazole miconazole fluconazole nystatin	Sporanox Monistat Diflucan Mycostatin	3. _____
antipruritics	agents that relieve or prevent itching	hydrocortisone hydroxyzine	Anusol-HC Atarax	4. _____
keratolytics	agents that soften the horny layer of the epidermis	tretinoin	Retin-A	5. _____
parasiticides	agents that destroy parasites	ivermectin (worms)	Mectizan	6. _____
topical anesthetics	agents used on the skin to abolish the sensation of pain	lidocaine topical benzocaine	Xylocaine, Solarcaine Ora-Jel	7. _____

 Pause CD

After practicing each word several times, use a sheet of paper to cover all columns except the Answer column. As each word is pronounced again on the CD, write it in the space provided.

 Start CD

Check the words you have written against the words in the left-hand column. If you have misspelled any words, practice writing them correctly.

Practice

LESSON 4-5

Drug Terminology Application

Without looking at your previous work, write the term that matches each definition.

Definition	Term
1. agents that destroy parasites	_____
2. agents that destroy fungus or suppress its growth	_____
3. agents that can kill infectious agents or prevent them from spreading	_____
4. agents used on the skin to abolish the sensation of pain	_____
5. agents that counteract or suppress inflammation	_____
6. agents that relieve or prevent itching	_____
7. agents that soften the horny layer of the epidermis	_____

Check your answers against the information given in this lesson's terminology presentation. If you have any errors, count them and write the number in the blank at the top of the page. Sign your work and give it to your instructor.

Practice

CHAPTER 4
Terminology Review

This is a review of the word parts and words you have learned in the preceding lessons. Some of the medical terms listed below may be new, but they are composed of the word parts and word roots that you have already learned. Read the words below as they are pronounced on the CD.

 Start CD

Word Element Review

Word	Word Part	Meaning of Word Part
1. histocyte	hist(o)	_____
histocyte	-cyte	_____
(his′to-sit)	Meaning of Word	_____
2. dermomycosis	derm(o)	_____
dermomycosis	myc(o)	_____
(der′mo-mi-ko′sis)	-osis	_____
	Meaning of Word	_____
3. trichalgia	trich(o)	_____
trichalgia	-algia	_____
(trik-al′je-ah)	Meaning of Word	_____
4. keratoma	kerat(o)	_____
keratoma	-oma	_____
(ker′ah-to′mah)	Meaning of Word	_____
5. sarcolysis	sarc(o)	_____
sarcolysis	-lysis	_____
(sar-kol′i-sis)	Meaning of Word	_____
6. onychophagia	onych(o)	_____
onychophagia	-phagia	_____
(on′i-ko-fa′je-ah)	Meaning of Word	_____
7. hidradenitis	hidr(o)	_____
hidradenitis	-aden(o)	_____
hidradenitis	-itis	_____
(hi′drad-e-ni-tis)	Meaning of word	_____

Word	Word Part	Meaning of Word Part
8. lipemia	lip(o)	_____
lipemia	-emia	_____
(li-pe'-me-ah)	Meaning of Word	_____
9. histology	hist(o)	_____
histology	-(o)logy	_____
(his-tol'o-je)	Meaning of Word	_____
10. dermatitis	dermat	_____
dermatitis	-itis	_____
(der'mah-ti'tis)	Meaning of Word	_____
11. histotoxic	hist(o)	_____
histotoxic	tox	_____
histotoxic	-ic	_____
(his'to-tok'sik)	Meaning of Word	_____
12. sarcosis	sarc(o)	_____
sarcosis	-osis	_____
(sar-ko'sis)	Meaning of Word	_____
13. onychomalacia	onych(o)	_____
onychomalacia	-malacia	_____
(on'i-ko-mah-la'she-ah)	Meaning of Word	_____

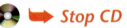 *Stop CD*

On the lines provided, write in the meanings of as many suffixes, prefixes, roots, and words as you can from memory. Check your definitions in the glossary or a medical dictionary, and make any needed corrections.

CHAPTER 4

Terminology Review

Complete this review, and turn it in to your instructor when you are finished.

Definition

Each phrase below defines one of the words you have just studied. Without looking at your previous work, write in the word that matches each definition.

Definition	Term
1. pain when the hair is touched	_____
2. inflammation of the skin	_____
3. an abnormal increase in flesh	_____
4. inflammation of a sweat gland	_____
5. obesity	_____
6. any fungal disease of the skin	_____
7. the study of tissue	_____
8. dissolution of flesh	_____
9. a tissue cell	_____
10. a tumor or growth of horny tissue	_____
11. forming flesh	_____
12. softening of the nails	_____
13. habitual biting of the nails	_____
14. a fatty tumor	_____
15. an agent that relieves or prevents itching	_____

continued

Matching

Match the following terms with the definitions given. Write the letter of the correct term to the left of the definition.

Definition	Term
_____ 16. producing cells that result in the formation of horny tissue such as the nails	**a.** adiposuria
_____ 17. the study of tissue	**b.** steatorrhea
_____ 18. splitting of the hair	**c.** dermatosis
_____ 19. the presence of fat in the urine	**d.** onychomycosis
_____ 20. a specialist in the treatment of skin diseases	**e.** keratogenous
_____ 21. a fungal condition of the nails	**f.** histology
_____ 22. excessive amounts of fats in the feces	**g.** trichoschisis
_____ 23. the study of the hair	**h.** sarcoma
_____ 24. tumor of fleshy or connective tissue	**i.** dermatologist
_____ 25. any generalized skin disease	**j.** trichology

CHAPTER 4

Terminology Review

Case Studies

Read the following brief case studies. In each case study, some terms are followed by a superscript letter. Write a brief definition for each of those terms on the corresponding lines below.

1. A.R., a retired office worker, has noticed several areas of redness on her lower right arm. She has a history of keratoderma[a] and several years ago had several sarcomas[b] removed; she suspects that this new redness is probably a type of dermatitis[c] but has decided to visit a dermatologist[d] to get an expert's opinion.

   a. _____

   b. _____

   c. _____

   d. _____

2. J.D. has noticed a drastic change in his fingernails. His doctor has diagnosed him with onychomycosis[a] and has recommended treatment with agents that include anti-fungals[b]. J.D. has a history of onychophagia[c] and does not take care of his nails as he should.

   a. _____

   b. _____

   c. _____

3. B.X. has had difficulty with hidradenitis[a]. Her doctor has suggested a series of tests to determine the extent of her illness.

   a. _____

4. C.J. has been diagnosed with adiposis[a] and has had lipedema[b]. Her doctor has recommended a change in diet and an exercise program to help C.J. learn to control her weight.

   a. _____

   b. _____

Labeling

Fill in the blanks with the correct terminology.

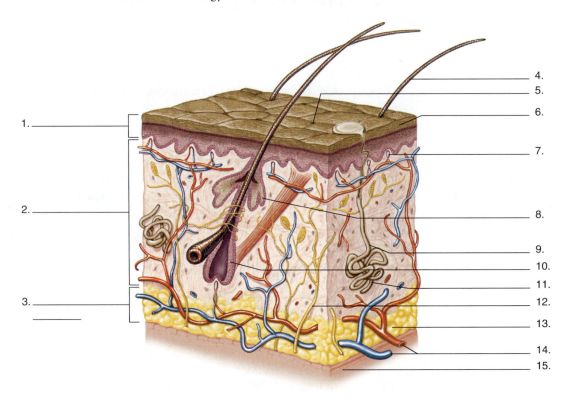

1. _____

2. _____

3. _____
   _____

4. _____

5. _____

6. _____

7. _____

8. _____

9. _____

10. _____

11. _____

12. _____

13. _____

14. _____

15. _____

FIGURE 4-3 Structure of skin: epidermis, dermis, subcutaneous layer, sebaceous gland, sudoriferous (sweat) gland, nerve endings, blood vessels, hair, and adipose tissue.

You may now go on to Chapter Test 4.

5

Respiratory System

Objectives

After completing Chapter 5, you should be able to do the following:

1. identify word roots pertaining to the nose;

2. identify word roots pertaining to the throat and the larynx;

3. identify word roots pertaining to the trachea and the bronchial passages;

4. understand the difference between a bronchus and a bronchiole;

5. identify the word root for the pleural sac;

6. understand several word roots that identify the lungs and chest cavity;

7. name and identify the parts of the upper respiratory tract;

8. name and identify the parts of the lower respiratory tract; and

9. identify several types of drugs associated with respiratory conditions and treatments.

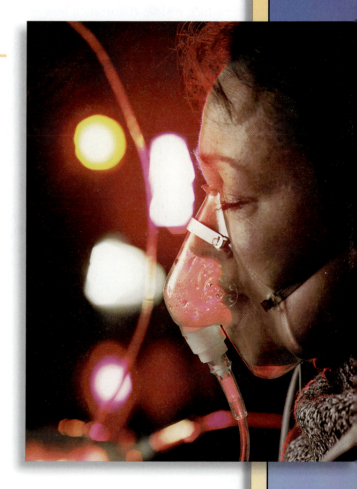

Orientation to the Respiratory System

The respiratory system is a continuous open passage from the mouth (the oral cavity) and nose through the head, neck, and chest to the lungs. Breathing in and out (inhalation and exhalation) allows oxygen (O_2) to enter and carbon dioxide (CO_2) to exit the body. The two main parts of the respiratory system are the upper respiratory tract (nose, mouth, pharynx, and larynx) and the lower respiratory tract (trachea, bronchi, bronchioles, pleura, lungs, and alveoli).

Air enters the nose through the nostrils (openings in the nose). The mucous membranes and numerous hairs in the nostrils filter dust and dirt from the air. The air then passes to the nasal cavities, which are separated from the mouth by the palate (roof of the mouth). The air then passes into the pharynx (throat) and into the larynx. Air travels from the larynx to the lungs via the trachea, which divides (bifurcates) into two branches called bronchi. After the bronchi enter the lungs, they branch into increasingly smaller tubes called bronchioles that extend deep into the lungs.

The lungs are membranous sacs on either side of the chest (thorax). Inside the lungs, at the tips of the bronchioles, are thin-walled alveolar sacs (alveoli) that are in close contact with blood capillaries. Gas exchange takes place at this level, as the red blood cells pick up inhaled oxygen to be distributed throughout the body. The surfaces of both lungs are lined with a membrane called the pleura.

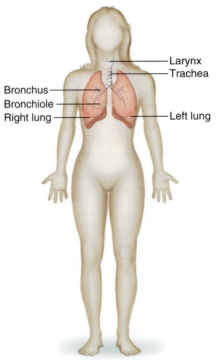

Respiratory system

5-1 Terminology Presentation

Nose

As you listen to the CD, read the words and notice the pronunciations given.

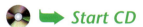 **Start CD**

Look at Figures 5-1 and 5-2

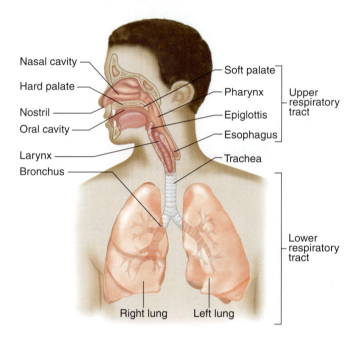

Figure 5-1 The upper and lower tracts of the respiratory system.

Nasal cavity

Hard palate

Nostril

Oral cavity

Larynx

Bronchus

Soft palate — Pharynx — Epiglottis — Esophagus } Upper respiratory tract

Trachea

Right lung   Left lung

Lower respiratory tract

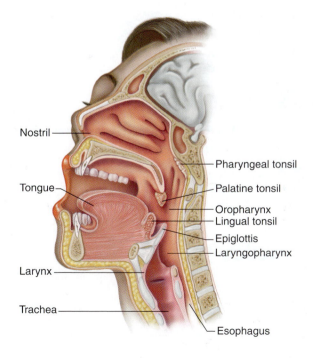

Nostril

Tongue

Larynx

Trachea

Pharyngeal tonsil

Palatine tonsil

Oropharynx

Lingual tonsil

Epiglottis

Laryngopharynx

Esophagus

Figure 5-2 The parts of the upper respiratory system.

rhin(o)	a combining form denoting the nose		
Word	**Word Part**	**Definition**	**Answer**
1. rhinodynia (ri′no -din′e-ah)	-dynia	pain	1. _____
2. rhinesthesia (ri′nes-the′ze-ah)	-esthesia	perception, sense	2. _____
3. rhinolith (ri′no-lith)	-lith(o)	stone	3. _____
4. rhinorrhagia (ri′no-ra′je-ah)	-rrhagia	excessive flow, bleeding	4. _____
5. rhinocheiloplasty (ri-no-ki′lo-plas′te)	cheil(o) -plasty	lip plastic surgery	5. _____
6. rhinitis (ri-ni′tis)	-itis	inflammation	6. _____
7. rhinomycosis (ri′no-mi-ko′sis)	myc(o) -osis	fungus abnormal condition	7. _____

nas(o)	a combining form denoting relationship to the nose		
Word	**Word Part**	**Definition**	**Answer**
8. nasal (na′zal)	-al	pertaining to	8. _____
9. nasopharynx (na′zo-far′inks)	pharynx	throat	9. _____
10. nasopharyngeal (na′zo-fah-rin′je-al)	pharyng(o) -eal	pharynx pertaining to	10. _____
11. nasoseptal (na′zo-sep′tal)	sept(a) -al	septum pertaining to	11. _____
12. nasoscope (na′zo-skop)	-scope	instrument for viewing	12. _____
13. nasogastric (na′zo-gas′trik)	gastr(o) -ic	stomach pertaining to	13. _____

 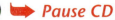 *Pause CD*

After practicing each word several times, use a sheet of paper to cover all columns except the Answer column. As each word is pronounced again on the CD, write it in the space provided.

  Start CD

Check the words you have written against the words in the left-hand column. If you have misspelled any words, practice writing them correctly.

Practice

_____

_____

LESSON 5-1

Terminology Application

Without looking at your previous work, write the word that matches each definition.

Definition	Term
1. a plastic surgery on the lip and nose	_____
2. nosebleed (also known as epistaxis)	_____
3. pertaining to the nose	_____
4. a stone or concretion of the nose	_____
5. part of the pharynx above the level of the soft palate	_____
6. pertaining to the sense of smell	_____
7. inflammation of the mucous membrane of the nose	_____
8. pertaining to the nasal septum	_____
9. fungus infection of the nose	_____
10. pertaining to the nasopharynx	_____
11. pertaining to the nose and stomach	_____
12. pain in the nose or nasal area	_____
13. lighted instrument used for examination of the nasal cavity	_____

Check your answers against the information given in this lesson's terminology presentation. If you have any errors, count them and write the number in the blank at the top of the page. Sign your work and give it to your instructor.

Practice

LESSON

5-2 Terminology Presentation

Throat and Larynx

As you listen to the CD, read the words and notice the pronunciations given.

 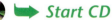 **Start CD**

Look at Figures 5-1 and 5-2 on pages 109

pharyng(o)	a combining form denoting relationship to the throat		
Word	**Word Part**	**Definition**	**Answer**
1. pharynx (far'inks)	pharynx	throat	1. _____
2. pharyngoplegia (far'ing-go-ple'je-ah)	-plegia	condition of paralysis	2. _____
3. pharyngomycosis (fah-ring'go-mi-ko'sis)	myc(o) -osis	fungus abnormal condition	3. _____
4. pharyngitis (far'in-ji'tis)	-itis	inflammation	4. _____
5. pharyngeal (fah-rin'je-al)	-eal	pertaining to	5. _____
6. pharyngectomy (far'in-jek'to-me)	-ectomy	excision, removal	6. _____
7. oropharynx (o'ro-far'inks)	or(o)	mouth	7. _____

laryng(o)	a combining form denoting the larynx (voice box)		
Word	**Word Part**	**Definition**	**Answer**
8. laryngitis (lar'in-ji'tis)	-itis	inflammation	8. _____
9. laryngeal (lah-rin'je-al)	-eal	of, pertaining to	9. _____
10. laryngoplegia (la-ring'go-ple'je-ah)	-plegia	paralysis	10. _____
11. laryngostenosis (lah-ring'go-ste-no'sis)	-stenosis	narrowing	11. _____

continued

Word	Word Part	Definition	Answer
12. laryngospasm (lah-ring'go-spazm)	-spasm	contraction	12. _____
13. laryngoscope (lah-ring'go-skop)	-scope	viewing instrument	13. _____
14. laryngectomy (lar'in-jek'to-me)	-ectomy	excision, removal	14. _____
15. laryngocentesis (lah-ring'go-sen-te'sis)	-centesis	surgical puncture	15. _____
16. laryngopharynx (lah-ring'go-far'inks)	-pharynx	throat	16. _____

 ➡ *Pause CD*

After practicing each word several times, use a sheet of paper to cover all columns except the Answer column. As each word is pronounced again on the CD, write it in the space provided.

 ➡ *Start CD*

Check the words you have written against the words in the left-hand column. If you have misspelled any words, practice writing them correctly.

Practice

_____

_____

_____

_____

_____

_____

_____

_____

_____

_____

_____

_____

_____

_____

LESSON 5-2

Terminology Application

Without looking at your previous work, write the word that matches each definition.

Definition	Term
1. paralysis of the larynx	_____
2. part of the pharynx above the level of the soft palate	_____
3. surgical puncture of the larynx	_____
4. paralysis of the muscles of the throat	_____
5. any fungal infection of the throat	_____
6. inflammation of the larynx	_____
7. inflammation of the throat	_____
8. spasmodic closure of the larynx	_____
9. musculo-membranous passage between the mouth and posterior nasal passage and the larynx and esophagus	_____
10. pertaining to the pharynx	_____
11. excision of the pharynx	_____
12. of or pertaining to the larynx	_____
13. division of pharynx below the upper edge of the epiglottis and opens into the larynx and esophagus	_____
14. narrowing of the larynx	_____
15. excision of the larynx	_____
16. instrument used to examine the larynx	_____

Check your answers against the information given in this lesson's terminology presentation. If you have any errors, count them and write the number in the blank at the top of the page. Sign your work and give it to your instructor.

Practice

5-3 Terminology Presentation

Trachea and Bronchi

As you listen to the CD, read the words and notice the pronunciations given.

  ➡ *Start CD*

Look at Figures 5-1 and 5-2 on page 109

trache(o)	a combining form denoting the trachea or windpipe		
Word	**Word Part**	**Definition**	**Answer**
1. tracheostomy (tra′ke-os′to-me)	-stomy	connection, opening	1. _____
2. tracheotomy (tra′ke-ot′o-me)	-tomy	incision, cutting into	2. _____
3. tracheoplasty (tra′ke-o-plas′te)	-plasty	plastic surgery	3. _____
4. tracheostenosis (tra′ke-o-ste-no′sis)	-stenosis	narrowing	4. _____
5. tracheopathy (tra′ke-op′ah-the)	-pathy	disease	5. _____
6. tracheorrhaphy (tra′ke-or′ah-fe)	-rrhaphy	suture, surgical repair	6. _____
7. tracheitis (tra′ke-i′tis)	-itis	inflammation	7. _____

bronch(i)	a combining form denoting the bronchi (plural) or bronchus (singular), the air passages within the lungs		
Word	**Word Part**	**Definition**	**Answer**
8. bronchorrhea (brong-ko-re′ah)	-rrhea	flow	8. _____
9. bronchiectasis (brong′ke-ek′tah-sis)	-ectasis	dilatation, expansion	9. _____
10. bronchitis (brong-ki′tis)	-itis	inflammation	10. _____
11. bronchoedema (brong′ko-e-de′mah)	-edema	swelling	11. _____

continued

Look at Figure 5-3

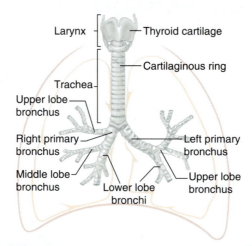

Figure 5-3   The larynx, trachea, and bronchi.

	Word	Word Part	Definition	Answer
12.	bronchoscopy (brong-kos′ko-pe)	-scopy	examine	12. _____
13.	bronchoplegia (brong′ko-ple′je-ah)	-plegia	paralysis	13. _____
14.	bronchopneumonitis (brong′ko-nu′mo-ni′tis)	pneum(o) -itis	lungs inflammation	14. _____
15.	bronchiole (brong′ke-ol)	-ole	diminutive spelling; refers to reduction in size	15. _____

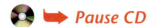 **Pause CD**

After practicing each word several times, use a sheet of paper to cover all columns except the Answer column. As each word is pronounced again on the CD, write it in the space provided.

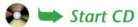 **Start CD**

Check the words you have written against the words in the left-hand column. If you have misspelled any words, practice writing them correctly.

Practice

_____

_____

_____

_____

LESSON 5-3

Terminology Application

Without looking at your previous work, write the word that matches each definition.

Definition	Term
1. excessive secretion of mucus from the bronchial mucous membrane	_____
2. surgical repair of the trachea	_____
3. dilatation (dilation) of the bronchi	_____
4. narrowing of the trachea	_____
5. plastic surgery of the trachea	_____
6. inspection or examination of the bronchi	_____
7. paralysis of the bronchi	_____
8. surgical creation of an opening into the trachea	_____
9. any disease of the trachea	_____
10. inflammation of the bronchi	_____
11. swelling of the mucosa of the bronchi	_____
12. incision into the trachea	_____
13. an inflammation of the lungs that originates at the bronchi	_____
14. inflammation of the trachea	_____
15. finer subdivisions of the bronchi	_____

Check your answers against the information given in this lesson's terminology presentation. If you have any errors, count them and write the number in the blank at the top of the page. Sign your work and give it to your instructor.

Practice

Terminology Presentation

Lungs, Chest, and Breathing

As you listen to the CD, read the words and notice the pronunciations given.

 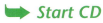 **Start CD**

pleura, pleur (o)	a term denoting the serous membrane surrounding the lungs and lining the chest cavity		
Word	**Word Part**	**Definition**	**Answer**
1. pleural (ploor'al)	-al	pertaining to	1. _____
2. pleurae (ploor'e)	-ae	more than one; plural ending	2. _____
3. pleuritis (ploo-ri'tis) (pleurisy) (ploor'i-se)	-itis	inflammation	3. _____
4. pleurectomy (ploor-ek'to-me)	-ectomy	excision, removal	4. _____
5. pleuralgia (ploor-al'je-ah)	-algia	pain	5. _____
6. pleurotomy (ploor-ot'o-me)	-tomy	incision, cutting	6. _____
7. pleurocentesis (ploor'o-sen-te'sis)	-centesis	surgical puncture	7. _____
8. pleurocele (ploor'o-sel)	-cele	tumor, swelling, hernia	8. _____

pneumon(o), pneum(o), pneumat(o), pneum(a)	combining forms denoting the lungs, respiration, air, or gas		
Word	**Word Part**	**Definition**	**Answer**
9. pneumonitis (nu'mo-ni'tis)	-itis	inflammation	9. _____
10. pneumonography (nu'mo-nog'rah-fe)	-graphy	recording	10. _____

continued

Look at Figure 5-1, on page 109, and Figure 5-4 here

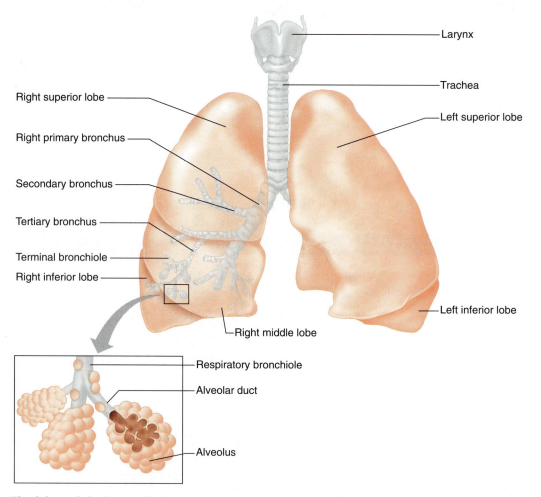

Larynx

Trachea

Right superior lobe

Left superior lobe

Right primary bronchus

Secondary bronchus

Tertiary bronchus

Terminal bronchiole

Right inferior lobe

Left inferior lobe

Right middle lobe

Respiratory bronchiole

Alveolar duct

Alveolus

Figure 5-4   The lobes of the lungs, the bronchi, the bronchioles, and the alveoli.

	Word	Word Part	Definition	Answer
11.	pneumomelanosis (nu'mo-mel'ah-no'sis)	melan(o) -osis	black abnormal condition	11. _____
12.	pneumodynamics (nu'mo-di-nam'iks)	-dynamics	force	12. _____
13.	pneumoencephalography (nu'mo-en-sef'ah-log'rah-fe)	encephal(o) -graphy	brain process of recording	13. _____
14.	pneumoconiosis (nu'mo-ko'ne-o'sis)	coni(o) -osis	dust abnormal condition	14. _____
15.	pneumothorax (nu'mo-tho'raks)	thorax	chest	15. _____
16.	pneumocentesis (nu'mo-sen-te'sis)	-centesis	surgical puncture	16. _____

pulmon(o)   a combining form denoting relationship to the lungs

	Word	Word Part	Definition	Answer
17.	pulmonectomy (pul'mo-nek'to-me)	-ectomy	excision, removal	17. _____
18.	pulmonitis (pul'mo-ni'tis)	-itis	inflammation	18. _____
19.	pulmonologist (pul'mo-nol'o-jist)	(o) -logist	specialist	19. _____
20.	pulmonic (pul-mon'ic)	-ic	pertaining to	20. _____

thorac(o)   a combining form denoting relationship to the thorax (chest)

	Word	Word Part	Definition	Answer
21.	thoracic (tho-ras'ik)	-ic	pertaining to	21. _____
22.	thoracotomy (tho'rah-kot'o-me)	-tomy	incision	22. _____
23.	thoracocentesis (tho'rah-ko-sen-te'sis) and thoracentesis (tho'rah-sen-te'sis)	-centesis -centesis	surgical puncture surgical puncture	23. _____

-pnea   a suffix denoting breathing or air or gas

	Word	Word Part	Definition	Answer
24.	eupnea (up-ne'ah)	eu-	well, normal	24. _____
25.	apnea (ap-ne'ah)	a-	without, lack of	25. _____
26.	dyspnea (disp'ne-ah)	dys-	abnormal, painful, difficult	26. _____
27.	orthopnea (or'thop-ne'ah)	orth(o)	straight, normal	27. _____
28.	tachypnea (tak'ip-ne'ah)	tachy-	fast	28. _____

continued

| | oxy, ox- | combining forms denoting the presence of oxygen | |
Word	Word Part	Definition	Answer
29. oximeter (ok-sim′e-ter)	meter	measurement	**29.** _____
30. hypoxemia (hi′pok-se′me-ah)	-emia	blood condition	**30.** _____

➡️ *Pause CD*

After practicing each word several times, use a sheet of paper to cover all columns except the Answer column. As each word is pronounced again on the CD, write it in the space provided.

➡️ *Start CD*

Check the words you have written against the words in the left-hand column. If you have misspelled any words, practice writing them correctly.

Practice

_____

_____

_____

_____

_____

_____

_____

_____

_____

_____

_____

_____

_____

_____

_____

_____

_____

LESSON 5-4

Terminology Application

Without looking at your previous work, write the word that matches each definition.

Definition	Term
1. pain in the pleura	_____
2. more than one pleura	_____
3. inflammation of the pleura	_____
4. pertaining to the chest	_____
5. X-ray of the lung	_____
6. incision into the chest	_____
7. herniation of the pleura	_____
8. photoelectric device used for determining the oxygen saturation in the blood	_____
9. inflammation of the lung	_____
10. difficult breathing	_____
11. the dynamics of the respiratory system	_____
12. easy, normal breathing	_____
13. pertaining to the lungs	_____
14. surgical puncture of the chest to aspirate fluid	_____
15. the blackening of the lungs as from coal dust	_____
16. abnormally fast rate of breathing	_____
17. pertaining to the pleura	_____
18. a lung specialist	_____
19. temporary absence of breathing	_____
20. inflammation of the lung	_____
21. inability to breathe unless in an upright position	_____

continued

22. a disease caused by dust or other particulates in the lungs

_____

23. radiographic films of the brain, created by utilizing injections of air or gas

_____

24. surgical puncture or tap of the pleura

_____

25. incision into the pleura

_____

26. excision of all or part of a lung

_____

27. accumulation of air in the chest cavity

_____

28. surgical puncture for aspiration of the lung

_____

29. excision of the pleura

_____

30. deficient oxygenation of the blood

_____

Check your answers against the information given in this lesson's terminology presentation. If you have any errors, count them and write the number in the blank at the top of the page. Sign your work and give it to your instructor.

LESSON
5-5 Drug Terminology Presentation

As you listen to the CD, read the words and notice the pronunciations given.

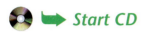 **Start CD**

Word	Definition	Example: Generic Name	Example: Brand/ Trade Name	Answer
antihistamines	agents that counter the effects of histamines; used to treat allergies	fexofenadine loratadine cetirizine promethazine diphenhydramine	Allegra Claritin Zyrtec Phenergan Benadryl	1. _____
antitussives	agents that relieve or prevent coughs	guaifenesin benzonatate promethazine hydrochloride	Robitussin Tessalon Perles Phenergan + codeine	2. _____
bronchodilators	agents that expand the air passages in the lungs	albuterol ipratropium salmeterol flunisolide (a corticosteroid) epinephrine triamcinolone (a corticosteroid) fluticason (a corticosteroid)	Proventil Atrovent Serevent Aerobid (various) Azmacort (various)	3. _____
decongestants	agents that reduce congestion and bronchial swelling	loratadine	Claritin	4. _____
expectorants	agents that promote the ejection of mucus or other fluids from the lower respiratory tract	guaifenesin benzonatate hydrocodone ammonium chloride codeine	Robitussin Tessalon Perles Hycodan (various) (various)	5. _____
mucolytics	agents that destroy or dissolve mucus	guaifenesin acetylcystein	Robitussin Mucomyst, Mucosil	6. _____

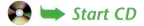 **Stop CD**

After practicing each word several times, use a sheet of paper to cover all columns except the Answer column. As each word is pronounced again on the CD, write it in the space provided.

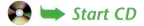 **Start CD**

Check the words you have written against the words in the left-hand column. If you have misspelled any words, practice writing them correctly.

Practice

LESSON
5-5
Drug Terminology Application

Without looking at your previous work, write the word that matches each definition.

Definition	Term
1. agents that promote the ejection of mucus or other fluids from the lower respiratory tract	_____
2. agents that destroy or dissolve mucus	_____
3. agents that counter the effects of histamines	_____
4. agents that expand the air passages in the lungs	_____
5. agents that reduce congestion and bronchial swelling	_____
6. agents that relieve or prevent coughs	_____

Check your answers against the information given in this lesson's terminology presentation. If you have any errors, count them and write the number in the blank at the top of the page. Sign your work and give it to your instructor.

Practice

CHAPTER
5
Terminology Review

This is a review of the word parts and words you have learned in the preceding lessons. Some of the medical terms listed below may be new, but they are composed of the word parts and word roots that you have already learned. Read the words below as they are pronounced on the CD.

 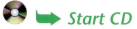 *Start CD*

Word Element Review

Word	Word Part	Meaning of Word Part
1. nasopharynx	nas(o)	_____
nasopharynx	pharynx	_____
(na′zo-far′inks)	Meaning of word	_____
2. laryngoscope	laryng(o)	_____
laryngoscope	-scope	_____
(lah-ring′go-skop)	Meaning of word	_____
3. rhinomycosis	rhin(o)	_____
rhinomycosis	myc(o)	_____
rhinomycosis	-osis	_____
(ri′no-mi-ko′sis)	Meaning of word	_____
4. bronchitis	bronch(o)	_____
bronchitis	-itis	_____
(brong-ki′tis)	Meaning of word	_____
5. oropharynx	or(o)	_____
oropharynx	pharynx	_____
(o′ro-far′inks)	Meaning of word	_____
6. tracheorrhaphy	trache(o)	_____
tracheorrhaphy	-rrhaphy	_____
(tra′ke-or′ah-fe)	Meaning of word	_____
7. pleurotomy	pleur(o)	_____
pleurotomy	-tomy	_____
(ploor-ot′o-me)	Meaning of word	_____

continued

Word	Word Part	Meaning of Word Part
8. pneumocentesis	pneum(o)	_____
pneumocentesis	-centesis	_____
(nu′mo-sen-te′sis)	Meaning of word	_____
9. thoracotomy	thorac(o)	_____
thoracotomy	-tomy	_____
(tho′rah-kot′o-me)	Meaning of word	_____
10. pulmonitis	pulmon(o)	_____
pulmonitis	-itis	_____
(pul′mo-ni′tis)	Meaning of word	_____
11. nasogastric	nas(o)	_____
nasogastric	gastr(o)	_____
nasogastric	-ic	_____
(na′zo-gas′trik)	Meaning of word	_____
12. bronchiole	bronch(i)	_____
bronchiole	-ole	_____
(brong′ke-ol)	Meaning of word	_____
13. pulmonectomy	pulmon(o)	_____
pulmonectomy	-ectomy	_____
(pul′mo-nek′to-me)	Meaning of word	_____
14. nasopharyngeal	nas(o)	_____
nasopharyngeal	pharyng(o)	_____
nasopharyngeal	-eal	_____
(na′zo-fah-rin′je-al)	Meaning of word	_____
15. thoracic	thorac(o)	_____
thoracic	-ic	_____
(tho-ras′ik)	Meaning of word	_____

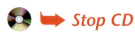 ➡ *Stop CD*

On the lines provided, write in the meanings of as many suffixes, prefixes, roots, and words as you can from memory. Check your definitions in the glossary or a medical dictionary, and make any needed corrections.

CHAPTER 5
Terminology Review

Complete this review, and turn it in to your instructor when you are finished.

Definition

Each phrase below defines one of the words you have just studied. Without looking at your previous work, write in the word that matches each definition.

Definition	Term
1. temporary absence of breathing	_____
2. pertaining to the chest	_____
3. excision of the larynx	_____
4. dilatation of the bronchi	_____
5. herniation of the pleura	_____
6. surgical puncture of the larynx	_____
7. pertaining to the nasal septum	_____
8. plastic surgery on the lip and nose	_____
9. the blackening of a lung, as from coal dust	_____
10. paralysis of a bronchus	_____
11. inability to breathe unless in an upright position	_____
12. radiographic films of the brain, created using injections of air or gas	_____
13. pain in the nose	_____
14. an inflammation of the lungs that originates at the bronchi	_____
15. nosebleed	_____
16. incision into the trachea	_____
17. lighted instrument used for examination of the nasal cavity	_____

continued

18. difficult breathing   _____

19. incision into the pleura   _____

20. inflammation of the pleura _____

Matching

Match the following definitions with the terms given. Write the letter of the correct definition to the left of the term.

Term	Definition
_____ **21.** laryngostenosis	**a.** difficult breathing
_____ **22.** tracheotomy	**b.** surgical repair or suture of the trachea
_____ **23.** thoracodynia	**c.** inflammation of the bronchi
_____ **24.** dyspnea	**d.** narrowing of the larynx
_____ **25.** rhinomycosis	**e.** fungus infection of the nose
_____ **26.** bronchoplegia	**f.** surgical procedure for aspiration of the lung
_____ **27.** thoracomyodynia	**g.** pain in the muscles of the chest
_____ **28.** tracheorrhaphy	**h.** incision into the trachea
_____ **29.** pneumocentesis	**i.** paralysis of the bronchi
_____ **30.** bronchitis	**j.** pain in the chest region

CHAPTER 5

Terminology Review

Case Studies

Read the following brief case studies. In each case study, some terms are followed by a superscript letter. Write a brief definition for each of those terms on the corresponding lines below.

1. J. is a former steelworker who has asthma and a variety of pulmonary[a] problems. Last year, he went to his pulmonologist[b] several times to be treated for pneumoconiosis[c] that resulted from his years working in a steel foundry. He usually has bronchitis[d] at least once a year, and he uses bronchodilators[e] on a regular basis.

   a. _____

   b. _____

   c. _____

   d. _____

   e. _____

2. P.N. works for a pediatrician and is familiar with the various types of children's respiratory[a] ailments and some of the common treatments. For example, one child recently diagnosed with allergies was treated with antihistamines[b]. Another child had considerable thoracic[c] congestion with a nagging cough; this child was treated with an antitussive[d], a decongestant[e], and a mucolytic[f].

   a. _____

   b. _____

   c. _____

   d. _____

   e. _____

   f. _____

3. A local hospital ER treated several elderly patients who had breathing difficulties. One patient had sleep apnea[a], another had tracheostenosis[b], and another had bronchopneumonitis[c]. All patients were admitted for 24-hour observation and were put on a regimen of appropriate medications and breathing treatments.

a. _____

b. _____

c. _____

4. T.Y. has been hospitalized for a stroke and suffers from laryngoplegia[a]. The patient in the adjoining hospital room has had surgery and currently has a temporary tracheostomy[b]. This second patient had been injured in a car accident and had to undergo thoracoplasty[c] to repair damage that he sustained.

a. _____

b. _____

c. _____

5. R.B. has a history of dyspnea[a] resulting from a nasoseptal[b] problem. She has had recurring nasal[c] and pharyngeal[d] infections caused by bacterial growth in her nasal cavities

a. _____

b. _____

c. _____

d. _____

Labeling

Fill in the blanks with the correct terminology.

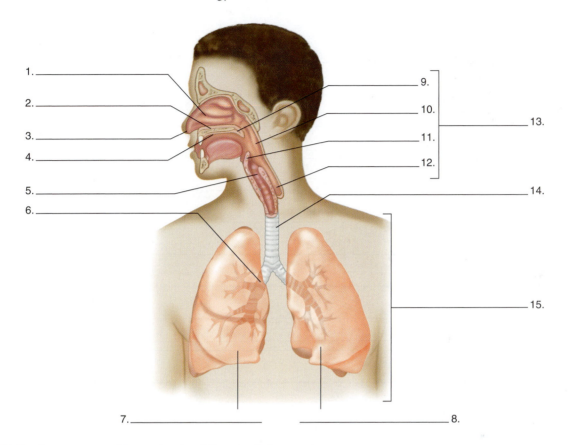

1. _____
2. _____
3. _____
4. _____
5. _____
6. _____

9. _____
10. _____
11. _____
12. _____
13. _____
14. _____
15. _____

7. _____   _____ 8.

Figure 5-5   The upper and lower tracts of the respiratory system.

You may now go on to Chapter Test 5.

Practice

6

Digestive System

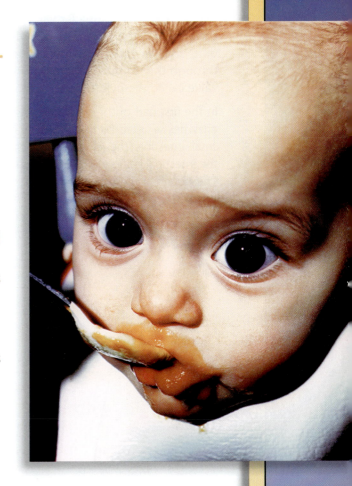

Objectives

After completing Chapter 6, you should be able to do the following:

1. identify word roots pertaining to the mouth and oral cavity;

2. identify word roots pertaining to the tongue and esophagus;

3. identify word roots pertaining to the stomach;

4. understand the differences among the main parts of the small intestine—the duodenum, the jejunum, and the ileum;

5. identify the word parts associated with the main parts of the large intestine;

6. understand the differences among the main parts of the colon, including the sigmoid, rectum, and anus;

7. identify the word parts associated with the main parts of the colon;

8. identify word parts for the accessory organs—the gallbladder and the liver;

9. name and identify the parts of the digestive system; and

10. identify several types of drugs associated with digestive conditions and treatments.

Orientation to the Digestive System

The digestive system carries out five important functions: (a) breaking up food into smaller pieces, (b) transporting food through the alimentary canal (digestive tract) by means of rhythmic muscular contractions (peristalsis), (c) secreting digestive enzymes, (d) promoting absorption of nutrients into the bloodstream, and (e) excreting the solid wastes of digestion.

The digestive system consists of the mouth, pharynx, esophagus, stomach, small intestine, large intestine, and secretory glands (salivary glands, liver, and pancreas); collectively these are referred to as the alimentary canal. Food is first broken up into smaller pieces by the teeth and mixed with saliva, a fluid that coats the pieces to make swallowing easier. It then passes through the pharynx, to and through the esophagus, which extends from the pharynx to the stomach.

The stomach has muscular valves, called sphincters, that keep the food flowing in one direction. In the stomach, the food is mixed with gastric juices. These juices are composed of acids and enzymes that dissolve food, destroy bacteria, and break down protein. Normally the food is processed through the stomach in 2 to 6 hours. Food passes from the stomach to the small intestine through a valve called the pyloric sphincter.

In the first part of the small intestine (the duodenum) the nutrients are mixed with very strong digestive enzymes secreted by the accessory organs (the liver, gallbladder, and pancreas). In the remainder of the small intestine (the jejunum and ileum) nutrients are further broken down and then absorbed through the intestinal lining into the bloodstream. Unabsorbed nutrients then pass into the colon (large intestine). The pouch at the beginning of the colon is known as the cecum. Attached to the cecum is a small tube called the vermiform appendix. The four parts of the colon are the ascending, transverse, descending, and sigmoid segments. Here, liquid is reabsorbed into the body, so that the solid waste product (fecal material) can leave the body through the rectum and its opening, the anus.

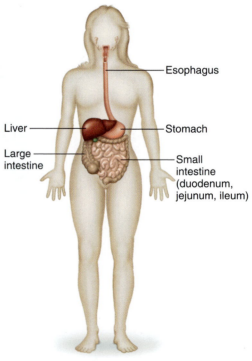

Digestive system

6-1 Terminology Presentation

Mouth, Throat, Tongue, and Esophagus

As you listen to the CD, read the words and notice the pronunciations given.

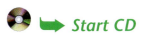 **Start CD**

Look at Figures 6-1 and 6-2

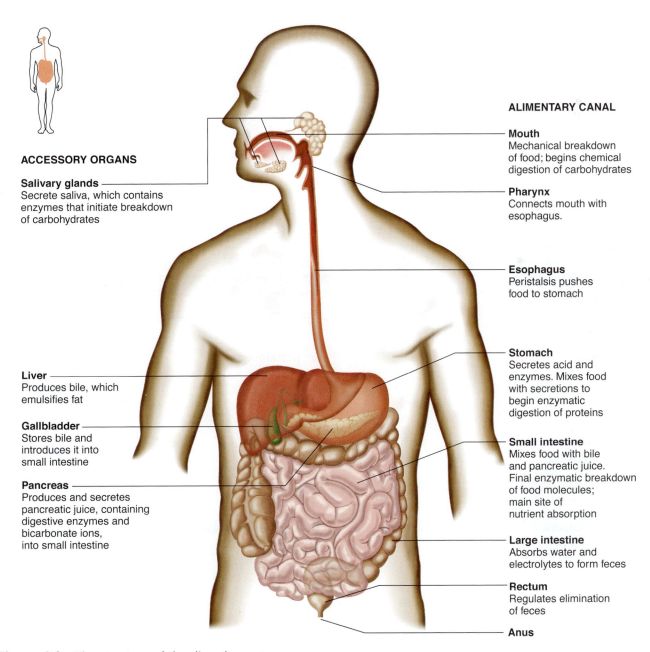

ACCESSORY ORGANS

Salivary glands
Secrete saliva, which contains enzymes that initiate breakdown of carbohydrates

Liver
Produces bile, which emulsifies fat

Gallbladder
Stores bile and introduces it into small intestine

Pancreas
Produces and secretes pancreatic juice, containing digestive enzymes and bicarbonate ions, into small intestine

ALIMENTARY CANAL

Mouth
Mechanical breakdown of food; begins chemical digestion of carbohydrates

Pharynx
Connects mouth with esophagus.

Esophagus
Peristalsis pushes food to stomach

Stomach
Secretes acid and enzymes. Mixes food with secretions to begin enzymatic digestion of proteins

Small intestine
Mixes food with bile and pancreatic juice. Final enzymatic breakdown of food molecules; main site of nutrient absorption

Large intestine
Absorbs water and electrolytes to form feces

Rectum
Regulates elimination of feces

Anus

Figure 6-1 The structure of the digestive system.

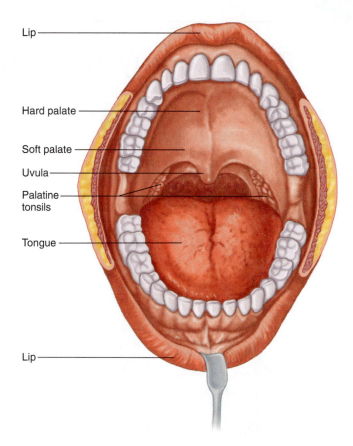

Lip

Hard palate

Soft palate

Uvula

Palatine tonsils

Tongue

Lip

Figure 6-2   The oral cavity—the mouth.

	stomat(o)	a combining form denoting relationship to the mouth		
Word	**Word Part**	**Definition**	**Answer**	
1. stomatitis (sto-mah-ti′tis)	**-itis**	inflammation	1. _____	
2. stomatic (sto-mat′ik)	-ic	of, pertaining to	2. _____	
3. stomatalgia (sto′mah-tal′je-ah)	-algia	pain	3. _____	
4. stomatopathy (sto′mah-top′ah-the)	-pathy	disease	4. _____	
5. stomatoplasty (sto′mah-to-plas′te)	-plasty	plastic surgery	5. _____	
6. stomatoscope (sto-mat′o-skop)	-scope	instrument for viewing	6. _____	

or(o)   a combining form denoting relationship to the mouth

Word	Word Part	Definition	Answer
7. oral (o′ral)	-al	pertaining to	7. _____
8. orolingual (o′ro-ling′gwal)	ling(a) -al	tongue pertaining to	8. _____

pharyng(o)   a combining form denoting the pharynx (throat)

Word	Word Part	Definition	Answer
9. pharyngonasal (fah-ring′go-na′sal)	nas(o) -al	nose of, pertaining to	9. _____
10. pharyngoscope (fah-ring′go-skop)	-scope	viewing instrument	10. _____
11. pharyngostenosis (fah-ring′go-ste-no′sis)	-stenosis	narrowing	11. _____

gloss(o), gloss(ia), lingu(a)   combining forms denoting the tongue

Word	Word Part	Definition	Answer
12. glossitis (glos-si′tis)	-itis	inflammation	12. _____
13. glossal (glos′al)	-al	pertaining to	13. _____
14. glossectomy (glos-sek′to-me)	-ectomy	excision, removal	14. _____
15. lingual (ling′gwal)	-al	pertaining to	15. _____
16. sublingual (sub-ling′gwal)	sub	under	16. _____

esophagus   a term denoting the musculo-membranous passage extending from the pharynx to the stomach

Word	Word Part	Definition	Answer
17. esophagoscopy (e-sof′ah-gos′ko-pe)	-scopy	visual examination	17. _____
18. esophagitis (e-sof′ah-ji′tis)	-itis	inflammation	18. _____
19. esophageal (e-sof′ah-je′al)	-eal	of, pertaining to	19. _____

continued

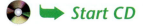 *Pause CD*

After practicing each word several times, use a sheet of paper to cover all columns except the Answer column. As each word is pronounced again on the CD, write it in the space provided.

Start CD

Check the words you have written against the words in the left-hand column. If you have misspelled any words, practice writing them correctly.

Practice

LESSON 6-1 Terminology Application

Without looking at your previous work, write the word that matches each definition.

Definition	Term
1. pertaining to under the tongue	_____
2. pertaining to the mouth and tongue	_____
3. pertaining to the esophagus	_____
4. inflammation of the esophagus	_____
5. narrowing of the throat (pharynx)	_____
6. pertaining to the mouth	**a.** _____
	b. _____
7. pertaining to the nose and throat	_____
8. inflammation of the tongue	_____
9. inflammation of the mouth (of the mucous membranes in the mouth)	_____
10. instrument used for examination of the mouth	_____
11. visual examination (endoscopy) of the esophagus	_____
12. instrument used for viewing the throat (pharynx)	_____
13. pain in the mouth	_____
14. excision of all or part of the tongue	_____
15. any disease of the mouth	_____
16. pertaining to the tongue	**a.** _____
	b. _____
17. plastic surgery of the mouth	_____

Check your answers against the information given in this lesson's terminology presentation. If you have any errors, count them and write the number in the blank at the top of the page. Sign your work and give it to your instructor.

Practice

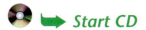

LESSON

6-2   Terminology Presentation

Stomach and Small Intestine

As you listen to the CD, read the words and notice the pronunciations given.

🔘 ➡ *Start CD*

Look at Figures 6-3 and 6-4

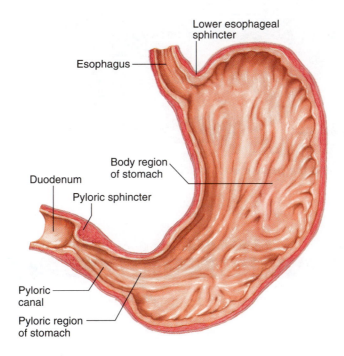

Figure 6-3   The stomach.

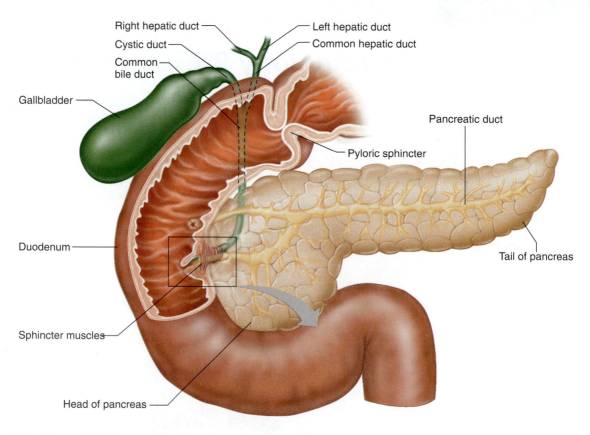

Figure 6-4 The gallbladder and the hepatic duct structures.

gastr(o)	a combining form denoting relationship to the stomach			
Word		**Word Part**	**Definition**	**Answer**
1. gastritis (gas-tri′tis)		-itis	inflammation	**1.** _____
2. gastrectomy (gas-trek′to-me)		-ectomy	excision, removal	**2.** _____
3. gastropathy (gas-trop′ah-the)		-pathy	disease	**3.** _____
4. gastrostomy (gas-tros′to-me)		-ostomy	surgical creation of a new opening	**4.** _____
duoden(o)	a combining form denoting relationship to the duodenum, the first portion of the small intestine			
Word		**Word Part**	**Definition**	**Answer**
5. duodenectomy (du′o-de-nek′to-me)		-ectomy	excision, removal	**5.** _____

Word	Word Part	Definition	Answer
6. duodenal (du'o-de'nal)	-al	of, pertaining to	6. _____
7. duodenostomy (du'od-e-nos'to-me)	-ostomy	surgical creation of a new opening	7. _____

jejun(o) a combining form denoting relationship to the jejunum, the middle section of the small intestine

Word	Word Part	Definition	Answer
8. jejunitis (je'joo-ni'tis)	-itis	inflammation	8. _____
9. jejunorrhaphy (je'joo-nor'ah-fe)	-rrhaphy	suturing	9. _____

ile(o) a combining part denoting relationship to the ileum, the third or distal portion of the small intestine

Word	Word Part	Definition	Answer
10. ileectomy (il'e-ek'to-me)	-ectomy	excision, removal	10. _____
11. ileocecal (il'e-o-se'kal)	cec(o) -al	cecum pertaining to	11. _____
12. ileotomy (il'e-ot'o-me)	-tomy	incision, cutting into	12. _____
13. ileitis (il'e-i'tis)	-itis	inflammation	13. _____
14. ileorrhaphy (il'e-or'ah-fe)	-rrhaphy	suturing	14. _____

enter(o) a word element indicating the intestines

Word	Word Part	Definition	Answer
15. enterorrhagia (en'ter-o-ra'je-ah)	-rrhagia	excessive flow, bleeding	15. _____
16. enterococcus (en'ter-o-kok'us)	-coccus	bacterium	16. _____
17. enterolithiasis (en'ter-o-li-thi'ah-sis)	-lithiasis	condition of stones	17. _____
18. enterostomy (en'ter-os'to-me)	-ostomy	surgical creation of a new opening	18. _____

continued

Word	Word Part	Definition	Answer
19. enterorrhexis (en'ter-o-rek'sis)	-rrhexis	rupture	**19.** _____
20. enterocleisis (en'ter-o-kli'sis)	-cleisis	closure	**20.** _____
21. enterokinesis (en'ter-o-ki-ne'sis)	-kinesis	movement	**21.** _____
22. enteroclysis (en'ter-ok'li-sis)	-clysis	wash out	**22.** _____

  Pause CD

After practicing each word several times, use a sheet of paper to cover all columns except the Answer column. As each word is pronounced again on the CD, write it in the space provided.

  Start CD

Check the words you have written against the words in the left-hand column. If you have misspelled any words, practice writing them correctly.

Practice

_____

_____

_____

_____

_____

_____

_____

_____

_____

_____

_____

_____

_____

_____

_____

_____

_____

LESSON 6-2

Terminology Application

Without looking at your previous work, write the word that matches each definition.

Definition	Term
1. blockage or closure of the intestine	_____
2. surgical creation of a new opening into the small intestine	_____
3. injection or introduction of liquid into the intestine	_____
4. muscular movement of the intestinal canal; peristalsis	_____
5. stones or calculi found in the intestine	_____
6. rupture of the intestinal wall	_____
7. hemorrhage from the intestine	_____
8. pertaining to the duodenum	_____
9. surgical creation of a new opening into the duodenum	_____
10. inflammation of the ileum	_____
11. any disease of the stomach	_____
12. suturing the ileum	_____
13. inflammation of the stomach	_____
14. incision into the ileum	_____
15. excision of all or part of the duodenum	_____
16. pertaining to the ileum and the cecum	_____
17. inflammation of the jejunum	_____
18. suturing the jejunum	_____
19. excision of all or part of the ileum	_____

continued

Definition	Term
20. surgical creation of a new opening into the stomach	_____
21. excision of all or part of the stomach	_____
22. a type of intestinal bacteria	_____

Check your answers against the information given in this lesson's terminology presentation. If you have any errors, count them and write the number in the blank at the top of the page. Sign your work and give it to your instructor.

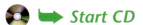

LESSON

6-3   Terminology Presentation

Large Intestine (Colon) and Anus

As you listen to the CD, read the words and notice the pronunciations given.

Start CD

Look at Figure 6-5

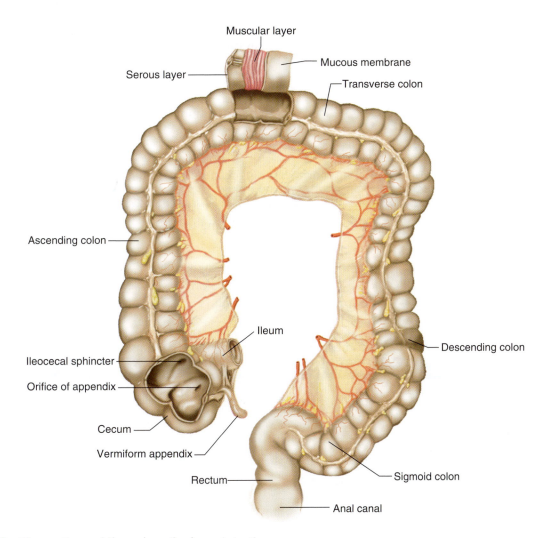

Figure 6-5   The sections of the colon; the large intestine.

colon	a term denoting the portion of the large intestine that extends from the cecum to the rectum		
Word	**Word Part**	**Definition**	**Answer**
1. colitis (ko-li′tis)	-itis	inflammation	1. _____
2. colectomy (ko-lek′to-me)	-ectomy	excision, removal	2. _____
3. colostomy (ko-los′to-me)	-ostomy	surgical creation of a new opening	3. _____

sigmoid	a word denoting the S-shaped portion of the colon		
Word	**Word Part**	**Definition**	**Answer**
4. sigmoidoscope (sig-moi′do-skop)	-scope	instrument for examination	4. _____
5. sigmoidectomy (sig′moi-dek′to-me)	-ectomy	excision	5. _____
6. sigmoiditis (sig′moi-di′tis)	-itis	inflammation	6. _____

rect(o)	a combining form denoting relationship to the rectum		
Word	**Word Part**	**Definition**	**Answer**
7. rectal (rek′tal)	-al	pertaining to	7. _____
8. rectosigmoidectomy (rek′to-sig′moi-dek′to-me)	sigmoid -ectomy	S-shaped portion of the colon excision	8. _____

proct(o)	a combining form denoting the rectum or anus		
Word	**Word Part**	**Definition**	**Answer**
9. proctologist (prok-tol′o-jist)	-logist	specialist	9. _____
10. proctatresia (prok′tah-tre′ze-ah)	a- -tresia	without, lack of opening, hole	10. _____
11. proctoptosis (prok′top-to′sis)	-ptosis	falling or prolapse	11. _____
12. proctocele (prok′to-sel)	-cele	tumor, swelling, hernia	12. _____
13. proctopexy (prok′to-pek′se)	-pexy	fix, fasten	13. _____

Word	Word Part	Definition	Answer
14. proctorrhea (prok'to-re'ah)	-rrhea	flow	14. _____
15. proctoscopy (prok-tos'ko-pe)	-scopy	examine	15. _____

anus   a word denoting the distal or terminal orifice of the alimentary canal

Word	Word Part	Definition	Answer
16. anal (a'nal)	-al	pertaining to	16. _____
17. anusitis (a-nus-i'tis)	-itis	inflammation	17. _____

 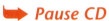 *Pause CD*

After practicing each word several times, use a sheet of paper to cover all columns except the Answer column. As each word is pronounced again on the CD, write it in the space provided.

 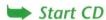 *Start CD*

Check the words you have written against the words in the left-hand column. If you have misspelled any words, practice writing them correctly.

Practice

_____

_____

_____

_____

_____

_____

_____

_____

_____

_____

_____

_____

_____

_____

Practice

LESSON 6-3

Terminology Application

Without looking at your previous work, write the word that matches each definition.

Definition	Term
1. specialist in the diagnosis and treatment of rectal disorders	_____
2. visual examination of the sigmoid	_____
3. pertaining to the rectum	_____
4. hernial protrusion of the rectum	_____
5. excision of all or part of the colon	_____
6. anal atresia, absence of a proper rectal opening	_____
7. removal of the sigmoid	_____
8. surgical creation of a new opening into the colon	_____
9. pertaining to the anus	_____
10. examination of the rectum by the use of a proctoscope	_____
11. inflammation of the sigmoid	_____
12. inflammation of the colon	_____
13. a mucoserous discharge from the rectum	_____
14. excision of the sigmoid and the rectum	_____
15. prolapse or falling of the rectum	_____
16. inflammation of the anus	_____
17. surgical fixing or fastening of the rectum	_____

Check your answers against the information given in this lesson's terminology presentation. If you have any errors, count them and write the number in the blank at the top of the page. Sign your work and give it to your instructor.

Practice

Terminology Presentation

Bile Duct, Gallbladder, and Liver

As you listen to the CD, read the words and notice the pronunciations given.

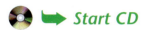 **Start CD**

Look at Figure 6-5, on page 153, and Figure 6-6 here

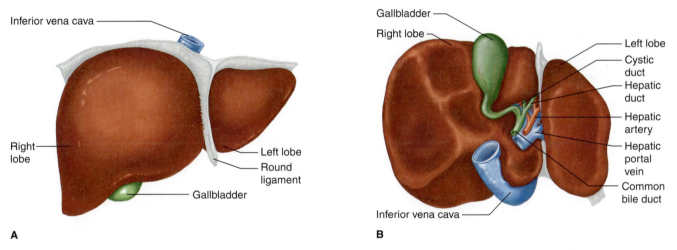

A   B

Figure 6-6   The lobes of the liver: (A) anterior view, (B) inferior view.

choledoch(o)   a combining form denoting the common bile duct
cholecyst(o)   a combining form to denote the gallbladder (a bile sac)

Word	Word Part	Definition	Answer
1. cholecystography (ko′le-sis-tog′rah-fe)	-graphy	recording	1. _____
2. cholecystectomy (ko′le-sis-tek′to-me)	-ectomy	excision, removal	2. _____
3. choledochotomy (ko-led′o-kot′o-me)	-tomy	incision, cutting into	3. _____
4. choledocholithotripsy (ko-led′o-ko-lith′o-trip′se)	lith(o) -tripsy	stone crush	4. _____
5. cholecystitis (ko′le-sis-ti′tis)	-itis	inflammation	5. _____

	Word	Word Part	Definition	Answer
6.	choledochogastrostomy (ko-led′o-ko-gas-tros′to-me)	gastr(o) -stomy	stomach connection, opening	6. _____
7.	cholelithiasis (ko′le-li-thi′ah-sis)	lith(o) -iasis	stone diseased condition	7. _____

hepat(o), hepat(ico)		word parts denoting the liver	

	Word	Word Part	Definition	Answer
8.	hepatic (he-pat′ik)	-ic	of, pertaining to	8. _____
9.	hepatatrophy (hep′ah-tat′ro-fe)	a- -trophy	without nourishment	9. _____
10.	hepatorenal (hep′ah-to-re′nal)	ren(o) -al	kidney of, pertaining to	10. _____
11.	hepatomegaly (hep′ah-to-meg′ah-le)	-megaly	abnormal enlargement	11. _____
12.	hepatitis (hep′ah-ti′tis)	-itis	inflammation	12. _____
13.	hepatorrhaphy (hep′ah-tor′ah-fe)	-rrhaphy	suturing	13. _____

 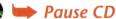 *Pause CD*

After practicing each word several times, use a sheet of paper to cover all columns except the Answer column. As each word is pronounced again on the CD, write it in the space provided.

 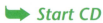 *Start CD*

Check the words you have written against the words in the left-hand column. If you have misspelled any words, practice writing them correctly.

Practice

_____

_____

_____

_____

_____

_____

_____

_____

LESSON
6-4

Terminology Application

Without looking at your previous work, write the word that matches each definition.

Definition	Term
1. suturing of the liver	_____
2. inflammation of the gallbladder	_____
3. the crushing of a stone in the common bile duct	_____
4. surgical connection between the stomach and the common bile duct	_____
5. pertaining to the liver and kidney	_____
6. X-ray examination of the gallbladder	_____
7. incision into the bile duct	_____
8. condition of gallstones	_____
9. atrophy of the liver	_____
10. abnormal enlargement of the liver	_____
11. inflammation of the liver	_____
12. pertaining to the liver	_____
13. excision or removal of the gallbladder	_____

Check your answers against the information given in this lesson's terminology presentation. If you have any errors, count them and write the number in the blank at the top of the page. Sign your work and give it to your instructor.

Practice

LESSON

6-5   Drug Terminology Presentation

As you listen to the CD, read the words and notice the pronunciations given.

 ➡ **Start CD**

Word	Definition	Example: Generic Name	Example: Brand Trade Name	Answer
antacids	agents that counteract or neutralize acidity, usually in the stomach	bismuth subsalicylate calcium carbonate famotidine ranitidine cimetidine esomeprazole omeprazole	Pepto-Bismol Rolaids, Tums Pepcid Zantac Tagamet Nexium Prilosec	1. _____
antidiarrheals	agents that counteract diarrhea	bismuth subsalicylate loperamide	Pepto-Bismol Imodium, Kaopectate	2. _____
antiemetics	agents that prevent or alleviate nausea and vomiting	promethazine dimenhydrinate prochlorperazine	Phenergan Dramamine Compazine	3. _____
emetics	agents that cause vomiting	ipecac	Ipecac Syrup	4. _____
laxatives	agents that promote peristalsis and bowel evacuation	bisacodyl docusate [stool softener] psyllium	Dulcolax Colace Metamucil	5. _____

 ➡ **Pause CD**

After practicing each word several times, use a sheet of paper to cover all columns except the Answer column. As each word is pronounced again on the CD, write it in the space provided.

 ➡ **Start CD**

Check the words you have written against the words in the left-hand column. If you have misspelled any words, practice writing them correctly.

Practice

LESSON
6-5

Drug Terminology Application

Without looking at your previous work, write the word that matches each definition.

Definition	Term
1. agents that prevent or alleviate nausea and vomiting	_____
2. agents that counteract or neutralize acidity, usually in the stomach	_____
3. agents that promote peristalsis and bowel evacuation	_____
4. agents that cause vomiting	_____
5. agents that counteract diarrhea	_____

Check your answers against the information given in this lesson's terminology presentation. If you have any errors, count them and write the number in the blank at the top of the page. Sign your work and give it to your instructor.

Practice

CHAPTER
6
Terminology Review

This is a review of the word parts and words you have learned in the preceding lessons. Some of the medical terms listed below may be new, but they are composed of the word parts and word roots that you have already learned. Read the words below as they are pronounced on the CD.

  Start CD

Word Element Review

Word	Word Part	Meaning of Word Part
1. proctatresia	proct	_____
proctatresia	-a	_____
proctatresia	-tresia	_____
(prok'tah-tre'ze-ah)	Meaning of the Word	_____
2. ileostomy	ile(o)	_____
ileostomy	-stomy	_____
(il'e-os'to-me)	Meaning of Word	_____
3. jejunitis	jejun(o)	_____
jejunitis	-itis	_____
(je'joo-ni'tis)	Meaning of Word	_____
4. hepatatrophy	hepat	_____
hepatatrophy	-a	_____
hepatatrophy	-trophy	_____
(hep'ah-tat'ro-fe)	Meaning of Word	_____
5. rectal	rect(o)	_____
rectal	-al	_____
(rek'tal)	Meaning of Word	_____
6. cholecystogram	cholecyst(o)	_____
cholecystogram	-gram	_____
(ko'le-sis'to-gram)	Meaning of Word	_____
7. ileotomy	ile(o)	_____
ileotomy	-tomy	_____
(il'e-ot'o-me)	Meaning of Word	_____

Word	Word Part	Meaning of Word Part
8. stomatitis stomatitis (sto-mah-ti′tis)	stomat(o) -itis Meaning of Word	_____ _____ _____
9. enterorrhagia enterorrhagia (en′ter-o-ra′je-ah)	enter(o) -rrhagia Meaning of Word	_____ _____ _____
10. proctoscopy proctoscopy (prok′tos′ko-pe)	proct(o) -scopy Meaning of Word	_____ _____ _____
11. pharyngeal pharyngeal (fah-rin′je-al)	pharyng(o) -eal Meaning of Word	_____ _____ _____
12. pharyngorhinitis pharyngorhinitis (fah-ring′go-ri-ni′tis)	pharyng(o) rhin(o) -itis Meaning of Word	_____ _____ _____ _____
13. enterococcus enterococcus (en′ ter-o-kok′ us)	enter(o) -coccus Meaning of Word	_____ _____ _____
14. hepatorenal hepatorenal (hep′ ah-to-re′ nal)	hepat(o) ren(o) -al Meaning of Word	_____ _____ _____ _____

➡ *Stop CD*

On the lines provided, write in the meanings of as many suffixes, prefixes, roots, and words as you can from memory. Check your definitions in the glossary or a medical dictionary, and make any needed corrections.

CHAPTER 6

Terminology Review

Complete this review, and turn it in to your instructor when you are finished.

Defintion

Each phrase below defines one of the words you have just studied. Without looking at your previous work, write in the word that matches each definition.

Definition	Term
1. pertaining to the mouth and the tongue	_____
2. anal atresia, absence of a proper anal opening	_____
3. a surgical opening into the ileum	_____
4. pertaining to the liver and the kidneys	_____
5. narrowing of the pharynx	_____
6. intestinal hemorrhage or bleeding	_____
7. X-ray examination of the gallbladder	_____
8. incision into the ileum	_____
9. a type of intestinal bacteria	_____
10. examination of the rectum via a proctoscope	_____
11. atrophy or wasting of the liver	_____
12. inflammation of the sigmoid	_____
13. pertaining to the pharynx and nose	_____
14. downward displacement of the gallbladder	_____
15. inflammation of the anus	_____
16. a surgical opening into the small intestine	_____
17. an incision into a bile duct	_____
18. pertaining to the tongue	_____
19. pertaining to the throat (pharynx)	_____
20. a specialist in the treatment of rectal disorders	_____

Matching

Match the following definitions with the terms given. Put the letter of the correct definition to the left of the term.

Term	Definition
_____ 21. pharyngonasal	a. suturing the jejunum
_____ 22. stomatoplasty	b. inflammation of the small intestines
_____ 23. jejunorrhaphy	c. excision of the rectum and the sigmoid colon
_____ 24. ileocecal	d. pertaining to the pharynx and the nose
_____ 25. enteritis	e. inflammation of the gallbladder
_____ 26. cholecystitis	f. pertaining to the anus
_____ 27. rectosigmoidectomy	g. having gallstones
_____ 28. anal	h. plastic surgery of the mouth
_____ 29. hepatic	i. pertaining to the liver
_____ 30. cholelithiasis	j. pertaining to the ileum and the cecum

CHAPTER 6

Terminology Review

Case Studies

Read the following brief case studies. In each case study, some terms are followed by a superscript letter. Write a brief definition for each of those terms on the corresponding lines below.

1. Patients who suffer from oral cancer many times have painful glossitis[a] and often have a partial glossectomy[b] to remove damaged tissue. Patients with stomach cancers often have a partial gastrectomy[c] combined with a gastrostomy[d] for drainage purposes.

   a. _____

   b. _____

   c. _____

   d. _____

2. N.D. has complained of extreme fatigue and has tested positive for melena[a]. He has had an esophagoscopy[b] and a gastroscopy[c], which have revealed an esophageal[d] bleed and severe gastritis[e]. In addition, he has had a colonoscopy[f] and a proctoscopy[g], which have revealed no other lower GI (gastrointestinal) problems.

   a. _____

   b. _____

   c. _____

   d. _____

   e. _____

   f. _____

   g. _____

3. G. was the victim of a gunshot wound to the abdomen, which caused gastric[a] and duodenal[b] damage in addition to damage to the jejunum[c] and the ileum[d] (the ileal damage resulted in severe enterorrhagia[e]). The surgeries she has had to repair the damage include a duodenectomy[f], jejunorrhaphy[g], and a partial ileectomy[h]. Surgeons have also given her a temporary colostomy[i] to aid in her healing process.

   a. _____

   b. _____

   c. _____

    d. _____

    e. _____

    f. _____

    g. _____

    h. _____

    i. _____

4. A.H. was having abdominal pain and suspected that he was experiencing acute cholecystitis[a]. Because he has had a history of GI problems, he assumed that he would be a candidate for a cholecystectomy[b]. However, when he was examined by his doctor, he was diagnosed with cholelithiasis[c]; his doctor recommended trying lithotripsy[d] rather than surgery.

    a. _____

    b. _____

    c. _____

    d. _____

5. S. suffers from gastric[a] ulcers and colitis[b]. The symptoms include abdominal pain, GI bleeding, nausea, and diarrhea. This patient needs to maintain a specific diet while taking a prescription antacid[c], a prescription antiemetic[d], and some type of antidiarrheal[e] to alleviate the symptoms.

    a. _____

    b. _____

    c. _____

    d. _____

    e. _____

Labeling

Fill in the blanks with the correct terminology.

ACCESSORY ORGANS   **ALIMENTARY CANAL**

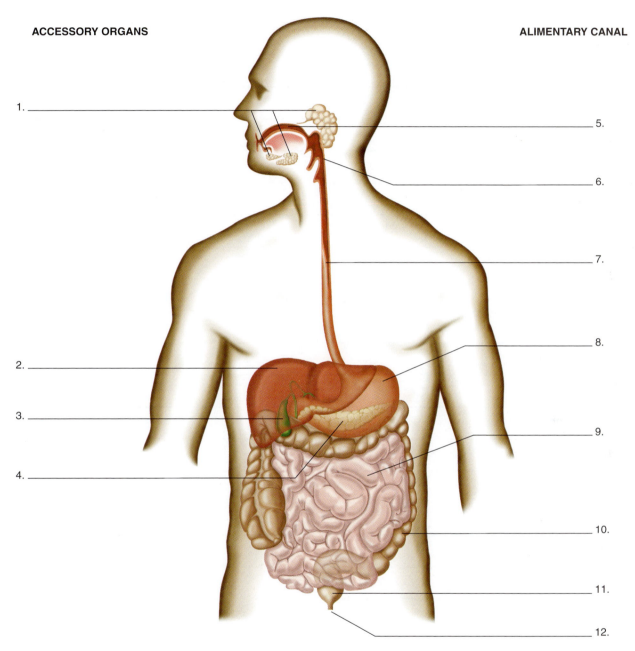

1. _____

2. _____

3. _____

4. _____

5. _____

6. _____

7. _____

8. _____

9. _____

10. _____

11. _____

12. _____

Figure 6-7 Major organs of the digestive system.

You may now go on to Chapter Test 6.

Practice

7

Cardiovascular System

Objectives

After completing Chapter 7, you should be able to do the following:

1. identify word roots pertaining to the heart and the major blood vessels;

2. know the three layers of the heart: the endocardium, the myocardium, and the epicardium;

3. identify the word roots associated with the arteries, veins, and blood vessels;

4. identify the word roots pertaining to blood pressure; and

5. identify several types of drugs associated with heart conditions and treatments.

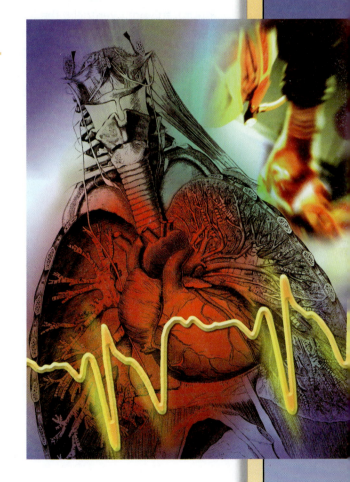

Orientation to the Cardiovascular System

The cardiovascular system consists of the heart and blood vessels. The heart is located between the lungs, somewhat to the left of the center of the body. There are three layers in the heart wall: the endocardium (the membrane that lines the inside of the heart), the myocardium (the heart muscle), and the epicardium (the outermost layer). Enclosing the heart is the pericardium, a fibroserous sac.

There are two types of blood vessels: arteries and veins. The arteries carry blood away from the heart, and the veins return the blood to the heart. Arteries and veins are connected by thin-walled vessels called capillaries, which form a network throughout the body. Some capillaries branch into small sacs called alveoli.

The heart is a hollow muscle about the size of a fist and is divided into four chambers: the right atrium, the right ventricle, the left atrium, and the left ventricle. The purpose of the atria is to collect blood, and the purpose of the ventricles is to pump blood. The right atrium collects deoxygenated blood, which the right ventricle pumps to the lungs. The left atrium collects oxygenated blood and the left ventricle pumps it to the rest of the body.

The heart functions as a pump that forces the blood to circulate, under pressure, through a series of blood vessels. Blood pressure is determined by the force of the heartbeat and by the condition of the walls of the vessels. The active phase of contraction (pumping) is known as systole (systolic pressure), and the resting phase (expansion) is known as diastole (diastolic pressure). An instrument called a sphygmomanometer is used to measure arterial blood pressure.

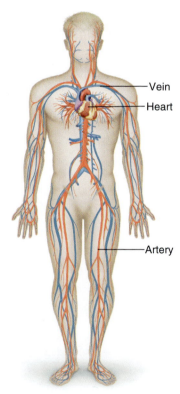

Cardiovascular system

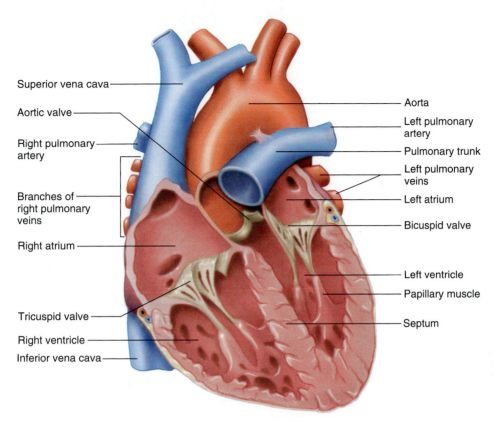

Superior vena cava

Aortic valve

Right pulmonary
artery

Branches of
right pulmonary
veins

Right atrium

Tricuspid valve

Right ventricle

Inferior vena cava

Aorta

Left pulmonary
artery

Pulmonary trunk

Left pulmonary
veins

Left atrium

Bicuspid valve

Left ventricle

Papillary muscle

Septum

Coronal section of the heart showing the connection between the left ventricle and the aorta as well as the four hollow chambers.

Practice

Heart and Aorta

As you listen to the CD, read the words and notice the pronunciations given.

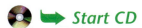 **Start CD**

Look at Figure 7-1

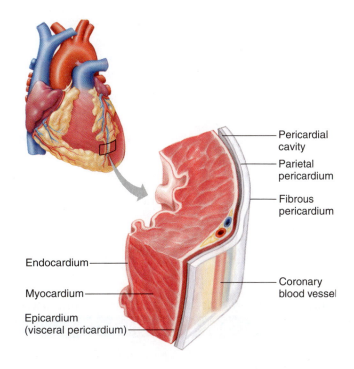

FIGURE 7-1 The endocardium, the myocardium, and the layers of the pericardium.

cardi(o) a combining form denoting the heart			
Word	**Word Part**	**Definition**	**Answer**
1. endocarditis (en'do-kar-di'tis)	endo- -itis	within inflammation	**1.** _____
2. myocarditis (mi'o-kar-di'tis)	my(o)- -itis	muscle inflammation	**2.** _____
3. pericarditis (per'i-kar-di'tis)	peri- -itis	surrounding, around inflammation	**3.** _____

continued

Word	Word Part	Definition	Answer
4. cardiology (kar-di-ol′o-je)	-logy	study of, science of	4. _____
5. cardiac (kar′de-ak)	-ac	pertaining to	5. _____
6. electrocardiograph (e-lek′tro-kar′de-o-graf′)	electro- -graph	pertaining to electricity instrument used for measurement	6. _____
7. electrocardiography (e-lek′tro-kar′de-og′rah fe)	electro- -graphy	pertaining to electricity process of recording	7. _____
8. electrocardiogram (e-lek′tro-kar′de- o- gram)	electro- -gram	pertaining to electricity something drawn, written, or recorded	8. _____
9. cardiomegaly (kar′de-o-meg′ah-le)	-megaly	enlargement	9. _____
10. cardiomyopathy (kar′de-o-mi-op′ah-the)	my(o) -pathy	muscle disease	10. _____
11. bradycardia (brad′e-kar′de- ah)	brady-	slow	11. _____
12. tachycardia (tak′e-kar′de-ah)	tachy-	fast	12. _____

aorta   a word denoting the main trunk from which the systemic arterial system proceeds

Word	Word Part	Definition	Answer
13. aortic (a-or′tik)	-ic	pertaining to	13. _____
14. aortitis (a′or-ti′tis)	-itis	inflammation	14. _____
15. aortosclerosis (a-or′to-skle-ro′sis)	scler(o) -osis	hard abnormal condition	15. _____

Pause CD

After practicing each word several times, use a sheet of paper to cover all columns except the Answer column. As each word is pronounced again on the CD, write it in the space provided.

Start CD

Check the words you have written against the words in the left-hand column. If you have misspelled any words, practice writing them correctly.

Practice

_____

_____

_____

_____

_____

_____

_____

_____

_____

_____

_____

_____

_____

_____

_____

_____

_____

_____

_____

_____

Practice

LESSON
7-1
Terminology Application

Without looking at your previous work, write the word that matches each definition.

Definition	Term
1. excessive rapidity in the action of the heart, usually in the pulse rate	_____
2. inflammation within the heart	_____
3. primary myocardial disease	_____
4. pertaining to the aorta	_____
5. the science or study of the heart	_____
6. the process of making a recording of the heart's activity	_____
7. pertaining to the heart	_____
8. inflammation of the membrane surrounding the heart	_____
9. enlargement of the heart	_____
10. the written record of the heart's activity	_____
11. inflammation of the aorta	_____
12. abnormally slow heartbeat	_____
13. inflammation of the heart muscle	_____
14. hardening of the aorta	_____
15. an instrument used for recording the heart's activity	_____

Check your answers against the information given in this lesson's terminology presentation. If you have any errors, count them and write the number in the blank at the top of the page. Sign your work and give it to your instructor.

Practice

Terminology Presentation

Arteries and Veins

As you listen to the CD, read the words and notice the pronunciations given.

Start CD

Look at Figure 7-2

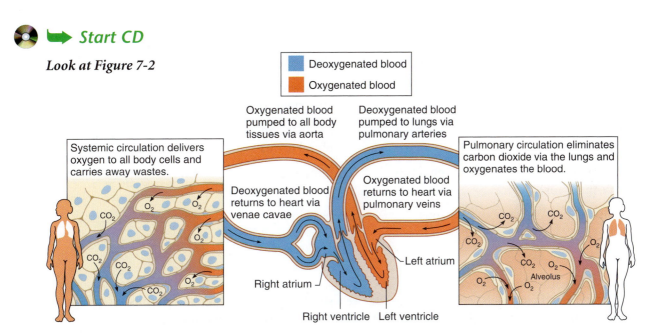

Deoxygenated blood
Oxygenated blood

Oxygenated blood pumped to all body tissues via aorta

Deoxygenated blood pumped to lungs via pulmonary arteries

Systemic circulation delivers oxygen to all body cells and carries away wastes.

Deoxygenated blood returns to heart via venae cavae

Oxygenated blood returns to heart via pulmonary veins

Pulmonary circulation eliminates carbon dioxide via the lungs and oxygenates the blood.

Left atrium

Right atrium

Right ventricle   Left ventricle

Alveolus

FIGURE 7-2   The circulatory system: the pathways for oxygenated and deoxygenated blood.

arteri(o) a combining form denoting relationship to an artery or arteries			
Word	**Word Part**	**Definition**	**Answer**
1. arterial (ar-te′re-al)	-al	pertaining to	1. _____
2. arteriectasis (ar′te-re-ek′tah-sis)	-ectasis	dilation, expansion	2. _____
3. arteriole (ar-te′re-ol)	-ole	tiny, minute, diminutive	3. _____
4. arteriosclerosis (ar-te′re-o-skle-ro′sis)	scler- -osis	hard abnormal condition,	4. _____
5. arteriostenosis (ar-te′re-o-ste-no′sis)	sten(o) -osis	narrowing abnormal condition	5. _____
6. arteritis (ar′te-ri′tis)	-itis	inflammation	6. _____
7. arteriorrhexis (ar-te′re-o-rek′sis)	-rrhexis	rupture	7. _____

continued

phleb(o), ven(o) combining forms denoting a vein or the veins			
Word	**Word Part**	**Definition**	**Answer**
8. phlebotomy (fle-bot′o-me)	-tomy	incision, cutting into	8. _____
9. phlebitis (fle-bi′tis)	-itis	inflammation	9. _____
10. phleborrhagia (fleb′o-ra′je-ah)	-rrhagia	excessive flow, bleeding	10. _____
11. phlebosclerosis (fleb′o-skle-ro′sis)	scler(o) -osis	hard abnormal condition	11. _____
12. phlebostenosis (fleb′o-sten-no′sis)	sten(o) -osis	narrowing abnormal condition	12. _____
13. vena, venae (ve′nah) (ve′ne)	-a, -ae	singular and plural forms	13. _____
14. venipuncture (ven′i-punk′tur)	puncture	puncture	14. _____
15. venous (ve′nus)	-ous	pertaining to	15. _____

  Pause CD

After practicing each word several times, use a sheet of paper to cover all columns except the Answer column. As each word is pronounced again on the CD, write it in the space provided.

  Start CD

Check the words you have written against the words in the left-hand column. If you have misspelled any words, practice writing them correctly.

Practice

_____

_____

_____

_____

_____

_____

_____

_____

LESSON
7-2

Terminology Application

Without looking at your previous work, write the word that matches each definition.

Definition	Term
1. excessive bleeding from a vein	_____
2. singular form of the term *vein*	_____
3. hardening of the arteries	_____
4. minute arterial branch	_____
5. dilation of an artery	_____
6. plural form of the term *vein*	_____
7. hardening of the walls of the veins	_____
8. rupture of an artery	_____
9. incision into a vein	_____
10. inflammation of a vein	_____
11. pertaining to an artery	_____
12. pertaining to the veins	_____
13. narrowing of a vein	_____
14. inflammation of an artery	_____
15. puncture of a vein	_____
16. narrowing of an artery	_____

Check your answers against the information given in this lesson's terminology presentation. If you have any errors, count them and write the number in the blank at the top of the page. Sign your work and give it to your instructor.

Practice

Terminology Presentation

Vessels and Ducts

As you listen to the CD, read the words and notice the pronunciations given.

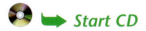

Start CD

Look at Figure 7-3

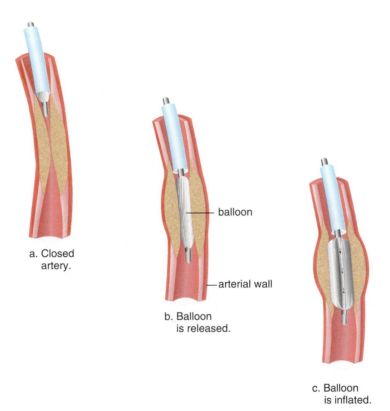

FIGURE 7-3 Arterial balloon angioplasty.

angi(o) a combining form denoting a relationship to a vessel, usually a blood vessel			
Word	**Word Part**	**Definition**	**Answer**
1. angiocarditis (an'je-o-kar-di'tis)	cardi(o) -itis	heart inflammation	1. _____
2. angiorrhaphy (an'je-or'ah-fe)	-rrhaphy	suturing	2. _____

continued

| | *vas(o)* | a combining form denoting a vessel or duct | | |

Word	Word Part	Definition	Answer
3. angioplasty (an′je-o-plas′te)	-plasty	plastic surgery	**3.** _____
4. vasorrhaphy (vas-or′ah-fe)	-rrhaphy	suturing	**4.** _____
5. vasography (vah-sog′rah-fe)	-graphy	process of recording	**5.** _____
6. vasospasm (vas′o-spazm)	-spasm	contraction	**6.** _____
7. vasodilator (vas′o-di-lat′or)	-dilator	something causing expansion	**7.** _____
8. vascular (vas′ku-lar)	-ar	pertaining to	**8.** _____
9. vasculitis (vas′ku-li′tis)	-itis	inflammation	**9.** _____
10. vasculopathy (vas′ku-lop′ah-the)	-pathy	disease	**10.** _____

  Pause CD

After practicing each word several times, use a sheet of paper to cover all columns except the Answer column. As each word is pronounced again on the CD, write it in the space provided.

  Start CD

Check the words you have written against the words in the left-hand column. If you have misspelled any words, practice writing them correctly.

Practice

_____

_____

_____

_____

_____

_____

_____

LESSON
7-3

Terminology Application

Without looking at your previous work, write the word that matches each definition.

Definition	Term
1. dilatation of a blood vessel by means of a balloon catheter	_____
2. contraction of a blood vessel	_____
3. inflammation of a blood vessel	_____
4. X-ray of the blood vessels	_____
5. pertaining to a blood vessel	_____
6. any disease of a blood vessel	_____
7. inflammation of the heart and major blood vessels	_____
8. agent that dilates a blood vessel	_____
9. suturing of a blood vessel	**a.** _____
	b. _____

Check your answers against the information given in this lesson's terminology presentation. If you have any errors, count them and write the number in the blank at the top of the page. Sign your work and give it to your instructor.

Practice

Terminology Presentation

Blood Pressure

As you listen to the CD, read the words and notice the pronunciations given.

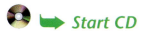 **Start CD**

Look at Figure 7-4

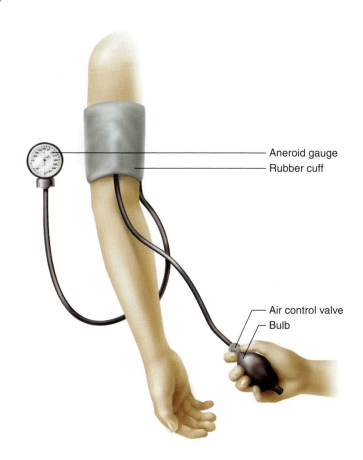

Aneroid gauge
Rubber cuff

Air control valve
Bulb

FIGURE 7-4 Sphygmomanometer.

sphygm(o) a combining form denoting the pulse or blood pressure			
Word	**Word Part**	**Definition**	**Answer**
1. sphygmoid (sfig′moid)	-oid	like, resembling	1. _____
2. sphygmology (sfig-mol′o-je)	-logy	study of, science of	2. _____

continued

Word	Word Part	Definition	Answer
3. sphygmopalpation (sfig′mo-pal-pa′shun)	-palpation	feeling	3. ________
4. sphygmomanometer (sfig′mo-mah-nom′e-ter)	manometer	instrument for measuring pressure of liquid or gas	4. ________
5. sphygmoscopy (sfig-mos′ko-pe)	-scopy	examination	5. ________
6. sphygmic (sfig′mik)	-ic	pertaining to	6. ________

diastole a word denoting dilatation of the ventricles of the heart

Word	Word Part	Definition	Answer
7. diastolic (di′ah-stol′ik)	-ic	pertaining to	7. ________

systole a word denoting the contraction of the ventricles of the heart

Word	Word Part	Definition	Answer
8. systolic (sis-tol′ik)	-ic	pertaining to	8. ________

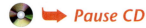

Pause CD

After practicing each word several times, use a sheet of paper to cover all columns except the Answer column. As each word is pronounced again on the CD, write it in the space provided.

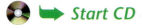

Start CD

Check the words you have written against the words in the left-hand column. If you have misspelled any words, practice writing them correctly.

Practice

LESSON 7-4

Terminology Application

Without looking at your previous work, write the word that matches each definition.

Definition	Term
1. an instrument used to measure blood pressure	_____
2. the study or science of the pulse	_____
3. resembling the pulse	_____
4. examination of the pulse	_____
5. palpating or feeling the pulse	_____
6. dilatation of the ventricles of the heart	_____
7. pertaining to the pulse	_____
8. contraction of the ventricles of the heart	_____

Check your answers against the information given in this lesson's terminology presentation. If you have any errors, count them and write the number in the blank at the top of the page. Sign your work and give it to your instructor.

Practice

Drug Terminology Presentation

As you listen to the CD, read the words and notice the pronunciations given.

 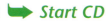 **Start CD**

Word	Definition	Example: Generic Name	Example: Brand/ Trade Name	Answer
antianginals	agents that alleviate angina pectoris by dilating coronary arteries to improve blood flow	nitroglycerin	Nitro-Bid (ointment)	1. _____
		nitroglycerin	Nitrogard (buccal tablets)	
		nitroglycerin	Nitrocine (transdermal)	
		nitroglycerin	Nitrolingual Translingual Spray	
		diltiazem hydrochloride	Cardizem (also for hypertension)	
antihypertensives	agents that counteract high blood pressure	nifedipine	Procardia	2. _____
		lisinopril	Prinivil, Zestril	
		hydrochlorothiazide/ triamterene	Maxzide	
antihypotensives	agents that counteract low blood pressure by causing contraction of blood vessels	phenylephrine	various	3. _____
antilipidemics	agents that counteract high levels of lipids (fats) in the bloood	simvastatin	Zocor	4. _____
		atorvastatin	Lipitor	
		lovastatin	Mevacor	
thrombolytics/ anticoagulants	agents that dissolve blood clots	heparin	(various)	5. _____
		warfarin	Coumadin	
		streptokinase	(various)	
vasodilators	agents that dilate blood vessels	isosorbide	Imdur	6. _____
		minoxidil	Loniten	
		amyl nitrite	(various)	
		hydralazine	(various)	
		nitroglycerin	(various)	

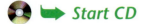 **Pause CD**

After practicing each word several times, use a sheet of paper to cover all columns except the Answer column. As each word is pronounced again on the CD, write it in the space provided.

Start CD

Check the words you have written against the words in the left-hand column. If you have misspelled any words, practice writing them correctly.

Practice

LESSON
7-5

Drug Terminology Application

Without looking at your previous work, write the word that matches each definition.

Definition	Term
1. agents that dilate blood vessels	_____
2. agents that counteract low blood pressure	_____
3. agents that counteract high levels of lipids (fats) in the blood	_____
4. agents that counteract high blood pressure	_____
5. agents that alleviate angina pectoris by dilating coronary arteries to improve blood flow	_____
6. agents that dissolve blood clots	a. _____
	b. _____

Check your answers against the information given in this lesson's terminology presentation. If you have any errors, count them and write the number in the blank at the top of the page. Sign your work and give it to your instructor.

Practice

CHAPTER 7
Terminology Review

This is a review of the word parts and words you have learned in the preceding lessons. Some of the medical terms listed below may be new, but they are composed of the word parts and word roots that you have already learned. Read the words below as they are pronounced on the CD.

 Start CD

Word Element Review

Word	Word Part	Meaning of Word Part
1. arteriosclerosis	arteri(o)	_____
arteriosclerosis	scler(o)	_____
arteriosclerosis	-osis	_____
(ar-te're-o'skle-ro'sis)	Meaning of Word	_____
2. angioplasty	angi(o)	_____
angioplasty	-plasty	_____
(an'je-o-plas'te)	Meaning of Word	_____
3. venous	ven(o)	_____
venous	-ous	_____
(ve'nus)	Meaning of Word	_____
4. phlebectomy	phleb(o)	_____
phlebectomy	-ectomy	_____
(fle-bek'to-me)	Meaning of Word	_____
5. sphygmomanometer	sphygm(o)	_____
sphygmomanometer	manometer	_____
(sfig'mo-mah-nom'e-ter)	Meaning of Word	_____
6. arteriospasm	arteri(o)	_____
arteriospasm	-spasm	_____
(ar-te're-o-spazm')	Meaning of Word	_____
7. cardiorrhaphy	cardi(o)	_____
cardiorrhaphy	-rrhaphy	_____
(kar'de-or'ah-fe)	Meaning of Word	_____

Word	Word Part	Meaning of Word Part
8. arteriostenosis	arteri(o)	_____
arteriostenosis	sten(o)	_____
arteriostenosis	-osis	_____
(ar-te′re-o-ste-no′sis)	Meaning of Word	_____
9. diastolic	diastole	_____
diastolic	-ic	_____
(di′ah-stol′ik)	Meaning of Word	_____
10. vasodilator	vas(o)	_____
vasodilator	-dilator	_____
(vas′o-di-lat′or)	Meaning of Word	_____
11. tachycardia	tachy-	_____
tachycardia	-cardi(a)	_____
(tak′e-kar-de-ah)	Meaning of Word	_____
12. arteriectasis	arteri(o)	_____
arteriectasis	-ectasis	_____
(ar′te-re-ek′tah-sis)	Meaning of Word	_____
13. arterial	arteri(o)	_____
arterial	-al	_____
(ar-te′re-al)	Meaning of Word	_____
14. vasculitis	vascul(o)	_____
vasculitis	-itis	_____
(vas′ku-li′tis)	Meaning of Word	_____
15. angiocarditis	angi(o)	_____
angiocarditis	cardi(o)	_____
angiocarditis	-itis	_____
(an′je-o-kar-di′tis)	Meaning of Word	_____

➡ *Stop CD*

On the lines provided, write in the meanings of as many suffixes, prefixes, roots, and words as you can from memory. Check your definitions in the glossary or a medical dictionary, and make any needed corrections.

CHAPTER
7
Terminology Review

Complete this review, and turn it in to your instructor when you are finished.

Definition

Each phrase below defines one of the words you have just studied. Without looking at your previous work, write in the word that matches each definition.

Definition	Term
1. dilation of an artery	_____
2. instrument used for measuring blood pressure	_____
3. narrowing of an artery	_____
4. pertaining to the contraction of the ventricles	_____
5. excessive rapidity in the action of the heart, especially in the pulse rate	_____
6. hardening of the arteries	_____
7. pertaining to the dilation of the ventricles	_____
8. suture or surgical repair of the heart	_____
9. excision or removal of a vein	_____
10. an agent that causes dilation of a blood vessel	_____
11. inflammation of the sac surrounding the heart	_____
12. palpating or feeling the pulse	_____
13. process of recording electrical impulses of the heart	_____
14. inflammation of the heart muscle	_____
15. abnormally slow heart rate	_____
16. pertaining to veins	_____
17. inflammation of the inner lining of the heart	_____
18. any disease of the blood vessels	_____
19. pertaining to the pulse	_____

Definition	Term
20. pertaining to the aorta	_____
21. inflammation of the heart and the major blood vessels	_____
22. the study of the science of the pulse	_____
23. inflammation of the aorta	_____
24. pertaining to the heart	_____
25. primary myocardial disease	_____

Matching

Match the following definitions with the terms given. Place the letter of the correct definition to the left of the term.

Term	Definition
_____ **26.** cardiomyopathy	**a.** abnormally slow heart rate
_____ **27.** arteriorrhexis	**b.** suturing blood vessels
_____ **28.** angiorrhaphy	**c.** the study or science of the pulse
_____ **29.** vasculopathy	**d.** rupture of an artery
_____ **30.** bradycardia	**e.** pertaining to the blood vessels
_____ **31.** sphygmology	**f.** incision into a vein
_____ **32.** vascular	**g.** enlargement of the heart
_____ **33.** phlebotomy	**h.** any disease of the blood vessels
_____ **34.** cardiomegaly	**i.** inflammation of the heart and great blood vessels
_____ **35.** angiocarditis	**j.** primary myocardial disease

Terminology Review

Case Studies

Read the following brief case studies. In each case study, some terms are followed by a superscript letter. Write a brief definition for each of those terms on the corresponding lines below.

1. M.K. is an elderly patient with cardiomyopathy[a] that has caused considerable endocarditis[b]. His arterial[c] flow is not good, and he has had two angioplasty[d] procedures within the past year. Since his last angioplasty, he has been on an antianginal[e], a thrombolytic[f], and an antilipidemic[g].

    a. _____

    b. _____

    c. _____

    d. _____

    e. _____

    f. _____

    g. _____

2. V. has had carditis[a] for several years and has recently experienced severe pain. She has recently met with her cardiologist[b], who first diagnosed her with this problem. The doctor has scheduled her for a battery of cardiac tests, and she will need to be hospitalized for a few days.

    a. _____

    b. _____

3. After suffering a stab wound to the chest, this ER patient underwent arteriorrhaphy[a] and phleborraphy[b] to repair damage. During the surgery, the patient suffered severe arterial[c] bleeding, after which the blood began to coagulate too quickly. Rather than have this patient risk thrombosis[d], the doctor put the patient on an IV (intravenous) blood thinner.

    a. _____

    b. _____

    c. _____

    d. _____

4. B. has a history of blocked arteries, and his doctor has prescribed a vasodilator[a] to alleviate stress on the heart. B. might be hypertensive[b] and might need to be on a strict regimen of antihypertensive[c] medication.

a. _____

b. _____

c. _____

Labeling

Fill in the blanks with the correct terminology.

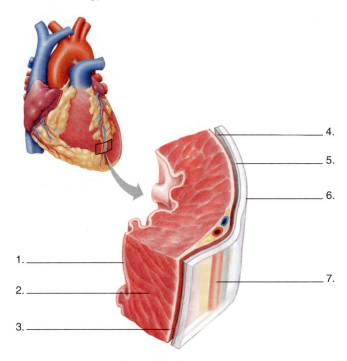

FIGURE 7-5   The endocardium, the myocardium, and the layers of the pericardium.

You may now go on to Chapter Test 7.

8

Hematic and Lymphatic Systems

Objectives

After completing Chapter 8, you should be able to do the following:

1. identify word roots and combining forms denoting the blood;

2. understand the terms associated with the three different types of blood cells;

3. identify the word root for a clotting cell or platelet;

4. identify word roots pertaining to the spleen;

5. identify word roots pertaining to the lymphatic system; and

6. identify several types of drugs associated with hematic and lymphatic conditions and treatments.

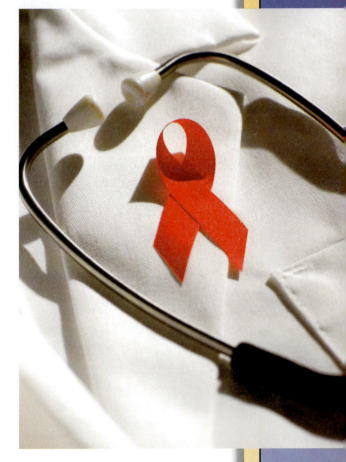

Orientation to the Hematic and Lymphatic Systems

The hematic and lymphatic systems include tissues made up of cells that are suspended in a liquid. Blood contains solid cells and a liquid called plasma. The three types of blood cells are erythrocytes (red blood cells), leukocytes (white blood cells), and thrombocytes (clotting cells, platelets). Blood is about 55 percent plasma, which in turn is about 90 percent water; the remaining part of plasma contains protein, including serum albumin, serum globulin, and fibrinogen.

The red blood cells (erythrocytes) contain the protein hemoglobin, which allows the cells to carry oxygen throughout the body. Erythrocytes are formed in the red bone marrow and contain iron.

There are several types of white blood cells (leukocytes). Some consume foreign particles such as bacteria and viruses, and others produce antibodies. An increased amount of leukocytes in the bloodstream is often a sign of infection.

The clotting cells (thrombocytes, or platelets) are important elements in the blood for coagulation (clotting). When a blood vessel is damaged or injured, the thrombocytes form and release fibrin (a protein) that promotes clotting in the damaged or injured area.

The lymphatic system drains fluid from tissues and transports it back to the blood. In addition, the lymphatic system carries nutrient materials, hormones, and oxygen to cells within the body and transports waste materials from tissues to the blood.

The lymphatic system includes structures that aid in the transporting of fluid (lymph) to the blood. The lymphatic vessels and nodes, the spleen, the thymus gland, and the tonsils aid in this process.

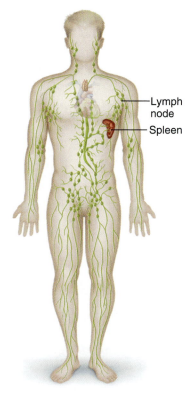

Lymphatic system

8-1 Terminology Presentation

Blood

As you listen to the CD, read the words and notice the pronunciations given.

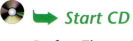 **Start CD**

Look at Figures 8-1 and 8-2

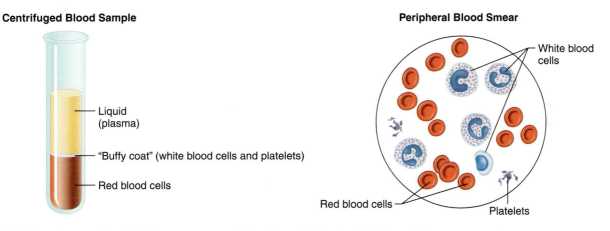

Centrifuged Blood Sample

Liquid (plasma)

"Buffy coat" (white blood cells and platelets)

Red blood cells

Peripheral Blood Smear

White blood cells

Red blood cells

Platelets

FIGURE 8-1 Plasma (the liquid component of blood) and blood cells (the solid components).

hem(o), hemat(o) combining forms denoting the blood			
Word	**Word Part**	**Definition**	**Answer**
1. hemarthrosis (hem'ar-thro'sis)	arthr(o) -osis	joint abnormal condition	1. _____
2. hemostat (he'mo-stat)	-stat	stop	2. _____
3. hematic (he-mat'ik)	-ic	pertaining to	3. _____
4. hematocrit (he-mat'o-krit)	-crit	separate	4. _____
5. hemolysis (he-mol'i-sis)	-lysis	dissolve, break down	5. _____
6. hematemesis (hem'ah-tem-e-sis)	-emesis	vomit	6. _____

continued

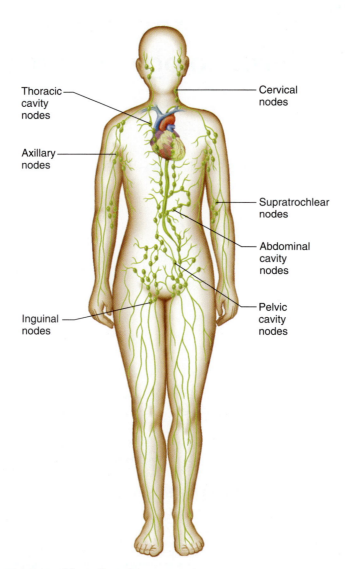

FIGURE 8-2 Lymphatic system and lymph nodes.

Labels on figure:
- Thoracic cavity nodes
- Cervical nodes
- Axillary nodes
- Supratrochlear nodes
- Abdominal cavity nodes
- Pelvic cavity nodes
- Inguinal nodes

Word	Word Part	Definition	Answer
7. hemangioma (he-man′je-o′ma)	angi(o) -oma	vessels tumor	**7.** _____
8. hemoptysis (he-mop′ti-sis)	-ptysis	cough up, spit up	**8.** _____

emia	a word element denoting relationship to the blood		

Word	Word Part	Definition	Answer
9. polycythemia (pol′e-si-the′me-ah)	poly cyt(o)	many, increase cell	**9.** _____
10. lipidemia (lip′i-de′me-ah)	lipid	fat	**10.** _____
11. hyperglycemia (hi′per-gli-se′me-ah)	hyper glyc(o)	above, over, abundant sugar	**11.** _____

Word	Word Part	Definition	Answer
12. anemia (ah-ne'me-ah)	an	without, lack of	12. _____
13. oligemia (ol'i-ge'me-ah)	olig(o)	few	13. _____
14. septicemia (sep'ti-se'me-ah)	sept(i)	toxin, poison	14. _____

  Pause CD

After practicing each word several times, use a sheet of paper to cover all columns except the Answer column. As each word is pronounced again on the CD, write it in the space provided.

  Start CD

Check the words you have written against the words in the left-hand column. If you have misspelled any words, practice writing them correctly.

Practice

_____

_____

_____

_____

_____

_____

_____

_____

_____

_____

_____

_____

_____

_____

_____

_____

Practice

LESSON
8-1

Terminology Application

Without looking at your previous work, write the word that matches each definition.

Definition	Term
1. accumulation of blood in a joint cavity	_____
2. spitting up or coughing up blood	_____
3. pertaining to or contained in the blood	_____
4. an instrument for stopping bleeding	_____
5. vomiting of blood	_____
6. systemic disease associated with the presence and persistence of microorganisms in the blood	_____
7. a benign tumor composed of newly formed blood vessels	_____
8. a deficiency in the volume of blood	_____
9. an abnormally high concentration of fat in the blood	_____
10. the volume percentage of red cells in whole blood	_____
11. an increase in the number of red blood cells in the blood	_____
12. excessive sugar in the blood	_____
13. breaking down or destroying blood cells	_____
14. a reduction in the number of red blood cells in the blood	_____

Check your answers against the information given in this lesson's terminology presentation. If you have any errors, count them and write the number in the blank at the top of the page. Sign your work and give it to your instructor.

Practice

LESSON

8-2   Terminology Presentation

Blood Cells—Red Blood Cells, White Blood Cells, and Thrombocytes (platelets)—and Blood Clots

As you listen to the CD, read the words and notice the pronunciations given.

  Start CD

erythr(o)	a word element denoting red or red blood cells		
Word	**Word Part**	**Definition**	**Answer**
1. erythrocyte (e-rith′ro-sit)	-cyte	cell	1. _____
2. erythropenia (e-rith′ro-pe′ne-ah)	-penia	decrease, deficiency	2. _____
3. erythropoiesis (e-rith′ro-poi-e′sis)	-poiesis	form, formation	3. _____
4. erythroclasis (er′e-throk′lah-sis)	-clasis	break, fracture	4. _____
5. erythrocytosis (e-rith′ro-si-to′sis)	-cytosis	an increase in cells	5. _____

leuk(o)	a combining form meaning white or denoting a relationship to a leukocyte		
Word	**Word Part**	**Definition**	**Answer**
6. leukocyte (loo′ko-sit)	-cyte	cell	6. _____
7. leukocytology (loo′ko-si-tol′o-je)	-cyte -logy	cell study of, science of	7. _____
8. leukopenia (loo′ko-pe′ne-ah)	-penia	reduction of, difficiency	8. _____
9. leukemia (loo-ke′me-ah)	-emia	blood condition	9. _____

continued

	Word	Word Part	Definition	Answer
thromb(o)	a combining form indicating a blood clot, or thrombus			
10.	thrombocyte (throm′bo-site)	-cyte	cell	10. _____
11.	thrombopoiesis (throm′bo-poi-e′sis)	-poiesis	form, formation	11. _____
12.	thrombosis (throm-bo′sis)	-osis	abnormal condition	12. _____
13.	thrombectomy (throm-bek′to-me)	-ectomy	excision, removal	13. _____
14.	thrombolytic (throm′bo-lit′ik)	-lysis -ic	dissolving, splitting pertaining to	14. _____
15.	thrombophlebitis (throm′bo-fle-bi′tis)	phleb(o) -itis	vein inflammation	15. _____
16.	thrombopathy (throm-bop′ah-the)	-pathy	disease	16. _____

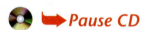 ➡ *Pause CD*

> After practicing each word several times, use a sheet of paper to cover all columns except the Answer column. As each word is pronounced again on the CD, write it in the space provided.

➡ *Start CD*

> Check the words you have written against the words in the left-hand column. If you have misspelled any words, practice writing them correctly.

Practice

_____

_____

_____

_____

_____

_____

_____

_____

_____

_____

LESSON 8-2

Terminology Application

Without looking at your previous work, write the word that matches each definition.

Definition	Term
1. the study of the science of white blood cells	_____
2. a deficiency of white blood cells	_____
3. a white blood cell	_____
4. any disease involving clotting cells	_____
5. a clotting cell; a platelet	_____
6. the formation of red blood cells	_____
7. the formation of clotting cells	_____
8. an increase in the number of red blood cells	_____
9. the formation of clots or thrombi	_____
10. a red blood cell	_____
11. an agent that dissolves a blood clot	_____
12. the breaking up or splitting of red blood cells	_____
13. inflammation of a vein in which a clot is present	_____
14. excision of a thrombus	_____
15. a decrease in the number of red blood cells	_____
16. a blood disease characterized by distorted proliferation and development of leukocytes	_____

Check your answers against the information given in this lesson's terminology presentation. If you have any errors, count them and write the number in the blank at the top of the page. Sign your work and give it to your instructor.

Practice

8-3 Terminology Presentation

Spleen

As you listen to the CD, read the words and notice the pronunciations given.

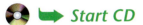 **Start CD**

Look at Figure 8-3

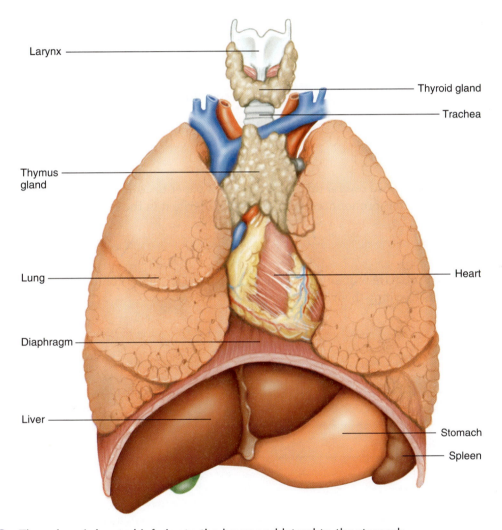

FIGURE 8-3 The spleen is located inferior to the lungs and lateral to the stomach.

	splen(o) a combining form denoting the spleen		
Word	**Word Part**	**Definition**	**Answer**
1. splenophrenic (splen-o-fren'ik)	phren(o) -ic	diaphragm pertaining to	1. _____
2. splenic (splen'ik)	-ic	pertaining to	2. _____
3. splenectomy (sple-nek'to-me)	-ectomy	excision, removal	3. _____
4. splenatrophy (splen-at'ro-fe)	a- -trophy	without nourishment	4. _____
5. splenohepatomegaly (sple'no-hep'ah-to-meg'ah-le)	hepat(o) -megaly	liver enlargement	5. _____
6. splenocele (sple'no-sel)	-cele	tumor, swelling, hernia	6. _____
7. splenorrhagia (sple'no-ra'je-ah)	-rrhagia	excessive flow, bleeding	7. _____

  ➡ *Pause CD*

After practicing each word several times, use a sheet of paper to cover all columns except the Answer column. As each word is pronounced again on the CD, write it in the space provided.

  ➡ *Start CD*

Check the words you have written against the words in the left-hand column. If you have misspelled any words, practice writing them correctly.

Practice

_____

_____

_____

_____

_____

_____

_____

_____

_____

LESSON
8-3

Terminology Application

Without looking at your previous work, write the word that matches each definition.

Definition	Term
1. bleeding or hemorrhage from the spleen	_____
2. pertaining to the spleen	_____
3. excision or removal of the spleen	_____
4. pertaining to the spleen and diaphragm	_____
5. atrophy or wasting of the spleen	_____
6. enlargement of the spleen and liver	_____
7. herniation or swelling of the spleen	_____

Check your answers against the information given in this lesson's terminology presentation. If you have any errors, count them and write the number in the blank at the top of the page. Sign your work and give it to your instructor.

Practice

8-4 Terminology Presentation

Lymphatic System

As you listen to the CD, read the words and notice the pronunciations given.

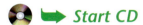

Start CD

Look at Figure 8-4

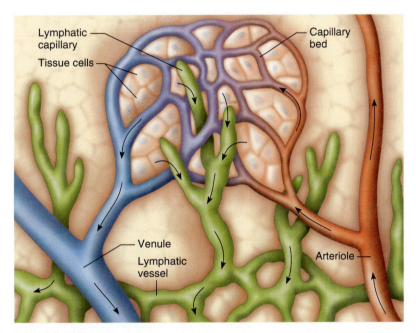

FIGURE 8-4 Lymphatic capillaries connected to blood vessels and tissue cells.

lymph(o)	a combining form indicating lymph or the lymphatic glands or vessels		
Word	**Word Part**	**Definition**	**Answer**
1. lymphadenitis (lim-fad′e-ni′tis)	aden(o) -itis	gland inflammation	1. _____
2. lymphopathy (lim-fop′ah-the)	-pathy	disease	2. _____
3. lymphangioma (lim-fan′je-o′mah)	angi(o) -oma	vessel tumor	3. _____
4. lymphocyte (lim′fo-sit)	-cyte	cell	4. _____

continued

Word	Word Part	Definition	Answer
5. lymphocytopenia (lim′fo-si′to-pe′ne-ah)	cyt(o) -penia	cell decrease	5. _____
6. lymphopoiesis (lim′fo-poi-e′sis)	-poiesis	form, formation	6. _____
7. lymphedema (lim′fe-de′mah)	-edema	swelling	7. _____
8. lymphostasis (lim-fos′tah-sis)	-stasis	stop	8. _____

 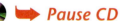 *Pause CD*

After practicing each word several times, use a sheet of paper to cover all columns except the Answer column. As each word is pronounced again on the CD, write it in the space provided.

 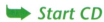 *Start CD*

Check the words you have written against the words in the left-hand column. If you have misspelled any words, practice writing them correctly.

Practice

_____

_____

_____

_____

_____

_____

_____

_____

_____

_____

_____

_____

_____

_____

_____

LESSON
8-4
Terminology Application

Without looking at your previous work, write the word that matches each definition.

Definition	Term
1. swelling of subcutaneous tissue due to excessive lymph fluid	_____
2. making or developing lymph	_____
3. inflammation of a lymph gland	_____
4. reduction in the number of lymphocytes in the blood	_____
5. stoppage of lymph flow	_____
6. a tumor in a lymphatic vessel	_____
7. any disease of the lymphatic system	_____
8. a white cell that is formed in the lymph glands	_____

Check your answers against the information given in this lesson's terminology presentation. If you have any errors, count them and write the number in the blank at the top of the page. Sign your work and give it to your instructor.

Practice

Drug Terminology Presentation

As you listen to the CD, read the words and notice the pronunciations given.

 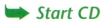 **Start CD**

Word	Definition	Example: Generic Name	Example: Brand Trade Name	Answer
anticoagulants	agents that prevent blood clotting	heparin warfarin	Heparin Coumadin	1. _____
hemostatics	agents that arrest the flow of blood	aminocaproic acid aprotinin tranexamic acid thrombin	Amicar Trasylol Biosaren	2. _____

 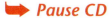 **Pause CD**

After practicing each word several times, use a sheet of paper to cover all columns except the Answer column. As each word is pronounced again on the CD, write it in the space provided.

 Start CD

Check the words you have written against the words in the left-hand column. If you have misspelled any words, practice writing them correctly.

Practice

_____

_____

_____

_____

_____

_____

_____

_____

_____

_____

Practice

LESSON 8-5 Drug Terminology Application

Without looking at your previous work, write the word that matches each definition.

Definition	Term
1. agents that arrest the flow of blood	_____
2. agents that prevent blood clotting	_____

Check your answers against the information given in this lesson's terminology presentation. If you have any errors, count them and write the number in the blank at the top of the page. Sign your work and give it to your instructor.

Practice

CHAPTER
8

Terminology Review

This is a review of the word parts and words you have learned in the preceding lessons. Some of the medical terms listed below may be new, but they are composed of the word parts and word roots that you have already learned. Read the words below as they are pronounced on the CD.

 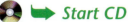 **Start CD**

Word Element Review

Word	Word Part	Meaning of Word Part
1. septicemia	sept(i)	_____
septicemia	-emia	_____
(sep′ti-se′me-ah)	Meaning of Word	_____
2. erythrocyte	erythr(o)	_____
erythrocyte	-cyte	_____
(e-rith′ro-sit)	Meaning of Word	_____
3. thrombolytic	thromb(o)	_____
thrombolytic	-lysis	_____
thrombolytic	-ic	_____
(throm′bo-lit′ik)	Meaning of Word	_____
4. erythropenia	erythr(o)	_____
erythropenia	-penia	_____
(e-rith′ro-pe′ne-ah)	Meaning of Word	_____
5. splenic	splen(o)	_____
splenic	-ic	_____
(splen′ik)	Meaning of Word	_____
6. hematemesis	hemat(o)	_____
hematemesis	-emesis	_____
(hem′ah-tem′-e-sis)	Meaning of Word	_____
7. leukocyte	leuk(o)	_____
leukocyte	-cyte	_____
(loo′ko-sit)	Meaning of Word	_____

Word	Word Part	Meaning of Word Part
8. <mark>hyper</mark>glycemia	hyper-	_____
hyper<mark>glyc</mark>emia	glyc(o)	_____
hyperglyc<mark>emia</mark>	-emia	_____
(hi′per-gli-se′me-ah)	Meaning of Word	_____
9. <mark>lympho</mark>pathy	lymph(o)	_____
lympho<mark>pathy</mark>	-pathy	_____
(lim-fop′ ah-the)	Meaning of Word	_____
10. <mark>lympho</mark>cyte	lymph(o)	_____
lympho<mark>cyte</mark>	-cyte	_____
(lim′ fo-sit)	Meaning of Word	_____
11. <mark>thromb</mark>ectomy	thromb(o)	_____
thromb<mark>ectomy</mark>	-ectomy	_____
(throm-bek′ to-me)	Meaning of Word	_____
12. <mark>lipid</mark>emia	lipid	_____
lipid<mark>emia</mark>	-emia	_____
(lip′ i-de′ me-ah)	Meaning of Word	_____
13. <mark>splen</mark>ectomy	splen(o)	_____
splen<mark>ectomy</mark>	-ectomy	_____
(sple-nek′ to-me)	Meaning of Word	_____
14. <mark>thrombo</mark>cyte	thromb(o)	_____
thrombo<mark>cyte</mark>	-cyte	_____
(throm′ bo-site)	Meaning of Word	_____
15. <mark>lympho</mark>poiesis	lymph(o)	_____
lympho<mark>poiesis</mark>	-poiesis	_____
(lim′ fo-poi-e′ sis)	Meaning of Word	_____

  Stop CD

On the lines provided, write in the meanings of as many suffixes, prefixes, roots, and words as you can from memory. Check your definitions in the glossary or a medical dictionary, and make any needed corrections.

CHAPTER 8

Terminology Review

Complete this review, and turn it in to your instructor when you are finished.

Definition

Each phrase below defines one of the words you have just studied. Without looking at your previous work, write in the word that matches each definition.

Definition	Term
1. vomiting of blood	_____
2. excessive sugar in the blood	_____
3. accumulation of blood in a joint cavity	_____
4. enlargement of the spleen and liver	_____
5. an instrument for stopping bleeding	_____
6. pertaining to the spleen	_____
7. a reduction of the number of lymphocytes in the blood	_____
8. an increase in the number of red blood cells in the blood	_____
9. pertaining to or contained in the blood	_____
10. removal of the spleen	_____
11. a tumor in a lymphatic vessel	_____
12. the formation of clots or thrombi	_____
13. a red blood cell	_____
14. atrophy or wasting of the spleen	_____
15. breaking up or splitting up of red blood cells	_____
16. any disease of the lymphatic system	_____
17. systemic disease associated with the presence and persistence of microorganisms and toxins in the blood	_____

18. a clotting cell   _____

19. a white blood cell   _____

20. inflammation of the lymph gland   _____

Matching

Match the following terms with the definitions given. Place the letter of the correct term to the left of the definition.

Definition	Term
_____ **21.** herniation or swelling of the spleen	**a.** hemostat
_____ **22.** stoppage of lymph flow	**b.** lymphocyte
_____ **23.** an increase in the number of red blood cells in the blood	**c.** hemoptysis
_____ **24.** spitting up or coughing up blood	**d.** erythrocytosis
_____ **25.** bleeding or hemorrhage from the spleen	**e.** lymphedema
_____ **26.** an instrument that stops bleeding	**f.** splenocele
_____ **27.** the formation of clotting cells	**g.** splenic
_____ **28.** pertaining to the spleen	**h.** lymphostasis
_____ **29.** a white cell that is formed in the lymph glands	**i.** splenorrhagia
_____ **30.** swelling of subcutaneous tissue due to excessive lymph fluid	**j.** thrombopoiesis

Terminology Review

Case Studies

Read the following brief case studies. In each case study, some terms are followed by a superscript letter. Write a brief definition for each of those terms on the corresponding lines below.

1. S.E. was in a construction accident and was rushed to a hospital. He had hematemesis[a] and needed immediate attention. Tests showed that he had internal injuries that were causing splenorrhagia[b]. He had an emergency splenectomy[c] and additional surgery to repair damage to his organs.

   a. _____

   b. _____

   c. _____

2. H. has been diagnosed with lymphatic cancer, a type of lymphopathy[a], and will need extensive chemotherapy. Apparently the increase in damaged lymphocytes[b] his body produces has caused severe lymphedema[c] and considerable pain.

   a. _____

   b. _____

   c. _____

3. W.N. has hyperglycemia[a] and must maintain a strict diet in order to stay healthy. She needs to monitor her blood sugar levels and be aware of recurring symptoms such as excessive thirst and excessive urination.

   a. _____

4. C.L. has anemia[a] exacerbated by erythropenia[b]. His doctor has him on iron therapy in an attempt to stimulate erythropoiesis[c].

   a. _____

   b. _____

   c. _____

Labeling

Fill in the blanks with the correct terminology.

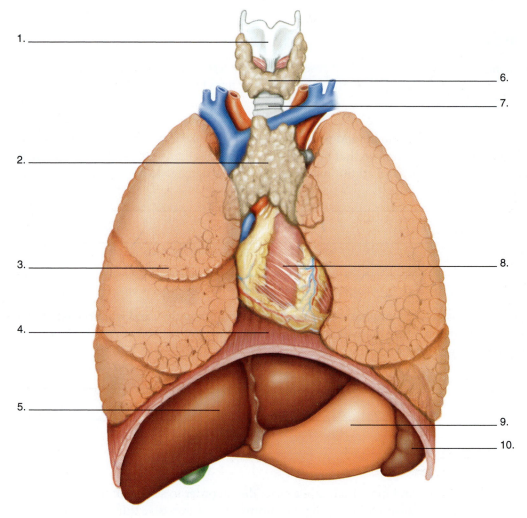

1. _____

2. _____

3. _____

4. _____

5. _____

6. _____

7. _____

8. _____

9. _____

10. _____

FIGURE 8-5   The endocardium, the myocardium, and the layers of the pericardium.

You may now go on to Chapter Test 8.

9

Urinary System

Objectives

After completing Chapter 9, you should be able to do the following:

1. identify word roots pertaining to the kidneys;

2. identify word roots pertaining to some parts of the kidney;

3. identify word roots pertaining to the urinary bladder;

4. understand the difference between the ureter and the urethra;

5. identify terms referring to urine; and

6. identify several types of drugs associated with urinary tract conditions and treatments.

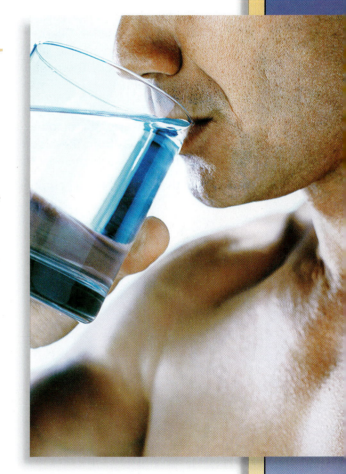

Orientation to the Urinary System

The urinary system is composed of two kidneys, two ureters, a urinary bladder, and the urethra. In the male, the prostate gland surrounds the first section of the urethra and secretes a substance that protects sperm cells from the acidity of vaginal secretions.

The urinary system is responsible for excreting wastes from the blood, regulating the amount of water in the body, and keeping the pH (relation of acids to bases) in balance. This system monitors and regulates body fluids, including plasma, lymph, and tissue fluid.

The blood is filtered in the kidneys, where certain fluids and minerals are reabsorbed. The remaining fluid wastes are collected in the urinary bladder. They pass out of the body through the urethra during urination.

Each kidney has a cortex (the outer layer) and a medulla (the inner layer) that produce hormones that will be discussed in Chapter 13. In addition, both layers function to filter waste material. Inside the kidney are microscopic structures called nephrons that help to maintain the correct chemical balance in the blood. The nephron has a renal corpuscle, a tuft of capillaries called the glomerulus, and a renal tubule.

The renal artery enters the kidney carrying blood that includes metabolic waste; once the kidney removes the waste, the blood exits the kidney through the renal vein. The waste material that the kidney has taken from the blood then goes through the renal pelvis into a tube called the ureter, which takes the waste material (urine) to the urinary bladder for storage.

When the urinary bladder empties, the urine exits through a single tube called the urethra.

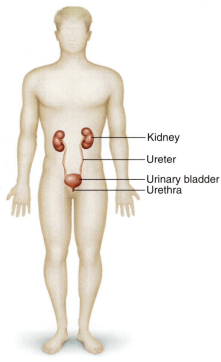

Urinary system

9-1   Terminology Presentation

Kidneys

As you listen to the CD, read the words and notice the pronunciations given.

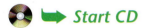 **Start CD**

Look at Figures 9-1 and 9-2

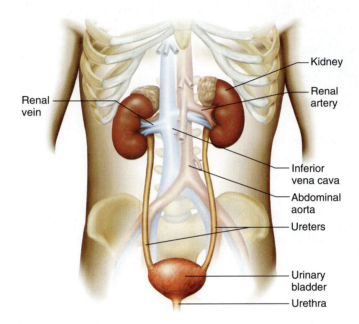

FIGURE 9-1   The urinary system.

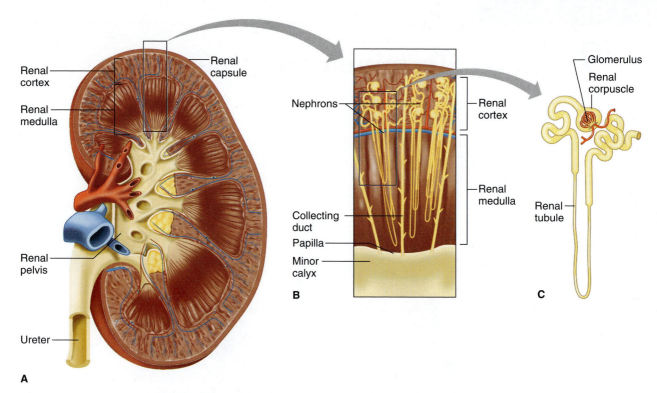

FIGURE 9-2   The kidney and the renal pelvis.

nephr(o) a combining form denoting relationship to the kidney			
Word	**Word Part**	**Definition**	**Answer**
1. nephritis (ne-fri′tis)	-itis	inflammation	1. _____
2. pyelonephritis (pi′e-lo-ne-fri′tis)	pyel(o) -itis	pelvis of the kidney inflammation	2. _____
3. nephrectomy (ne-frek′to-me)	-ectomy	excision, removal	3. _____
4. nephrolithiasis (nef′ro-li-thi′ah-sis)	-lithiasis	condition of stones	4. _____
5. nephropathy (nef-frop′ah-the)	-pathy	disease	5. _____
6. nephroptosis (nef′rop-to′sis)	-ptosis	falling	6. _____
7. nephrology (ne-frol′o-je)	-logy	study of, science of	7. _____

ren(o)	a combining form denoting relationship to the kidneys		
Word	**Word Part**	**Definition**	**Answer**
8. renal (re′nal)	-al	pertaining to	8. _____
9. reniform (ren′i-form)	-form	resembling	9. _____
10. renocortical (re′no-kor′ti-kal)	cortic(o) -al	cortex pertaining to	10. _____
11. suprarenal (soo′prah-re′nal)	supra- -al	above pertaining to	11. _____

pyel(o)	a combining form denoting the pelvis of the kidney		
Word	**Word Part**	**Definition**	**Answer**
12. pyelography (pi′e-log′rah-fe)	-graphy	process of recording using a roentgenograph (X-ray)	12. _____
13. pyelitis (pi′e-li′tis)	-itis	inflammation	13. _____
14. pyeloscopy (pi′e-los′ko-pe)	-scopy	visual examination	14. _____
15. pyelectasis (pi′e-lek′tah-sis)	-ectasis	dilatation, expansion	15. _____
16. pyelolithotomy (pi′e-lo-li-thot′o-me)	lith(o) -tomy	stone incision, cutting into	16. _____

glomerul(o)	a combining form denoting relationship to the renal glomeruli; a tuft/cluster of capillaries		
Word	**Word Part**	**Definition**	**Answer**
17. glomerular (glo-mer′u-lar)	-ar	pertaining to	17. _____
18. glomerulitis (glo-mer′u-li-tis)	-itis	inflammation	18. _____
19. glomerulopathy (glo-mer′u-lop′ah-the)	-pathy	disease	19. _____

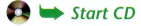

Pause CD

After practicing each word several times, use a sheet of paper to cover all columns except the Answer column. As each word is pronounced again on the CD, write it in the space provided.

Start CD

Check the words you have written against the words in the left-hand column. If you have misspelled any words, practice writing them correctly.

Practice

_____

_____

_____

_____

_____

_____

_____

_____

_____

_____

_____

_____

_____

_____

_____

_____

_____

_____

_____

_____

_____

_____

LESSON
9-1
Terminology Application

Without looking at your previous work, write the word that matches each definition.

Definition	Term
1. pertaining to the cortex of the kidney	_____
2. inflammation of the pelvis of the kidney	_____
3. located above the kidney; adrenal gland	_____
4. examination or observation of the kidney pelvis via a fluoroscope	_____
5. kidney-shaped	_____
6. excision of a kidney	_____
7. any disease of the glomerulus	_____
8. dilatation of the kidney pelvis	_____
9. pertaining to the glomerulus	_____
10. downward displacement of the kidney	_____
11. inflammation of the kidney	_____
12. roentgenographic (X-ray) study of the kidney and renal collecting system	_____
13. pertaining to the kidney	_____
14. inflammation of the kidney and its pelvis	_____
15. the operation of removing a renal calculus from the pelvis of the kidney	_____
16. inflammation of the glomerulus	_____
17. any kidney disease	_____
18. kidney stones	_____
19. study of the science of the kidney	_____

Check your answers against the information given in this lesson's terminology presentation. If you have any errors, count them and write the number in the blank at the top of the page. Sign your work and give it to your instructor.

Practice

LESSON

9-2 Terminology Presentation

Urinary Bladder

As you listen to the CD, read the words and notice the pronunciations given.

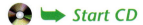 **Start CD**

Look at Figure 9-3

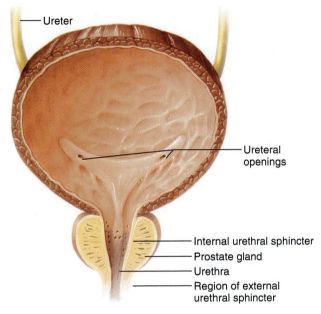

FIGURE 9-3 The urinary bladder, the ureters, and the urethra.

cyst(o), cyst(i) combining forms denoting a relationship to a sac or bladder, most frequently the urinary bladder			
Word	**Word Part**	**Definition**	**Answer**
1. cystic (sis′tik)	-ic	pertaining to	1. _____
2. cystitis (sis-ti′tis)	-itis	inflammation	2. _____
3. cystoscope (sis′to-skop′)	-scope	instrument used for viewing	3. _____

continued

Word	Word Part	Definition	Answer
4. cystoscopy (sis-tos'ko-pe)	-scopy	visual examination	4. _____
5. cystostomy (sis-tos'to-me)	-stomy	formation of an opening	5. _____
6. cystoptosis (sis'top-to'sis)	-ptosis	a falling	6. _____
7. cystorrhagia (sis'to-ra'je-ah)	-rrhagia	excessive flow, bleeding	7. _____
8. cystospasm (sis'to-spazm)	-spasm	spasm, contraction	8. _____

  ➡ *Pause CD*

After practicing each word several times, use a sheet of paper to cover all columns except the Answer column. As each word is pronounced again on the CD, write it in the space provided.

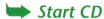 ➡ *Start CD*

Check the words you have written against the words in the left-hand column. If you have misspelled any words, practice writing them correctly.

Practice

_____

_____

_____

_____

_____

_____

_____

_____

_____

_____

_____

_____

_____

LESSON
9-2

Terminology Application

Without looking at your previous work, write the word that matches each definition.

Definition	Term
1. hemorrhage from the bladder	_____
2. prolapse of the bladder into the urethra	_____
3. surgical formation of an opening into the urinary bladder	_____
4. an endoscope for visual examination of the urinary bladder	_____
5. visual examination of the urinary bladder	_____
6. pertaining to a cyst or bladder	_____
7. spasm of the urinary bladder	_____
8. inflammation of the urinary bladder	_____

Check your answers against the information given in this lesson's terminology presentation. If you have any errors, count them and write the number in the blank at the top of the page. Sign your work and give it to your instructor.

Practice

Terminology Presentation

Ureter and Urethra

As you listen to the CD, read the words and notice the pronunciations given.

  Start CD

Look at Figure 9-1 on page 239

ureter(o)	a combining form denoting relationship to the ureter		
Word	**Word Part**	**Definition**	**Answer**
1. ureteral (u-re′ter-al)	-al	pertaining to	1. _____
2. ureteropathy (u-re′ter-op′ah-the)	-pathy	disease	2. _____
3. ureterolith (u-re′ter-o-lith′)	-lith(o)	stone, calculus	3. _____
4. ureterectomy (u′re-ter-ek′to-me)	-ectomy	excision, removal	4. _____
5. ureterectasis (u-re′ter-ek′tah-sis)	-ectasis	distension	5. _____
6. ureteralgia (u′re-ter-al′je-ah)	-algia	pain	6. _____
7. ureterolithiasis (u-re′ter-o-li-thi′ah-sis)	-lith(o) -iasis	stone, calculus condition	7. _____
8. ureteroplasty (u-re′ter-o-plas′te)	-plasty	plastic surgery	8. _____

urethr(o)	a combining form denoting relationship to the urethra		
Word	**Word Part**	**Definition**	**Answer**
9. urethral (u-re′thral)	-al	pertaining to	9. _____
10. urethrophraxis (u-re′thro-frak′sis)	-phraxis	obstruction	10. _____
11. urethritis (u′re-thri′tis)	-itis	inflammation	11. _____
12. urethrorrhaphy (u′re-thror′ah-fe)	-rrhaphy	suturing	12. _____

Word	Word Part	Definition	Answer
13. urethrorrhagia (u-re′thro-ra′je-ah)	-rrhagia	excessive flow, bleeding	13. _____
14. urethrectomy (u′re-threk′to-me)	-ectomy	excision, removal	14. _____
15. urethroplasty (u-re′thro-plas′te)	-plasty	plastic surgery	15. _____
16. urethrospasm (u-re′thro-spazm)	-spasm	spasm, contraction	16. _____

 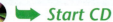 ***Pause CD***

After practicing each word several times, use a sheet of paper to cover all columns except the Answer column. As each word is pronounced again on the CD, write it in the space provided.

 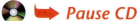 ***Start CD***

Check the words you have written against the words in the left-hand column. If you have misspelled any words, practice writing them correctly.

Practice

_____

_____

_____

_____

_____

_____

_____

_____

_____

_____

_____

_____

_____

_____

_____

_____

LESSON 9-3

Terminology Application

Without looking at your previous work, write the word that matches each definition.

Definition	Term
1. pertaining to the urethra	_____
2. pertaining to the ureter	_____
3. any disease of the ureter	_____
4. an obstruction of the urethra	_____
5. an excision of the urethra	_____
6. a stone or calculus in a ureter	_____
7. formation of stones in the ureter	_____
8. plastic surgery of the urethra	_____
9. pain in the ureter	_____
10. removal of the ureter	_____
11. spasm of the urethra	_____
12. suturing of the urethra	_____
13. distension of the ureter	_____
14. inflammation of the urethra	_____
15. excessive bleeding from the urethra	_____
16. plastic surgery of the ureter	_____

Check your answers against the information given in this lesson's terminology presentation. If you have any errors, count them and write the number in the blank at the top of the page. Sign your work and give it to your instructor.

Practice

Terminology Presentation

Urine

As you listen to the CD, read the words and notice the pronunciations given.

  Start CD

	-uria a suffix denoting urine or urination		
Word	**Word Part**	**Definition**	**Answer**
1. melanuria (mel'an-u're-ah)	melan(o)	black	1. _____
2. dysuria (dis-u're-ah)	dys-	difficult, painful	2. _____
3. anuria (ah-nu're-ah)	an-	not, without	3. _____
4. glycosuria (gli'ko-su're-ah)	glyc(o)	sugar	4. _____
5. polyuria (pol'e-u're-ah)	poly-	much, many	5. _____
6. oliguria (ol'i-gu're-ah)	olig(o)	scanty, few	6. _____
7. albuminuria (al'bu-mi-nu're-ah)	albumin	white (protein)	7. _____
8. hematuria (hem'ah-tu're-ah)	hemat(o)	blood	8. _____
9. nocturia (nok-tu're-ah)	noct(i)	night	9. _____
10. bacteriuria (bak-te're-u're-ah)	bacter(i)	bacteria	10. _____
11. pyuria (pi-u're-ah)	py(o)	pus, suppuration	11. _____
12. azoturia (as'o-tu're-ah)	azote	nitrogen	12. _____

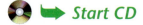 ➡ *Stop CD*

After practicing each word several times, use a sheet of paper to cover all columns except the Answer column. As each word is pronounced again on the CD, write it in the space provided.

➡ *Start CD*

Check the words you have written against the words in the left-hand column. If you have misspelled any words, practice writing them correctly.

Practice

LESSON
9-4

Terminology Application

Without looking at your previous work, write the word that matches each definition.

Definition	Term
1. painful or difficult urination	_____
2. presence of pus in the urine	_____
3. absence of secretion of urine	_____
4. excessive urination at night	_____
5. presence of glucose in the urine	_____
6. excessive nitrogen in the urine	_____
7. scanty production of urine	_____
8. presence of bacteria in the urine	_____
9. black or dark discoloration of the urine	_____
10. presence of blood in the urine	_____
11. excessive production of urine	_____
12. presence of serum albumin in the urine	_____

Check your answers against the information given in this lesson's terminology presentation. If you have any errors, count them and write the number in the blank at the top of the page. Sign your work and give it to your instructor.

Practice

LESSON

9-5

Drug Terminology Presentation

As you listen to the CD, read the words and notice the pronunciations given.

 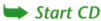 **Start CD**

Word	Definition	Example: Generic Name	Example: Brand/ Trade Name	Answer
anti-infectives	agents that can kill infectious agents or prevent them from spreading	ciprofloxacin cefepime cefaclor ofloxacin enoxacin	Cipro Maxipime Ceclor Floxin Penetrex	1. _____
diuretics	agents that promote and increase the excretion of urine	furosemide chlorothiazide triamterine (potassium sparing)	Lasix Diuril Dyrenium	2. _____
nonopioid analgesics	agents (not derived from opium) that provide an analgesic, anesthetic effect on the urinary tract and eliminate urinary spasms	phenazpyridine	Pyridium, Baridium, Urogesic	3. _____
uricosurics	agents that promote the excretion of uric acid in the urine; used in the treatment of gout	allopurinol probenecid sulfinpyrazone	Zyloprim, Alloprim Benemid Anturane	4. _____

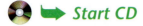 *Pause CD*

After practicing each word several times, use a sheet of paper to cover all columns except the Answer column. As each word is pronounced again on the CD, write it in the space provided.

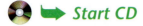 *Start CD*

Check the words you have written against the words in the left-hand column. If you have misspelled any words, practice writing them correctly.

Practice

_____

_____

_____

_____

_____

_____

_____

_____

_____

_____

_____

_____

_____

_____

_____

_____

_____

_____

_____

_____

_____

LESSON
9-5

Drug Terminology Application

Without looking at your previous work, write the word that matches each definition.

Definition	Term
1. agents that promote and increase the excretion of urine	1. _____
2. agents that provide an analgesic, anesthetic effect on the urinary tract and eliminate urinary spasms	2. _____
3. agents that promote the excretion of uric acid in the urine; used in the treatment of gout	3. _____
4. agents that can kill infectious agents or prevent them from spreading	4. _____

Check your answers against the information given in this lesson's terminology presentation. If you have any errors, count them and write the number in the blank at the top of the page. Sign your work and give it to your instructor.

Practice

CHAPTER 9

Terminology Review

This is a review of the word parts and words you have learned in the preceding lessons. Some of the medical terms listed below may be new, but they are composed of the word parts and word roots that you have already learned. Read the words below as they are pronounced on the CD.

  Start CD

Word Element Review

Word	Word Part	Meaning of Word Part
1. nephrology	nephr(o)	_____
nephrology	-logy	_____
(ne-frol′o-je)	Meaning of Word	_____
2. pyelitis	pyel(o)	_____
pyelitis	-itis	_____
(pi′e-li′tis)	Meaning of Word	_____
3. ureteropathy	ureter(o)	_____
ureteropathy	-pathy	_____
(u-re′ter-op′ah-the)	Meaning of Word	_____
4. cystoptosis	cyst(o)	_____
cystoptosis	-ptosis	_____
(sis′top-to′sis)	Meaning of Word	_____
5. azoturia	azote-	_____
azoturia	-uria	_____
(as′o-tu′re-ah)	Meaning of Word	_____
6. urethrophraxis	urethr(o)	_____
urethrophraxis	-phraxis	_____
(u-re′thro-frak′sis)	Meaning of Word	_____
7. ureterectasis	ureter(o)	_____
ureterectasis	-ectasis	_____
(u-re′ter-ek′tah-sis)	Meaning of Word	_____

Word	Word Part	Meaning of Word Part
8. cystorrhagia	cyst(o)	_____
cystorrhagia	-rrhagia	_____
(sis'to-ra'je-ah)	Meaning of Word	_____
9. pyelonephritis	pyel(o)	_____
pyelonephritis	nephr(o)	_____
pyelonephritis	-itis	_____
(pi'e-lo-ne-fri'tis)	Meaning of Word	_____
10. nephrapostasis	nephr(o)	_____
nephrapostasis	-apostasis	_____
(nef'rah-pos'tah-sis)	Meaning of Word	_____
11. pyelocystitis	pyel(o)	_____
pyelocystitis	cyst(o)	_____
pyelocystitis	-itis	_____
(pi'e-lo-sis-ti'tis)	Meaning of Word	_____
12. nephroptosis	nephr(o)	_____
nephroptosis	-ptosis	_____
(nef'rop-to'sis)	Meaning of Word	_____
13. urethritis	urethr(o)	_____
urethritis	-itis	_____
(u're-thri'tis)	Meaning of Word	_____
14. renocortical	ren(o)	_____
renocortical	cortic(o)	_____
renocortical	-al	_____
(re'no-kort'ti-kal)	Meaning of Word	_____
15. glomerulopathy	glomerul(o)	_____
glomerulopathy	-pathy	_____
(glo-mer'u-lop'ah-the)	Meaning of Word	_____

 ➡ *Stop CD*

On the lines provided, write in the meanings of as many suffixes, prefixes, roots, and words as you can from memory. Check your definitions in the glossary or a medical dictionary, and make any needed corrections.

CHAPTER 9 Terminology Review

Complete this review, and turn it in to your instructor when you are finished.

Defintion

Write the definition for each of the following terms to the right of the term.

Term	Definition
1. ureterolith	_____
2. renal	_____
3. polyuria	_____
4. pyelitis	_____
5. azoturia	_____
6. urethrectomy	_____
7. glomerular	_____
8. nephrology	_____
9. pyuria	_____
10. urethrorrhagia	_____
11. melanuria	_____
12. oliguria	_____
13. hematuria	_____
14. glomerulitis	_____
15. urethroplasty	_____
16. anuria	_____
17. ureterolithiasis	_____
18. nocturia	_____
19. suprarenal	_____
20. glomerulopathy	_____

Matching

Match the following definitions with the terms given. Put the letter of the correct definition to the left of the term.

Term	Definition
_____ 21. pyelolithotomy	a. plastic surgery of the ureter
_____ 22. renal	b. painful, difficult urination
_____ 23. urethrorrhaphy	c. suturing of the urethra
_____ 24. polyuria	d. pus in the urine
_____ 25. ureteroplasty	e. spasm of the urethra
_____ 26. glycosuria	f. excision of a stone from the pelvis of the kidney
_____ 27. nephrology	g. presence of sugar in the urine
_____ 28. dysuria	h. pertaining to the kidney
_____ 29. urethrospasm	i. study of the science of the kidney
_____ 30. pyuria	j. excessive urination

CHAPTER 9
Terminology Review

Case Studies

Read the following brief case studies. In each case study, some terms are followed by a superscript letter. Write a brief definition for each of those terms on the corresponding lines below.

1. K.R. has chronic cystitis[a] that often causes him to have cystorrhagia[b]. He has a cystoscopy[c] every 6 months, and he has recently been diagnosed with ureterolithiasis[d], which has resulted in considerable ureteralgia[e]. His doctor has scheduled him for surgery to locate the source of the problem.

   a. _____

   b. _____

   c. _____

   d. _____

   e. _____

2. B. has a urinary tract infection and is being treated with an anti-infective[a] and a nonopioid analgesic[b]. Her symptoms include dysuria[c], hematuria[d], urethrospasms[e], and urethritis[f].

   a. _____

   b. _____

   c. _____

   d. _____

   e. _____

   f. _____

3. A.J. takes a diuretic[a] each day to control her blood pressure. In addition, she must take an uricosuric[b] because she has gout.

   a. _____

   b. _____

4. L. was injured in a fall and suffered damage to a kidney that resulted in nephritis[a]. He had to have a nephrectomy[b] of the right kidney and is recuperating from the surgery.

a. _____

b. _____

Labeling

Fill in the blanks with the correct terminology.

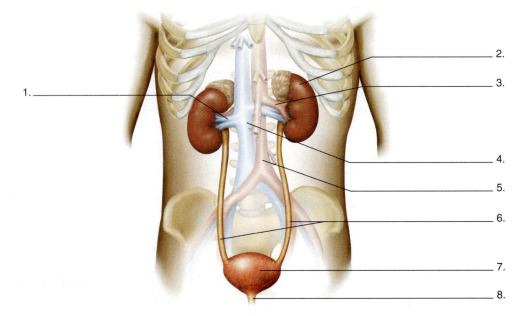

1. _____

2. _____

3. _____

4. _____

5. _____

6. _____

7. _____

8. _____

FIGURE 9-4   The urinary system.

You may now go on to Chapter Test 9.

10

Male Reproductive System

Objectives

After completing Chapter 10, you should be able to do the following:

1. identify word roots pertaining to the male reproductive system;

2. know the sections of the tubes and ducts that transport sperm as it becomes semen;

3. identify the word roots associated with the parts of the external male genitalia; and

4. identify several types of drugs associated with male reproductive disorders and treatments.

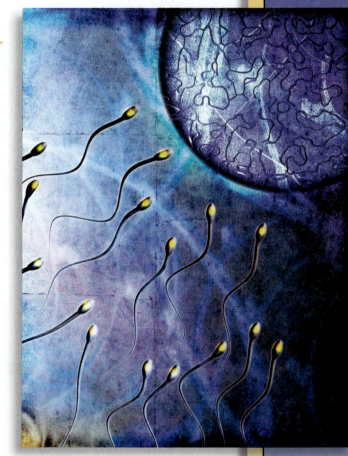

Orientation to the Male Reproductive System

The genitourinary system is really two systems: the urinary system (see Chapter 9) and the reproductive system, which consists of the male and female organs of reproduction (genitalia). The female reproductive system is discussed in Chapter 11.

The male genitalia consist of the testes, epididymis, vas deferens, ejaculatory duct, urethra, and penis. The male testes are located outside the body and are contained in a sac called the scrotum. The testes produce spermatozoa (sperm) inside small, coiled tubes called seminiferous tubules. They also produce the male hormone testosterone, which causes body hair, muscle development, and the deepening of the male voice.

Once sperm is produced in the testes, it is transported through a series of structures that maintain the sperm's viability.

The seminal vesicle provides most of the fluid component of semen. This fluid, containing nutrients, helps maintain the viability of the sperm.

The external male genitalia include the scrotum and the penis, a structure of erectile tissue that surrounds the urethra that expels urine and semen. The tip of the penis is called the glans penis, and the foreskin is called the prepuce. The area extending from the base of the scrotum to the opening of the anus is called the perineum.

There are several sexually transmitted diseases (STDs) that are contagious and easily transmitted via sexual activity with a person infected with the disease. See Appendix D for a chart that provides general information regarding several common STDs in men.

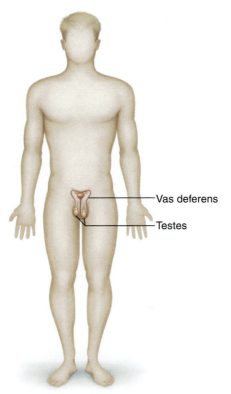

Male reproductive system

10-1 Terminology Presentation

Prostate, Testes, and Scrotum

As you listen to the CD, read the words and notice the pronunciations given.

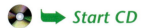 **Start CD**

Look at Figure 10-1

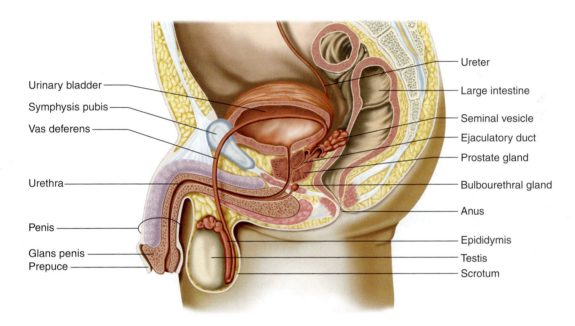

FIGURE 10-1 The structure of the male reproductive system.

	prostate a word denoting the gland in the male that surrounds the neck of the bladder and the urethra		
Word	**Word Part**	**Definition**	**Answer**
1. prostatectomy (pros'tah-tek'to-me)	-ectomy	excision, removal	**1.** _____
2. prostatitis (pros'tah-ti'tis)	-itis	inflammation	**2.** _____
3. prostatic (pros-tat'ik)	-atic	pertaining to	**3.** _____
4. prostatotomy (pros'tah-tot'o-me)	-tomy	incision	**4.** _____

	orchi(o), orchid(o) combining forms denoting relationship to the testes		
Word	**Word Part**	**Definition**	**Answer**
5. orchitis (or-ki′tis)	-itis	inflammation	5. _____
6. orchiopathy (or′ke-op′ah-the)	-pathy	disease	6. _____
7. orchiditis (or′ki-di′tis)	-itis	inflammation	7. _____
8. orchidoplasty (or′ki-do-plas′te)	-plasty	plastic surgery	8. _____
9. orchiopexy (or′ke-o-pek′se)	-pexy	surgical fixation	9. _____

	testis a word denoting the male gonad		
Word	**Word Part**	**Definition**	**Answer**
10. testicular (tes-tik′u-lar)	-ar	pertaining to	10. _____
11. testitis (tes-ti′tis)	-itis	inflammation	11. _____

	osche(o) a combining form denoting relationship to the scrotum		
Word	**Word Part**	**Definition**	**Answer**
12. oscheal (os′ke-al)	-al	pertaining to	12. _____
13. oscheitis (os′ke-i′tis)	-itis	inflammation	13. _____
14. oscheoma (os′ke-o′mah)	-oma	tumor	14. _____
15. oscheoplasty (os′ke-o-plas′te)	-plasty	plastic surgery	15. _____

 ➡ *Pause CD*

After practicing each word several times, use a sheet of paper to cover all columns except the Answer column. As each word is pronounced again on the CD, write it in the space provided.

 ➡ *Start CD*

Check the words you have written against the words in the left-hand column. If you have misspelled any words, practice writing them correctly.

Practice

_____

_____

LESSON
10-1

Terminology Application

Without looking at your previous work, write the word that matches each definition.

Definition	Term
1. any disease of the testes	_____
2. inflammation of the scrotum	_____
3. pertaining to the testis	_____
4. plastic surgery of the scrotum	_____
5. pertaining to the scrotum	_____
6. pertaining to the prostate gland	_____
7. inflammation of a testis	**a.** _____
	b. _____
	c. _____
8. a tumor of the scrotum	_____
9. inflammation of the prostate gland	_____
10. plastic surgery of the testis	_____
11. excision of the prostate gland	_____
12. surgical fixation in the scrotum of an undescended testis	_____
13. incision into the prostate gland	_____

Check your answers against the information given in this lesson's terminology presentation. If you have any errors, count them and write the number in the blank at the top of the page. Sign your work and give it to your instructor.

Practice

Glans Penis and Terms Indicating the Male Gender

As you listen to the CD, read the words and notice the pronunciations given.

 Start CD

Look at Figure 10-1 on page 269

balan(o)	a combining form indicating relationship to the glans penis		
Word	**Word Part**	**Definition**	**Answer**
1. balanoplasty (bal'ah-no-plas'te)	-plasty	plastic surgery	1. _____
2. balanitis (bal'ah-ni'tis)	-itis	inflammation	2. _____
3. balanorrhagia (bal'ah-no-ra'je-ah)	-rrhagia	excessive flow, bleeding	3. _____

andr(o)	a combining form denoting relationship to the male gender		
Word	**Word Part**	**Definition**	**Answer**
4. androgen (an'dro-jen)	-gen	producing	4. _____
5. andropathy (an-drop'ah-the)	-pathy	disease	5. _____
6. androgenic (an'dro-jen'ik)	-gen -ic	producing pertaining to	6. _____
7. androcyte (an'dro-sit)	-cyte	cell	7. _____
8. andrology (an-drol'o-je)	-logy	study of, science of	8. _____

continued

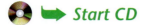

Pause CD

After practicing each word several times, use a sheet of paper to cover all columns except the Answer column. As each word is pronounced again on the CD, write it in the space provided.

Start CD

Check the words you have written against the words in the left-hand column. If you have misspelled any words, practice writing them correctly.

Practice

Glans Penis and Terms Indicating the Male Gender

As you listen to the CD, read the words and notice the pronunciations given.

 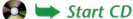 **Start CD**

Look at Figure 10-1 on page 269

balan(o) a combining form indicating relationship to the glans penis			
Word	**Word Part**	**Definition**	**Answer**
1. balanoplasty (bal'ah-no-plas'te)	-plasty	plastic surgery	1. _____
2. balanitis (bal'ah-ni'tis)	-itis	inflammation	2. _____
3. balanorrhagia (bal'ah-no-ra'je-ah)	-rrhagia	excessive flow, bleeding	3. _____

andr(o) a combining form denoting relationship to the male gender			
Word	**Word Part**	**Definition**	**Answer**
4. androgen (an'dro-jen)	-gen	producing	4. _____
5. andropathy (an-drop'ah-the)	-pathy	disease	5. _____
6. androgenic (an'dro-jen'ik)	-gen -ic	producing pertaining to	6. _____
7. androcyte (an'dro-sit)	-cyte	cell	7. _____
8. andrology (an-drol'o-je)	-logy	study of, science of	8. _____

continued

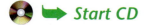 ➡️ *Pause CD*

After practicing each word several times, use a sheet of paper to cover all columns except the Answer column. As each word is pronounced again on the CD, write it in the space provided.

➡️ *Start CD*

Check the words you have written against the words in the left-hand column. If you have misspelled any words, practice writing them correctly.

Practice

_____

_____

_____

_____

_____

_____

_____

_____

_____

_____

_____

_____

_____

_____

_____

_____

_____

_____

_____

_____

LESSON
10-2

Terminology Application

Without looking at your previous work, write the word that matches each definition.

Definition	Term
1. any substance that conduces to masculinization	_____
2. any disease peculiar to men	_____
3. pertaining to producing male characteristics	_____
4. inflammation of the glans penis	_____
5. scientific study of the masculine constitution and the diseases of the male organs	_____
6. plastic surgery of the glans penis	_____
7. male sex cell	_____
8. balanitis with free discharge of pus	_____

Check your answers against the information given in this lesson's terminology presentation. If you have any errors, count them and write the number in the blank at the top of the page. Sign your work and give it to your instructor.

Practice

10-3 Terminology Presentation

Epididymis, Vas Deferens, and Seminal Vesicle

As you listen to the CD, read the words and notice the pronunciations given.

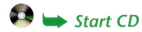 **Start CD**

Look at Figure 10-1, on page 269, and Figure 10-2

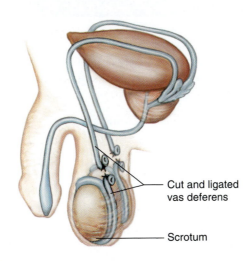

Cut and ligated
vas deferens

Scrotum

FIGURE 10-2   Surgical vasectomy.

epididymis a word denoting the elongated cordlike structure along the posterior border of the testis; for transit of spermatozoa			
Word	**Word Part**	**Definition**	**Answer**
1. epididymitis (ep′i-did′i-mi′tis)	-itis	inflammation	1. _____
2. epididymal (ep′i-did′i-mal)	-al	pertaining to	2. _____
3. epididymectomy (epi-did′i-mek′to-me)	-ectomy	excision, removal	3. _____
4. epididymotomy (ep′i-did′i-mot′o-me)	-tomy	incision	4. _____

vas(o) a combining form denoting a relationship to a vessel or duct			
Word	**Word Part**	**Definition**	**Answer**
5. vasorrhaphy (vas-or'ah-fe)	-rrhaphy	suture	5. _____
6. vasectomy (vah-sek'to-me)	-ectomy	excision, removal	6. _____
7. vasotomy (vah-sot'o-me)	-tomy	incision	7. _____

vesicul(o) a combining form denoting relationship to a vesicle or to the seminal vesicle			
Word	**Word Part**	**Definition**	**Answer**
8. vesiculitis (ve-sik'u-li'tis)	-itis	inflammation	8. _____
9. vesiculectomy (ve-sik'u-lek'to-me)	-ectomy	excision, removal	9. _____
10. vesiculotomy (ve-sik'u-lot'o-me)	-tomy	incision	10. _____

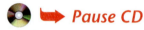 **Pause CD**

After practicing each word several times, use a sheet of paper to cover all columns except the Answer column. As each word is pronounced again on the CD, write it in the space provided.

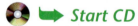 **Start CD**

Check the words you have written against the words in the left-hand column. If you have misspelled any words, practice writing them correctly.

Practice

_____

_____

_____

_____

_____

_____

_____

_____

LESSON 10-3

Terminology Application

Without looking at your previous work, write the word that matches each definition.

Definition	Term
1. surgical removal of all or part of the ductus (vas) deferens	_____
2. pertaining to the epididymis	_____
3. inflammation of a vesicle, especially the seminal vesicle	_____
4. excision of a vesicle, especially the seminal vesicle	_____
5. excision of the epididymis	_____
6. suture of a vessel, especially the ductus (vas) deferens	_____
7. incision into the epididymis	_____
8. incision into a vesicle, especially the seminal vesicle	_____
9. inflammation of the epididymis	_____
10. incision into a vessel, especially the ductus (vas) deferens	_____

Check your answers against the information given in this lesson's terminology presentation. If you have any errors, count them and write the number in the blank at the top of the page. Sign your work and give it to your instructor.

Practice

10-4

Terminology Presentation

Sperm and Semen

As you listen to the CD, read the words and notice the pronunciations given.

 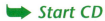 **Start CD**

spermat(o), sperm(a), sperm(i) combining forms denoting relationship to spermatozoa

Word	Word Part	Definition	Answer
1. spermatic (sper-mat′ik)	-ic	pertaining to	1. _____
2. spermatogenesis (sper′mah-to-jen′e-sis)	-genesis	production of	2. _____
3. spermatolysis (sper′mah-tol′i-sis)	-lysis	dissolution of, destruction of	3. _____
4. spermatorrhea (sper′mah-to-re′ah)	-rrhea	flow	4. _____
5. spermatopoietic (sper′mah-to-poi-et′ik)	-poiesis -ic	form, formation pertaining to	5. _____
6. spermatocyte (sper′mah-to-sit)	-cyte	cell	6. _____
7. spermicide (sper′mi-sid)	-cide	death, killer	7. _____

semen a word denoting spermatozoa in their nutrient plasma

Word	Word Part	Definition	Answer
8. seminal (sem′i-nal)	-al	pertaining to	8. _____
9. seminiferous (se′mi-nif′er-us)	-ferous	carrying, bearing	9. _____
10. seminoma (se′mi-no′mah)	-oma	tumor	10. _____
11. seminology (se′mi-nol′o-je)	-logy	study of, science of	11. _____

continued

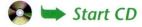

Pause CD

After practicing each word several times, use a sheet of paper to cover all columns except the Answer column. As each word is pronounced again on the CD, write it in the space provided.

Start CD

Check the words you have written against the words in the left-hand column. If you have misspelled any words, practice writing them correctly.

Practice

_____

_____

_____

_____

_____

_____

_____

_____

_____

_____

_____

_____

_____

_____

_____

_____

_____

_____

_____

_____

_____

LESSON
10-4

Terminology Application

Without looking at your previous work, write the word that matches each definition.

Definition	Term
1. pertaining to semen	a. _____
	b. _____
2. the scientific study of semen and spermatozoa	_____
3. an involuntary discharge of semen without orgasm	_____
4. conveying semen	_____
5. a sperm cell	_____
6. promoting the secretion of semen	a. _____
	b. _____
7. an agent that is destructive to spermatozoa	_____
8. malignant neoplasm of the testis	_____
9. spermatozoa in their nutrient plasma	_____
10. the process of destroying sperm	_____

Check your answers against the information given in this lesson's terminology presentation. If you have any errors, count them and write the number in the blank at the top of the page. Sign your work and give it to your instructor.

Practice

Drug Terminology Presentation

As you listen to the CD, read the words and notice the pronunciations given.

  Start CD

Word	Definition	Example: Generic Name	Example: Brand/ Trade Name	Answer
erectile agents	agents that enhance the erectile function of the penis	sildenafil	Viagra	1. _____
estrogen hormones	agents used in the treatment of prostatic cancer	bicalutamide flutamide	Casodex Eulexin	2. _____

  Stop CD

After practicing each word several times, use a sheet of paper to cover all columns except the Answer column. As each word is pronounced again on the CD, write it in the space provided.

  Start CD

Check the words you have written against the words in the left-hand column. If you have misspelled any words, practice writing them correctly.

Practice

_____

_____

_____

_____

_____

_____

_____

_____

_____

_____

Practice

LESSON 10-5
Drug Terminology Application

Without looking at your previous work, write the word that matches each definition.

Definition	Term
1. agents that enhance the erectile function of the penis	_____
2. agents used in the treatment of prostatic cancer	_____

Check your answers against the information given in this lesson's terminology presentation. If you have any errors, count them and write the number in the blank at the top of the page. Sign your work and give it to your instructor.

Practice

CHAPTER 10
Terminology Review

This is a review of the word parts and words you have learned in the preceding lessons. Some of the medical terms listed below may be new, but they are composed of the word parts and word roots that you have already learned. Read the words below as they are pronounced on the CD.

  Start CD

Word Element Review

Word	Word Part	Meaning of Word Part
1. balanorrhagia	balan(o)	_____
balanorrhagia	-rrhagia	_____
(bal′ah-no-ra′je-ah)	Meaning of Word	_____
2. epididymitis	epididymis	_____
epididymitis	-itis	_____
(ep′i-did′i-mi′tis)	Meaning of Word	_____
3. prostatectomy	prostate	_____
prostatectomy	-ectomy	_____
(pros′tah-tek′to-me)	Meaning of Word	_____
4. vasectomy	vas(o)	_____
vasectomy	-ectomy	_____
(vah-sek′to-me)	Meaning of Word	_____
5. vesiculitis	vesicul(o)	_____
vesiculitis	-itis	_____
(ve-sik′u-li′tis)	Meaning of Word	_____
6. spermatic	spermat(o)	_____
spermatic	-ic	_____
(sper-mat′ik)	Meaning of Word	_____
7. orchiditis	orchid(o)	_____
orchiditis	-itis	_____
(or′ki-di′tis)	Meaning of Word	_____

8. **balan**itis   balan(o)   _____

    bala**nitis**   -itis   _____

    (bal′ah-ni′tis)   Meaning of Word   _____

9. **semin**al   semen   _____

    semin**al**   -al   _____

    (sem′i-nal)   Meaning of Word   _____

10. **osche**itis   osche(o)   _____

    osche**itis**   -itis   _____

    (os′ke-i′tis)   Meaning of Word   _____

11. **andr**opathy   andr(o)   _____

    andro**pathy**   -pathy   _____

    (an-drop′ah-the)   Meaning of Word   _____

12. **spermat**orrhea   spermat(o)   _____

    spermato**rrhea**   -rrhea   _____

    (sper′mah-to-re′ah)   Meaning of Word   _____

13. **testi**cular   testis   _____

    testic**ul**ar   -ar   _____

    (tes-tik′u-lar)   Meaning of Word   _____

14. **prosta**titis   prostate   _____

    prosta**titis**   -itis   _____

    (pros′tah-ti′tis)   Meaning of Word   _____

15. **orchi**opexy   orchi(o)   _____

    orchio**pexy**   -pexy   _____

    (or′ke-o-pek′se)   Meaning of Word   _____

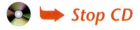 *Stop CD*

On the lines provided, write in the meanings of as many suffixes, prefixes, roots, and words as you can from memory. Check your definitions in the glossary or a medical dictionary, and make any needed corrections.

CHAPTER 10

Terminology Review

Complete this review, and turn it in to your instructor when you are finished.

Definition

Each term below is defined in the terminology presentations you have just studied. Without looking at your previous work, write the definition that matches each word.

Term	Definition
1. epididymectomy	_____
2. andropathy	_____
3. vesiculitis	_____
4. prostatotomy	_____
5. vesiculotomy	_____
6. spermatogenesis	_____
7. androcyte	_____
8. vasotomy	_____
9. oscheal	_____
10. oscheoma	_____
11. epididymal	_____
12. orchiditis	_____
13. spermatolysis	_____
14. andrology	_____
15. orchiopathy	_____
16. prostatitis	_____
17. testicular	_____
18. balanorrhagia	_____
19. vasectomy	_____
20. epididymotomy	_____

Matching

Match the following terms with the definitions given. Put the letter of the correct definition to the left of the term.

Term	Definition
_____ **21.** balanoplasty	**a.** scientific study of semen and spermatozoa
_____ **22.** oscheoplasty	**b.** inflammation of the scrotum
_____ **23.** epididymitis	**c.** plastic surgery of the glans penis
_____ **24.** seminoma	**d.** plastic surgery of the scrotum
_____ **25.** oscheitis	**e.** inflammation of the epididymis
_____ **26.** orchiopexy	**f.** malignant neoplasm of the testis
_____ **27.** spermatic	**g.** pertaining to spermatozoa
_____ **28.** balanitis	**h.** inflammation of the glans penis
_____ **29.** prostatectomy	**i.** surgical fixation in the scrotum of an undescended testis
_____ **30.** seminology	**j.** excision, removal of the prostate gland

CHAPTER 10

Terminology Review

Case Studies

Read the following brief case studies. In each case study, some terms are followed by a superscript letter. Write a brief definition for each of those terms on the corresponding lines below.

1. C.K. has a history of orchitis[a] and has been diagnosed with testicular[b] cancer. His doctor has removed both testes and has also performed an epididymectomy[c]. In addition, C.K. will need an extensive program of radiation therapy or chemotherapy.

   a. _____

   b. _____

   c. _____

2. R.T., a retired 70-year-old, has suffered from prostatitis[a] for several years. He was worried about his potential for prostate[b] cancer, and he has made an appointment with his doctor to discuss the possibility of a prostatectomy[c].

   a. _____

   b. _____

   c. _____

3. B.R. and his wife have had several children, and he has decided to have a vasectomy[a]. During his recent visit to his doctor, he had several questions regarding the function of the epididymis[b] and the vas deferens.

   a. _____

   b. _____

4. L.J. has had a variety of physical problems that include vesiculitis[a], balanitis[b], and balanorrhagia[c]. Recently, he was diagnosed with a seminoma[d] and will need to schedule surgery for the condition.

a. _____

b. _____

c. _____

d. _____

Labeling

Fill in the blanks with the correct terminology.

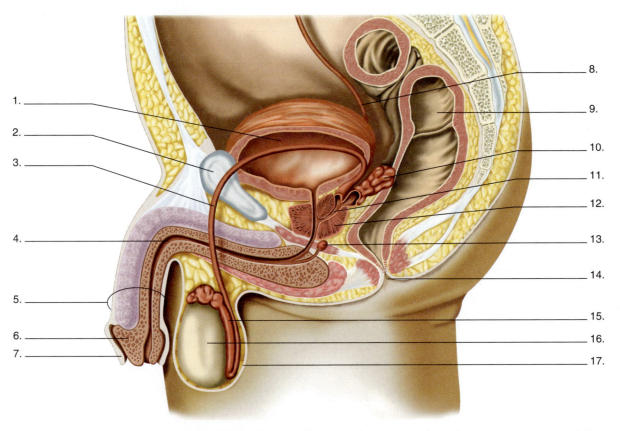

FIGURE 10-3 Male reproductive organs (sagittal view). The paired testes are the primary sex organs, and the other structures, both internal and external, are accessory sex organs.

You may now go on to Chapter Test 10.

11

Female Reproductive System

Objectives

After completing Chapter 11, you should be able to do the following:

1. identify word roots pertaining to the female reproductive system;

2. recognize word roots for the internal and external female genitalia;

3. understand terms used in reference to the number of pregnancies a female has had;

4. understand terms used in reference to the number of viable offspring a female has had; and

5. identify several types of drugs associated with female reproductive disorders and treatments.

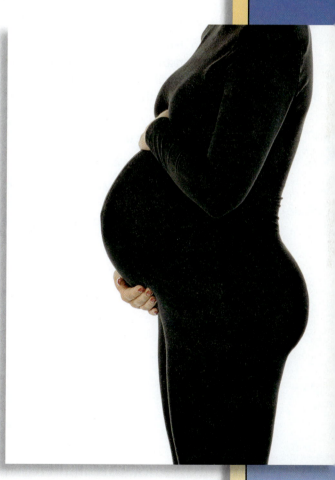

Orientation to the Female Reproductive System

The female reproductive system includes internal and external genitalia. The internal female genitalia consist of two ovaries, one on each side of the uterus, which produce the female sex cells (ovum, ova); two uterine or fallopian tubes (oviducts) that convey the ovum (egg) to the uterus (a pear-shaped organ designed to hold and to nourish a developing fetus); and the vagina, which provides access to the uterus.

The external female genitalia, known as the vulva, include the labia (lips) minora and majora and the clitoris. The area between the base of the vulva and the anus is called the perineum.

The ovaries produce the ova (eggs). When an ovum is released, it moves through the fallopian tube toward the uterus. If the ovum does not unite with a spermatozoon, it does not become fertilized and dies.

In females, the development of the body during puberty includes the onset of the menses, the menstrual cycle. The inner portion of the uterus, the endometrium, develops a layer of nutrient material used for nourishing a developing fetus; if an ovum does not become fertilized, the uterus releases this nutrient material and blood.

When an ovum does unite with a spermatozoon and becomes fertilized, the fertilized ovum implants itself in the uterine wall for nourishment and development.

Most females experience menopause (the cessation of menses) at about age 50.

There are several sexually transmitted diseases (STDs) that are contagious and easily transmitted via sexual activity with a person infected with the disease. See Appendix D for a chart that provides general information regarding several common STDs in women.

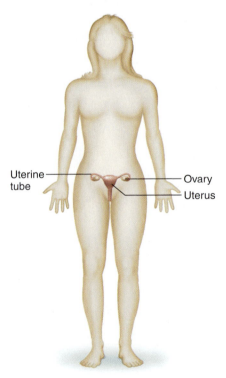

Uterine tube — Ovary — Uterus

Female reproductive system

11-1 Terminology Presentation

Uterus

As you listen to the CD, read the words and notice the pronunciations given.

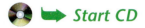 **Start CD**

Look at Figures 11-1 and 11-2

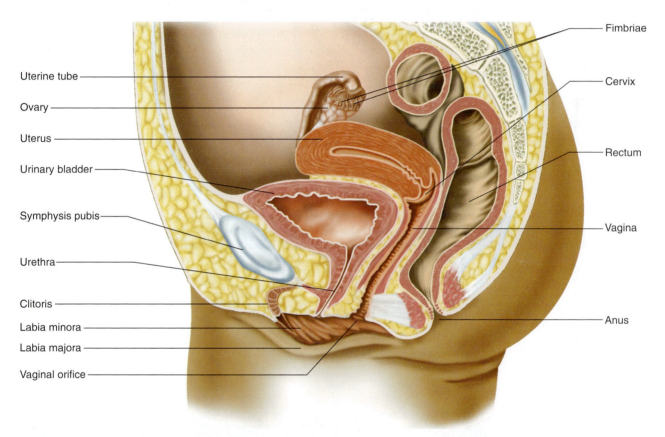

FIGURE 11-1 Side view of the female reproductive organs.

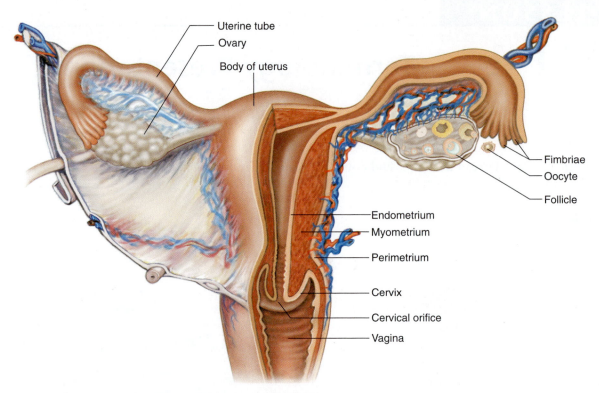

FIGURE 11-2 The uterus, the uterine (fallopian) tubes, and the ovaries.

uter(o) a combining form denoting relationship to the uterus			
Word	**Word Part**	**Definition**	**Answer**
1. uterocervical (u′ter-o-ser′vi-kal)	cervix	neck	1. _____
2. uteroplasty (u′ter-o-plas′te)	-plasty	surgical repair	2. _____
3. uterogenic (u′ter-o-jen′ik)	genic	formed	3. _____

hyster(o) a combining form denoting the uterus			
Word	**Word Part**	**Definition**	**Answer**
4. hysterectomy (his′te-rek′to-me)	-ectomy	excision, removal	4. _____
5. hysterocleisis (his′ter-o-kli′sis)	-cleisis	closure	5. _____
6. hysteralgia (his′te-ral′je-ah)	-algia	pain	6. _____

Word	Word Part	Definition	Answer
7. hysterospasm (his′ter-o-spaszm′)	-spasm	contraction	**7.** _____
8. hysterolith (his′ter-o-lith′)	lith(o)	stone	**8.** _____
9. hysteropexy (his′ter-o′-pek-se)	-pexy	fix, fasten	**9.** _____
10. hysteropathy (his′te-rop′ah-the)	-pathy	disease	**10.** _____
11. hysteroptosis (his′ter-op-to′sis)	-ptosis	falling	**11.** _____

metr(o), metr(a) combining forms denoting the uterus		

Word	Word Part	Definition	Answer
12. metritis (me-trl′tis)	-itis	inflammation	**12.** _____
13. metrocolpocele (me′tro-kol′po-sel)	colp(o) -cele	vagina tumor, hernia, swelling	**13.** _____
14. metrorrhea (me′tro-re′ah)	-rrhea	flow	**14.** _____
15. metropathy (me-trop′ah-the)	-pathy	disease	**15.** _____
16. metrostenosis (me′tro-ste-no′sis)	-stenosis	narrowing	**16.** _____
17. metroptosis (me′tro-to′sis)	-ptosis	falling	**17.** _____
18. metrorrhagia (me′tro-ra′je-ah)	-rrhagia	excessive flow, bleeding	**18.** _____
19. endometriosis (en′do-me′tre-o′sis)	endo- -osis	within abnormal condition	**19.** _____

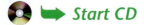

Pause CD

After practicing each word several times, use a sheet of paper to cover all columns except the Answer column. As each word is pronounced again on the CD, write it in the space provided.

Start CD

Check the words you have written against the words in the left-hand column. If you have misspelled any words, practice writing them correctly.

Practice

Terminology Application

Without looking at your previous work, write the word that matches each definition.

Definition	Term
1. a narrowing of the uterine cavity	_____
2. plastic surgery of the uterus	_____
3. inflammation of the uterus	_____
4. uterine bleeding	_____
5. excision, removal of the uterus	_____
6. prolapse of the uterus	a. _____
	b. _____
7. contraction, spasm of the uterus	_____
8. relating to the cervix of the uterus	_____
9. uterine calculus	_____
10. surgical fixation of the uterus	_____
11. any uterine disease	a. _____
	b. _____
12. formed in the uterus	_____
13. abnormal uterine discharge	_____
14. uterine pain	_____
15. condition in which tissue resembling endometrial tissue occurs aberrantly in the pelvic cavity	_____
16. surgical closure of the ostium uteri	_____
17. hernia of the uterus and vagina	_____

Check your answers against the information given in this lesson's terminology presentation. If you have any errors, count them and write the number in the blank at the top of the page. Sign your work and give it to your instructor.

Practice

Terminology Presentation

Ovaries and Fallopian Tubes

As you listen to the CD, read the words and notice the pronunciations given.

  Start CD

Look at Figures 11-1 and 11-2 on pages 297 and 298

ovari(o) a combining form denoting relationship to the ovary			
Word	**Word Part**	**Definition**	**Answer**
1. ovariopathy (o-va′re-op′ah-the)	-pathy	disease	1. _____
2. ovariectomy (o′va-re-ek′to-me)	-ectomy	excision, removal	2. _____
3. ovariorrhexis (o-va′re-o-rek′sis)	-rrhexis	rupture	3. _____
4. ovaritis (o′vah-ri′tis)	-itis	inflammation	4. _____
5. ovaricentesis (o-va′re-o-sen-te′sis)	-centesis	surgical puncture	5. _____
6. ovariopexy (o-va′re-o-pek′se)	-pexy	surgical reattachment	6. _____

oophor(o) a combining form denoting the ovaries			
Word	**Word Part**	**Definition**	**Answer**
7. oophoroma (o-of′o-ro′ma)	-oma	tumor	7. _____
8. oophoritis (o′of-o-ri′tis)	-itis	inflammation	8. _____
9. oophorectomy (o′-of-o-rek′to-me)	-ectomy	excision, removal	9. _____
10. oophorostomy (o-of′-o-ros′to-me)	-ostomy	opening	10. _____
11. oophoroplasty (o-of′o-ro-plas′te)	-plasty	plastic surgery	11. _____
12. oophorrhagia (o-of′o-ra′je-ah)	-rrhagia	excessive flow, bleeding	12. _____

continued

| | | salping(o) | a word element denoting the uterine (fallopian) tube or auditory (eustachian) tube |

	Word	Word Part	Definition	Answer
13.	salpingitis (sal′pin-ji′tis)	-itis	inflammation	13. _____
14.	salpingocele (sal′ping′go-sel)	-cele	tumor, swelling, hernia	14. _____
15.	salpingopexy (sal-ping′go-pek-se)	-pexy	fixing fastening	15. _____
16.	salpingo-oophorectomy (sal-ping′go-o′of-o-rek′to-me)	oophor(o) -ectomy	ovaries excision, removal	16. _____
17.	salpingotomy (sal-ping-got′o-me)	-tomy	incision, cutting into	17. _____
18.	salpingorrhagia (sal-ping′go-ra′je-ah)	-rrhagia	excessive flow, bleeding	18. _____
19.	salpingography (sal′ping-gog′rah-fe)	-graphy	recording	19. _____
20.	salpingoscopy (sal′ping-gos′ko-pe)	-scopy	examine	20. _____
21.	salpingorrhaphy (sal′ping-gor′ah-fe)	-rrhaphy	suture, surgical repair	21. _____

 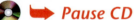 ➡ *Pause CD*

After practicing each word several times, use a sheet of paper to cover all columns except the Answer column. As each word is pronounced again on the CD, write it in the space provided.

 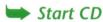 ➡ *Start CD*

Check the words you have written against the words in the left-hand column. If you have misspelled any words, practice writing them correctly.

Practice

_____

_____

_____

_____

_____

_____

_____

LESSON
11-2

Terminology Application

Without looking at your previous work, write the word that matches each definition.

Definition	Term
1. visual examination of the uterine tube	_____
2. surgically reattaching an ovary to the abdominal wall	_____
3. inflammation of the uterine tube (canal) or auditory tube (canal)	_____
4. excision or removal of an ovary	**a.** _____ **b.** _____
5. hernial protrusion of a uterine tube	_____
6. rupture of an ovary	_____
7. tumor of the ovary	_____
8. surgical incision into the uterine tube	_____
9. hemorrhage or bleeding from an ovary	_____
10. ovarian disease	_____
11. plastic surgery on the ovary	_____
12. making an opening into an ovarian cyst to provide drainage	_____
13. surgical puncture of an ovary	_____
14. excision of the ovary and the uterine tube	_____
15. inflammation of an ovary	**a.** _____ **b.** _____
16. hemorrhage from a fallopian tube	_____
17. surgical fixing or fastening of a uterine tube	_____

continued

Definition	Term

18. roentgenogram or X-ray picture of the uterine tube or tubes

_____

19. suture or surgical repair of the uterine tube

_____

Check your answers against the information given in this lesson's terminology presentation. If you have any errors, count them and write the number in the blank at the top of the page. Sign your work and give it to your instructor.

Terminology Presentation

Vagina and Breasts

As you listen to the CD, read the words and notice the pronunciations given.

 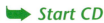 **Start CD**

Look at Figures 11-1 and 11-2 on pages 297 and 298

	vagin(o) a combining form denoting relationship to the canal in the female extending from the vulva to the cervix uteri		
Word	**Word Part**	**Definition**	**Answer**
1. vaginal (vaj'i-nal)	-al	pertaining to	1. _____
2. vaginitis (vaj'i-ni'tis)	-itis	inflammation	2. _____
3. vaginopathy (vaj'i-nop'ah-the)	-pathy	disease	3. _____
4. vaginoscopy (vaj'i-nos'ko-pe)	-scopy	visual examination	4. _____

	colp(o) a combining form denoting relationship to the vagina		
Word	**Word Part**	**Definition**	**Answer**
5. colporrhagia (kol'po-ra'je-ah)	-rrhagia	excessive flow, bleeding	5. _____
6. colpocele (kol'po-sel)	-cele	tumor, hernia, swelling	6. _____
7. colposcopy (kol-pos'ko-pe)	-scopy	visual examination	7. _____
8. colporrhaphy (kol-por'ah-fe)	-rrhaphy	suturing	8. _____

	mast(o), mamm(o) combining forms denoting relationship to the breast or to the mammary gland		
Word	**Word Part**	**Definition**	**Answer**
9. mastitis (mas-ti'tis)	-itis	inflammation	9. _____
10. mastectomy (mas-tek'to-me)	-ectomy	excision, removal	10. _____

continued

Look at Figure 11-3

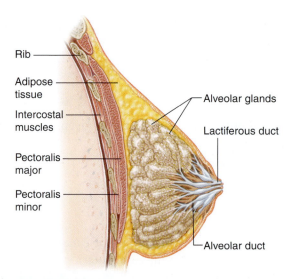

Rib
Adipose tissue
Intercostal muscles
Pectoralis major
Pectoralis minor
Alveolar glands
Lactiferous duct
Alveolar duct

FIGURE 11-3 Side view of the female breast.

	Word	Word Part	Definition	Answer
11.	mastoplasty (mas′to-plas′te)	-plasty	plastic surgery	11. _____
12.	mastopexy (mas′to-pek-se)	-pexy	fix, fasten	12. _____
13.	mastoid (mas′toid)	-oid	like, resembling	13. _____
14.	mammary (mam′er-e)	-ary	pertaining to	14. _____
15.	mammogram (mam′o-gram)	-gram	written, recorded	15. _____
16.	mammaplasty (mam′ah-plas′te)	-plasty	plastic surgery	16. _____

  ➡ *Pause CD*

After practicing each word several times, use a sheet of paper to cover all columns except the Answer column. As each word is pronounced again on the CD, write it in the space provided.

 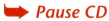 ➡ *Start CD*

Check the words you have written against the words in the left-hand column. If you have misspelled any words, practice writing them correctly.

Practice

_____

_____

LESSON
11-3

Terminology Application

Without looking at your previous work, write the word that matches each definition.

Definition	Term
1. herniation of the vagina	_____
2. pertaining to the vagina	_____
3. a roentgenography (X-ray) of the breast	_____
4. visual examination of the vagina	a. _____
	b. _____
5. inflammation of the breast	_____
6. breast-shaped	_____
7. inflammation of the vagina	_____
8. suturing the vagina	_____
9. surgical reattachment of the breast	_____
10. excessive flow, bleeding from the vagina	_____
11. excision of the breast	_____
12. any disease of the vagina	_____
13. pertaining to the breast	_____
14. plastic surgery of the breast	a. _____
	b. _____

Check your answers against the information given in this lesson's terminology presentation. If you have any errors, count them and write the number in the blank at the top of the page. Sign your work and give it to your instructor.

Practice

11-4 Terminology Presentation

Menstruation, Terms Indicating the Female Gender, Pregnancy, and Birth

As you listen to the CD, read the words and notice the pronunciations given.

  Start CD

men(o)	a combining form denoting relationship to the menses		
Word	**Word Part**	**Definition**	**Answer**
1. menses (men'sez)	plural of mensis	the monthly flow of blood from the genital tract of women	1. _____
2. menarche (me-nar'ke)	-arche	beginning	2. _____
3. menorrhea (men'o-re'ah)	-rrhea	flow	3. _____
4. menorrhagia (men'o-ra'je-ah)	-rrhagia	excessive flow, bleeding	4. _____
5. menopause (men'o-pawz)	-pause	cessation	5. _____
6. menstrual (men'stroo-al)	-al	pertaining to	6. _____
7. dysmenorrhea (dis'men-o-re'ah)	dys- -rrhea	difficult, painful flow	7. _____
8. dysmenorrhagia (dis'men-o-ra'je-ah)	dys- -rrhagia	difficult, painful excessive flow, bleeding	8. _____

gyn(o), gynec(o)	word elements denoting women or the female gender		
Word	**Word Part**	**Definition**	**Answer**
9. gynecology (gi'ne-kol'o-je)	-logy	study of, science of	9. _____
10. gynecologist (gi'ne-kol'o-jist)	-logist	specialist	10. _____
11. gynecopathy (jin'e-kop'ah-the)	-pathy	disease	11. _____
12. gynoplasty (ji'no-plas'te)	-plasty	plastic surgery	12. _____

gravida a word denoting a pregnant woman; used with Roman numerals to indicate the number of pregnancies a woman has had			
Word	**Word Part**	**Definition**	**Answer**
13. gravida I (grav′i-dah)	gravida I	pregnancy one	13. _____
14. gravida II (grav′i-dah)	gravida II	pregnancy two	14. _____
15. gravida III (grav′i-dah)	gravida III	pregnancy three	15. _____

para a word denoting a woman who has produced a viable offspring regardless of whether the child was living at birth; used with Roman numerals to designate the number of viable offspring a woman has had			
Word	**Word Part**	**Definition**	**Answer**
16. para V (par′ah)	para V	viable offspring five	16. _____
17. para I (par′ah)	para I	viable offspring one	17. _____
18. parturition (par′tu-rish′un)	-ion	process	18. _____
19. prepartal (pre-par′tal)	pre- -al	before pertaining to	19. _____
20. postpartum (post-par′tum)	post-	after	20. _____

NOTE: *gravida* and *para* can be used together to indicate the number of pregnancies as well as the number of viable offspring a woman has.

 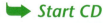 **Pause CD**

> After practicing each word several times, use a sheet of paper to cover all columns except the Answer column. As each word is pronounced again on the CD, write it in the space provided.

 Start CD

> Check the words you have written against the words in the left-hand column. If you have misspelled any words, practice writing them correctly.

Practice

_____

_____

_____

LESSON 11-4

Terminology Application

Without looking at your previous work, write the word that matches each definition.

Definition	Term
1. painful menses	_____
2. the study of the science of the female anatomy	_____
3. normal discharge of the menses	_____
4. pertaining to the menses	_____
5. the monthly flow of blood from the genital tract of women	_____
6. specialist in treating female disorders	_____
7. excessive bleeding during the menses	_____
8. the branch of medicine treating the diseases of women	_____
9. the beginning of the menstrual function	_____
10. plastic surgery of the female organs	_____
11. painful and excessive bleeding during the menses	_____
12. cessation of the menses	_____
13. the act or process of giving birth to a child	_____
14. a woman who has had two pregnancies	_____
15. occurring before labor	_____
16. a woman who has had six viable offspring	_____
17. a woman who has had four pregnancies	_____
18. occurring after childbirth	_____

continued

Definition	Term
19. a woman who has had three pregnancies and four viable offspring	_____
20. a woman who has had one pregnancy	_____

Check your answers against the information given in this lesson's terminology presentation. If you have any errors, count them and write the number in the blank at the top of the page. Sign your work and give it to your instructor.

Drug Terminology Presentation

As you listen to the CD, read the words and notice the pronunciations given.

 Start CD

Word	Definition	Example: Generic Name	Example: Brand/ Trade Name	Answer
contraceptives	agents that prevent conception or impregnation	estrogen (ethinyl estradiol) and progestin (norethindrone)	Ortho-Novum, Tri-Norinyl, Estrostep 21	1.
estrogen hormones	agents used in the treatment of menopause, prostatic cancer, osteoporosis, and abnormal menses	estrogen estradiol estradiol cypionate bicalutamide flutamide	Premarin, Cenestin Estrace Depogen, Estragyn Casodex Eulexin	2.
oxytocins	agents that promote uterine contractions and promote labor	oxytocin	Pitocin	3.

 Stop CD

After practicing each word several times, use a sheet of paper to cover all columns except the Answer column. As each word is pronounced again on the CD, write it in the space provided.

 Start CD

Check the words you have written against the words in the left-hand column. If you have misspelled any words, practice writing them correctly.

Practice

_____

_____

_____

_____

_____

_____

Practice

LESSON
11-5
Drug Terminology Application

Without looking at your previous work, write the word that matches each definition.

Definition	Term
1. agents that promote uterine contractions and promote labor	_____
2. agents used in the treatment of menopause, prostatic cancer, osteoporosis, and abnormal menses	_____
3. agents that prevent contraception or impregnation	_____

Check your answers against the information given in this lesson's terminology presentation. If you have any errors, count them and write the number in the blank at the top of the page. Sign your work and give it to your instructor.

Practice

CHAPTER 11
Terminology Review

This is a review of the word parts and words you have learned in the preceding lessons. Some of the medical terms listed below may be new, but they are composed of the word parts and word roots that you have already learned. Read the words below as they are pronounced on the CD.

  Start CD

Word Element Review

Word	Word Part	Meaning of Word Part
1. endometriosis	endo-	_____
endometriosis	metri-	_____
endometriosis	-osis	_____
(en′do-me′tre-o′sis)	Meaning of Word	_____
2. hysteroptosis	hyster(o)-	_____
hysteroptosis	-ptosis	_____
(his′ter-op-to′sis)	Meaning of Word	_____
3. salpingo-oophorectomy	salping(o)-	_____
salpingo-oophorectomy	oophor(o)-	_____
salpingo-oophorectomy	-ectomy	_____
(sal-ping′go-o′of-o-rek′to-me)	Meaning of Word	_____
4. mastectomy	mast(o)-	_____
mastectomy	-ectomy	_____
(mas-tek′to-me)	Meaning of Word	_____
5. menorrhagia	meno-	_____
menorrhagia	-rrhagia	_____
(men′o-ra′je-ah)	Meaning of Word	_____
6. prepartal	pre-	_____
prepartal	par(a)-	_____
prepartal	-al	_____
(pre-par′tal)	Meaning of Word	_____
7. ovariopexy	ovari(o)-	_____
ovariopexy	-pexy	_____
(o-va′re-o-pek′se)	Meaning of Word	_____

Word	Word Part	Meaning of Word Part
8. colposcopy	colp(o)-	_____
colposcopy	-scopy	_____
(kol-pos′ko-pe)	Meaning of Word	_____
9. oophoroplasty	oophor(o)-	_____
oophoroplasty	-plasty	_____
(o-of′o-ro-plas′te)	Meaning of Word	_____
10. para V	par(a)-	_____
para V	V	_____
(par′ah fiv′)	Meaning of Word	_____
11. gravida I	gravida	_____
gravida I	I	_____
(grav′i-dah wun′)	Meaning of Word	_____
12. uterocervical	uter(o)-	_____
uterocervical	cervic(o)-	_____
uterocervical	-al	_____
(u′ter-o-ser′vi-kal)	Meaning of Word	_____
13. vaginitis	vagin(o)-	_____
vaginitis	-itis	_____
(vaj′i-ni′tis)	Meaning of Word	_____
14. salpingocele	salping(o)-	_____
salpingocele	-cele	_____
(sal′ping′go-sel)	Meaning of Word	_____
15. metrorrhagia	metr(o)-	_____
metrorrhagia	-rrhagia	_____
(me′tro-ra′je-ah)	Meaning of Word	_____

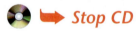 *Stop CD*

On the lines provided, write in the meanings of as many suffixes, prefixes, roots, and words as you can from memory. Check your definitions in the glossary or a medical dictionary, and make any needed corrections.

CHAPTER 11

Terminology Review

Complete this review, and return it to your instructor when you are finished.

Definition

Below are definitions of terms you learned in this chapter's terminology presentations. Without looking at your previous work, write the term that matches each definition.

Definition	Term
1. a condition in which tissue resembling endometrial tissue occurs aberrantly in the pelvic cavity	_____
2. surgical incision into the uterine tube	_____
3. visual examination of the vagina	_____
4. the act or process of giving birth to a child	_____
5. an X-ray of the breast	_____
6. making an opening into an ovarian cyst to provide drainage	_____
7. a woman who has had one pregnancy	_____
8. hernia of the uterus and vagina	_____
9. prolapse of the uterus	_____
10. a woman who has had two pregnancies and three viable offspring	_____
11. inflammation of an ovary	_____
12. painful and excessive bleeding during menses	_____
13. surgical fixation of an ovary	_____
14. uterine calculus	_____
15. any disease of the vagina	_____
16. agents that promote uterine contractions and labor	_____

17. hemorrhage from a fallopian tube   _____

18. the monthly flow of blood from the   _____
    genital tract of women

19. a woman who has had two viable offspring   _____

20. a visual examination of the fallopian tube _____

Matching

Match the following definitions with the terms given. Put the letter of the correct definition to the left of the term.

Term	Definition
_____ 21. vaginoscopy/colposcopy	a. plastic surgery of the uterus
_____ 22. oophorectomy	b. painful menses
_____ 23. uterocervical	c. visual examination of the vagina
_____ 24. dysmenorrhea	d. occurring before labor
_____ 25. menopause	e. pertaining to the cervix (neck) of the uterus
_____ 26. uteroplasty	f. surgical puncture of an ovary
_____ 27. ovaricentesis	g. cessation of the menses
_____ 28. postpartum	h. excision of an ovary
_____ 29. menstrual	i. occurring after childbirth
_____ 30. prepartal	j. pertaining to the menses

CHAPTER 11
Terminology Review

Case Studies

Read the following brief case studies. In each case study, some terms are followed by a superscript letter. Write a brief definition for each of those terms on the corresponding lines below.

1. R. has a history of vaginitis[a] and endometriosis[b]. During her regular menses[c] she has dysmenorrhea[d], which sometimes results in her absence from work. Her doctor has recommended a complete hysterectomy[e].

   a. _____

   b. _____

   c. _____

   d. _____

   e. _____

2. Z. was treated for ovaritis[a] several years ago. Just recently, she was hospitalized with ovariorrhexis[b] and had to undergo an oophorectomy[c]. The surgery was successful, and her recovery is going well.

   a. _____

   b. _____

   c. _____

3. M.R. is a gravida III[a], para I[b] who is in the early stages of menopause[c]. Her gynecologist has recommended estrogen hormone[d] therapy to alleviate the major symptoms of menopause.

   a. _____

   b. _____

   c. _____

   d. _____

4. C. has a family history of uterine[a] cancer, so she has regular gynecological examinations and tries to stay healthy. Her sister and her mother both suffer from endometriosis[b] as well as dysmenorrhagia[c]. To date, C. has shown no symptoms of these difficulties.

a. _____

b. _____

c. _____

Labeling

Fill in the blanks with the correct terminology.

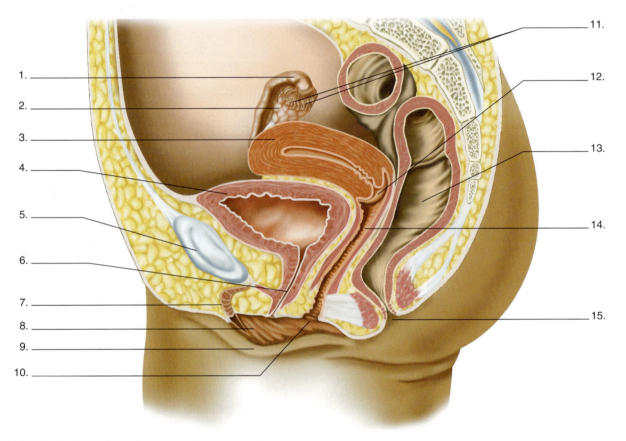

FIGURE 11-4 Side view of the female reproductive organs.

You may now go on to Chapter Test 11.

12

Nervous System

Objectives

After completing Chapter 12, you should be able to do the following:

1. identify word roots pertaining to the nerves;
2. identify word roots pertaining to the head and the brain;
3. recognize word parts that identify the spinal cord; and
4. identify several types of drugs associated with nervous system disorders and treatments.

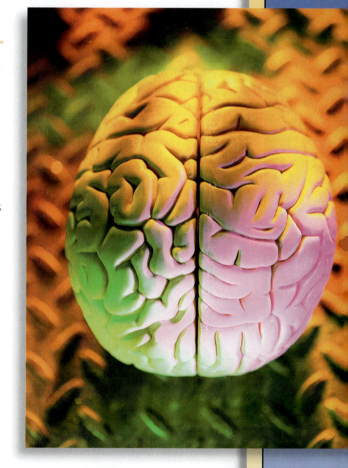

Orientation to the Nervous System

The nervous system is a very complex structure composed of neurons (sensory neurons and motor neurons) and neuroglia (literally "nerve glue"). The sensory neurons (referred to as afferent nerves) send impulses to the brain and spinal cord; the motor neurons (referred to as efferent nerves) send the impulses from the brain and spinal cord to the glands and muscles throughout the body.

The nervous system is divided into the central nervous system (CNS) and the peripheral nervous system (PNS). The central nervous system consists of the brain and the spinal cord. The brain is divided into three parts—the brain stem, cerebellum, and cerebrum. The brain stem (the midbrain, the medulla oblongata, and the pons) is connected to the lower part of the brain. The central nervous system coordinates the actions of the voluntary muscles and the conscious thought processes. The brain and the spinal cord are each covered by a membrane called the meninges, which has three layers: the dura mater, the tough outer layer; the arachnoid, the weblike middle layer; and the pia mater, the inner layer, which contains blood vessels.

The peripheral nervous system is divided into the somatic nervous system (SNS), which governs voluntary activities, and the autonomic nervous system (ANS), which governs involuntary activities such as circulation and digestion. The autonomic nervous system is further divided into sympathetic and parasympathetic nerves. The sympathetic nerves prepare the body for stress and action in times of emergency by slowing digestion and increasing the heart rate, respiration, and blood pressure. Once the emergency is over, the parasympathetic nerves restore the body's systems to normal by lowering blood pressure, slowing breathing, decreasing the heart rate, and stimulating digestion.

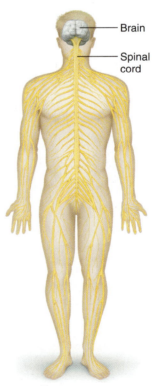

Brain

Spinal cord

Nervous system

Terminology Presentation

Brain

As you listen to the CD, read the words and notice the pronunciations given.

 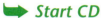 **Start CD**

Look at Figures 12-1 and 12-2

FIGURE 12-1   The nervous system: neurons carry impulses that allow body systems to communicate.

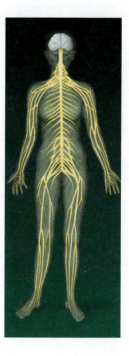

FIGURE 12-2   Side view of the brain.

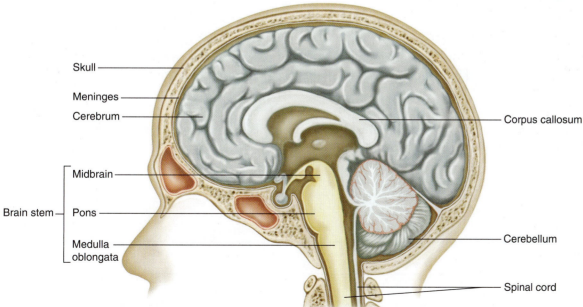

Skull
Meninges
Cerebrum
Corpus callosum
Midbrain
Brain stem — Pons
Medulla oblongata
Cerebellum
Spinal cord

cerebr(o)	a combining form denoting relationship to the cerebrum		
Word	**Word Part**	**Definition**	**Answer**
1. cerebral (ser′e-bral)	-al	pertaining to	1. _____
2. cerebrospinal (ser′e-bro-spi′nal)	spine -al	the spine pertaining to	2. _____
3. cerebromalacia (ser′e-bro-mah-la′she-ah)	-malacia	softening	3. _____

cerebell(o)	a combining form denoting relationship to the cerebellum		
Word	**Word Part**	**Definition**	**Answer**
4. cerebellar (ser′e-bel′ar)	-ar	pertaining to	4. _____
5. cerebellitis (ser′e-bel-li′tis)	-itis	inflammation	5. _____

encephal(o)	a combining form denoting relationship to the brain		
Word	**Word Part**	**Definition**	**Answer**
6. encephaloma (en′sef-ah-lo′mah)	-oma	tumor	6. _____
7. encephalomalacia (en-sef′ah-lo-mah-la′she-ah)	-malacia	softening	7. _____
8. encephalitis (en′sef-ah-li′tis)	-itis	inflammation	8. _____
9. encephalic (en′se-fal′ik)	-ic	pertaining to	9. _____

 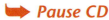 **Pause CD**

After practicing each word several times, use a sheet of paper to cover all columns except the Answer column. As each word is pronounced again on the CD, write it in the space provided.

  Start CD

Check the words you have written against the words in the left-hand column. If you have misspelled any words, practice writing them correctly.

Practice

_____

_____

_____

Name _____ Date_____ Errors _____

LESSON
LESSON
12-1

Terminology Application

Without looking at your previous work, write the word that matches each definition.

Definition	Term
1. inflammation of the brain	_____
2. tumor of the brain	_____
3. abnormal softening of the cerebrum	_____
4. pertaining to the cerebellum	_____
5. pertaining to the cerebrum	_____
6. pertaining to the brain and the spinal cord	_____
7. abnormal softening of the brain	_____
8. pertaining to the brain	_____
9. inflammation of the cerebellum	_____

Check your answers against the information given in this lesson's terminology presentation. If you have any errors, count them and write the number in the blank at the top of the page. Sign your work and give it to your instructor.

Practice

Spinal Cord and Meninges

As you listen to the CD, read the words and notice the pronunciations given.

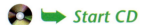 **Start CD**

Look at Figure 12-3

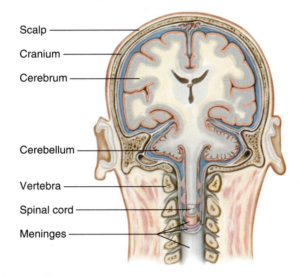

| Scalp |
| Cranium |
| Cerebrum |
| Cerebellum |
| Vertebra |
| Spinal cord |
| Meninges |

FIGURE 12-3   The brain and the meninges.

myel(o)	a combining form denoting relationship to the spinal cord, myelin (electrical insulator), or bone marrow		
Word	**Word Part**	**Definition**	**Answer**
1. myelitis (mi′e-li′tis)	-itis	inflammation	1. _____
2. myelogram (mi′e-lo-gram)	-gram	a recording	2. _____
3. myelopathy (mi′e-lop′ah-the)	-pathy	disease	3. _____
4. myeloneuritis (mi′e-lo-nu-ri′tis)	neur(o) -itis	nerve inflammation	4. _____
5. poliomyelitis (po′le-o-mi′e-ll-tis)	poli(o) -itis	gray inflammation	5. _____

continued

| | **mening(o)** a combining form denoting relationship to a membrane, especially the meninges | | |
| | | | |

	Word	Word Part	Definition	Answer
6.	meningorrhagia (me-ning′go-ra′je-ah)	-rrhagia	excessive flow, bleeding	6. _____
7.	meningomyelitis (me-ning′go-mi′e-li′tis)	myel(o) -itis	spinal cord inflammation	7. _____
8.	meningeal (me-nin′je-al)	-al	pertaining to	8. _____
9.	meningioma (me-nin′je-o′mah)	-oma	tumor	9. _____
10.	meningopathy (men′in-gop′ah-the)	-pathy	disease	10. _____
11.	meningocele (me-ning′go-sele)	-cele	herniation	11. _____
12.	meningitis (men′in-ji′tis)	-itis	inflammation	12. _____

 Pause CD

After practicing each word several times, use a sheet of paper to cover all columns except the Answer column. As each word is pronounced again on the CD, write it in the space provided.

 Start CD

Check the words you have written against the words in the left-hand column. If you have misspelled any words, practice writing them correctly.

Practice

_____

_____

_____

_____

_____

_____

_____

_____

_____

Terminology Presentation

Spinal Cord and Meninges

As you listen to the CD, read the words and notice the pronunciations given.

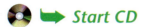 **Start CD**

Look at Figure 12-3

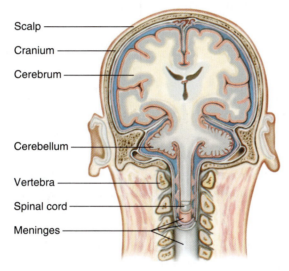

Scalp
Cranium
Cerebrum
Cerebellum
Vertebra
Spinal cord
Meninges

FIGURE 12-3 The brain and the meninges.

myel(o) a combining form denoting relationship to the spinal cord, myelin (electrical insulator), or bone marrow			
Word	**Word Part**	**Definition**	**Answer**
1. myelitis (mi′e-li′tis)	-itis	inflammation	1. _____
2. myelogram (mi′e-lo-gram)	-gram	a recording	2. _____
3. myelopathy (mi′e-lop′ah-the)	-pathy	disease	3. _____
4. myeloneuritis (mi′e-lo-nu-ri′tis)	neur(o) -itis	nerve inflammation	4. _____
5. poliomyelitis (po′le-o-mi′e-ll-tis)	poli(o) -itis	gray inflammation	5. _____

continued

	Word	Word Part	Definition	Answer
6.	meningorrhagia (me-ning′go-ra′je-ah)	-rrhagia	excessive flow, bleeding	6. _____
7.	meningomyelitis (me-ning′go-mi′e-li′tis)	myel(o) -itis	spinal cord inflammation	7. _____
8.	meningeal (me-nin′je-al)	-al	pertaining to	8. _____
9.	meningioma (me-nin′je-o′mah)	-oma	tumor	9. _____
10.	meningopathy (men′in-gop′ah-the)	-pathy	disease	10. _____
11.	meningocele (me-ning′go-sele)	-cele	herniation	11. _____
12.	meningitis (men′in-ji′tis)	-itis	inflammation	12. _____

mening(o)   a combining form denoting relationship to a membrane, especially the meninges

 Pause CD

After practicing each word several times, use a sheet of paper to cover all columns except the Answer column. As each word is pronounced again on the CD, write it in the space provided.

 Start CD

Check the words you have written against the words in the left-hand column. If you have misspelled any words, practice writing them correctly.

Practice

_____

_____

_____

_____

_____

_____

_____

_____

_____

LESSON 12-2

Terminology Application

Without looking at your previous work, write the word that matches each definition.

Definition	Term
1. sheath surrounding some nerve cells; electrical insulator	_____
2. herniation of the meninges	_____
3. excessive bleeding from the meninges	_____
4. inflammation of the meninges	_____
5. inflammation of the spinal cord and the peripheral nerves	_____
6. tumor of the meninges	_____
7. inflammation of the spinal cord	_____
8. inflammation of the meninges and the spinal cord	_____
9. pertaining to the meninges	_____
10. roentgenogram (X-ray) of the spinal cord	_____
11. any disease of the meninges	_____
12. any disease of the spinal cord	_____
13. membrane that surrounds the brain and the spinal cord	_____
14. viral inflammation of the gray matter of the spinal cord	_____

Check your answers against the information given in this lesson's terminology presentation. If you have any errors, count them and write the number in the blank at the top of the page. Sign your work and give it to your instructor.

Practice

Terminology Presentation

Nervous System

As you listen to the CD, read the words and notice the pronunciations given.

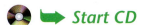 **Start CD**

Look at Figure 12-4

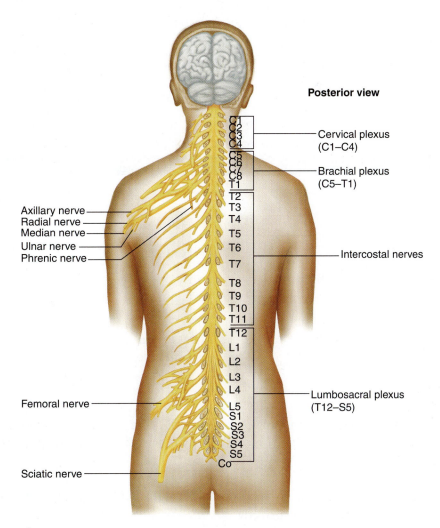

Posterior view

Cervical plexus (C1–C4)

Brachial plexus (C5–T1)

Axillary nerve
Radial nerve
Median nerve
Ulnar nerve
Phrenic nerve

Intercostal nerves

Lumbosacral plexus (T12–S5)

Femoral nerve

Sciatic nerve

FIGURE 12-4 Nerve plexuses.

neur(o) a combining form denoting the nerves or the nervous system			
Word	**Word Part**	**Definition**	**Answer**
1. neuritis (nu-ri′tis)	-itis	inflammation	1. _____

Word	Word Part	Definition	Answer
2. neuralgia (nu-ral′je-ah)	-algia	pain	**2.** _____
3. neural (nu′ral)	-al	pertaining to	**3.** _____
4. neuroglia (nu-rog′le-ah)	-glia	glue	**4.** _____
5. neuropathy (nu-rop′ah-the)	-pathy	disease	**5.** _____
6. neurology (nu-rol′o-je)	-logy	science of, study of	**6.** _____
7. neuroplasty (nu′ro-plas′te)	-plasty	plastic surgery	**7.** _____
8. intercostal nerves (in′ter-kos′tal)	inter- cost(o) -al	between ribs pertaining to	**8.** _____

plexus a general term for a network

Word	Word Part	Definition	Answer
9. neuroplexus (nu′ro-plek′sis)	neur(o)	nerve	**9.** _____
10. cervical plexus (ser′vi-kal plek′sis)	cervic(o) -al	neck pertaining to	**10.** _____
11. brachial plexus (bra′ke-al plek′sis)	brachi(o) -al	arm pertaining to	**11.** _____
12. lumbosacral plexus (lum′bo-sa′kral plek′sis)	lumb(o) sacr(o) -al	loin sacral region pertaining to	**12.** _____

 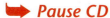 *Pause CD*

After practicing each word several times, use a sheet of paper to cover all columns except the Answer column. As each word is pronounced again on the CD, write it in the space provided.

 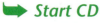 *Start CD*

Check the words you have written against the words in the left-hand column. If you have misspelled any words, practice writing them correctly.

Practice

_____

_____

LESSON 12-3

Terminology Application

Without looking at your previous work, write the word that matches each definition.

Definition	Term
1. network of nerves in the shoulders between the neck and the armpits	_____
2. the study of the science of the nervous system	_____
3. network of nerves in the loin region	_____
4. plastic surgery of the nerves	_____
5. nerve glue	_____
6. network of nerves in the neck	_____
7. any disease of the nervous system	_____
8. nerve pain	_____
9. network of nerves	_____
10. inflammation of the nerves	_____
11. pertaining to the nerves	_____
12. a network	_____
13. pertaining to the nerves between the ribs	_____

Check your answers against the information given in this lesson's terminology presentation. If you have any errors, count them and write the number in the blank at the top of the page. Sign your work and give it to your instructor.

Practice

12-4

Terminology Presentation

Nervous System Disorders

As you listen to the CD, read the words and notice the pronunciations given.

  Start CD

	Word	Word Part	Definition	Answer
	-lepsy a suffix denoting a seizure			
1.	epilepsy (ep'i-lep'se)	epi-	above	1. _____
2.	epileptic (ep'i-lep'tik)	epi- -ic	above pertaining to	2. _____
3.	narcolepsy (nar'ko-lep'se)	narc(o)	stupor	3. _____
4.	narcoleptic (nar'ko-lep'tik)	narc(o) -ic	stupor pertaining to	4. _____

	Word	Word Part	Definition	Answer
	-phasia a suffix denoting speech			
5.	aphasia (ah fa'ze-ah)	a-	not, without	5. _____
6.	aphasiology (a-fa'ze-ol'o-je)	a- -logy	not, without science of, study **of**	6. _____
7.	aphasic (ah-fa'zik)	a- -ic	not, without pertaining to	7. _____

	Word	Word Part	Definition	Answer
	-plegia a suffix denoting a blow or a stroke; paralysis			
8.	quadriplegia (kwod'ri-ple'je-ah)	quadri-	four	8. _____
9.	hemiplegia (hem'e-ple'je-ah)	hemi-	half	9. _____
10.	hemiplegic (hem'e-ple'jik)	hemi- -ic	half pertaining to	10. _____
11.	paraplegia (par'ah-ple'je-ah)	para-	beside, near, accessory to	11. _____

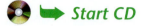 *Pause CD*

After practicing each word several times, use a sheet of paper to cover all columns except the Answer column. As each word is pronounced again on the CD, write it in the space provided.

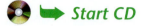 *Start CD*

Check the words you have written against the words in the left-hand column. If you have misspelled any words, practice writing them correctly.

Practice

LESSON
12-4

Terminology Application

Without looking at your previous work, write the word that matches each definition.

Definition	Term
1. paroxysmal transient disturbances of brain function with episodic impairment or loss of consciousness	_____
2. loss of speech capabilities	_____
3. recurrent, uncontrollable, brief episodes of sleep	_____
4. paralysis in all four limbs	_____
5. paralysis of the legs and lower part of the body	_____
6. pertaining to someone with narcolepsy	_____
7. the study of the science of speech	_____
8. paralysis on one side of the body	_____
9. pertaining to someone with epilepsy	_____
10. pertaining to someone with paralysis on one side of the body	_____
11. pertaining to the loss of speech capabilities	_____

Check your answers against the information given in this lesson's terminology presentation. If you have any errors, count them and write the number in the blank at the top of the page. Sign your work and give it to your instructor.

Practice

Drug Terminology Presentation

As you listen to the CD, read the words and notice the pronunciations given.

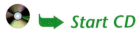 **Start CD**

Word	Definition	Example: Generic Name	Example: Brand/ Trade Name	Answer
analgesics	agents that relieve pain	hydrocodone meperidine acetominophen oxycodone codeine morphine	Vicodin Demerol Tylenol (various) (various) (various)	1. _____
anesthetics	agents that reduce or eliminate the perception of sensation	lidocaine procaine midazolam droperidol propofol thiopental sodium	Xylocaine Novocain Versed Inapsine Diprivan Pentothal	2. _____
antianxiety drugs (psychotropics)	agents that reduce or eliminate anxiety	diazepam alprazolam lorazepam	Valium Xanax Ativan	3. _____
anticonvulsants	agents that prevent or relieve convulsions	diazepam phenobarbital primidone phenytoin	Valium Solfoton, Luminal Sertan Dilantin	4. _____
antidepressants	agents that prevent or relieve depression	venlafaxine sertraline fluoxetine paroxetine	Effexor Zoloft Prozac Paxil	5. _____
antipsychotics	agents that are effective in the treatment of psychoses	lithium haloperidol chlorpromazine	Lithotabs Haldol Thorazine	6. _____
sedatives (hypnotics)	agents that allay activity and excitement; used for short-term treatment of insomnia	zolpidem diphenhydramine chloral hydrate lorazepam pentobarbital secobarbital	Ambien Benadryl, Sominex 2, Nytol, Allerdryl Aquachloral Ativan Nembutal Seconal	7. _____
tranquilizers (major)	agents that have a calm, soothing effect, antipsychotic agents	lithium haloperidol chlorpromazine	Lithotabs Haldol Thorazine	8. _____
tranquilizers (minor)	agents that have a calm, soothing effect; antianxiety drugs	diazepam alprazolam lorazepam	Valium Xanax Ativan	9. _____

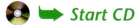

Pause CD

After practicing each word several times, use a sheet of paper to cover all columns except the Answer column. As each word is pronounced again on the CD, write it in the space provided.

Start CD

Check the words you have written against the words in the left-hand column. If you have misspelled any words, practice writing them correctly.

Practice

LESSON 12-5

Drug Terminology Application

Without looking at your previous work, write the word that matches each definition.

Definition	Term
1. agents that are effective in the treatment of psychoses	_____
2. agents that allay activity and excitement; used for the short-term treatment of insomnia	_____
3. agents that prevent or relieve depression	_____
4. agents that have a calm, soothing effect; antianxiety drugs	_____
5. agents that prevent or relieve convulsions	_____
6. agents that relieve pain	_____
7. agents that reduce or eliminate anxiety	_____
8. agents that have a calm, soothing effect; antipsychotic agents	_____
9. agents that reduce or eliminate the perception of sensation	_____

Check your answers against the information given in this lesson's terminology presentation. If you have any errors, count them and write the number in the blank at the top of the page. Sign your work and give it to your instructor.

Practice

CHAPTER 12

Terminology Review

This is a review of the word parts and words you have learned in the preceding lessons. Some of the medical terms listed below may be new, but they are composed of the word parts and word roots that you have already learned. Read the words below as they are pronounced on the CD.

 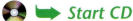 *Start CD*

Word Element Review

Word	Word Part	Meaning of Word Part
1. cerebral	cerebr(o)	_____
cerebral	-al	_____
(ser'e-bral)	Meaning of Word	_____
2. meningitis	mening(o)	_____
meningitis	-itis	_____
(men'in-ji'tis)	Meaning of Word	_____
3. cerebellar	cerebell(o)	_____
cerebellar	-ar	_____
(ser'e-bel'ar)	Meaning of Word	_____
4. poliomyelitis	poli(o)	_____
poliomyelitis	myel(o)	_____
poliomyelitis	-itis	_____
(po'le-o-mi'e-li-tis)	Meaning of Word	_____
5. neuroplexus	neur(o)	_____
neuroplexus	plexus	_____
(nu'ro-plek'sis)	Meaning of Word	_____
6. neuropathy	neur(o)	_____
neuropathy	-pathy	_____
(ne-rop'ah-the)	Meaning of Word	_____
7. encephalitis	encephal(o)	_____
encephalitis	-itis	_____
(en'sef-ah-li'tis)	Meaning of Word	_____

Word	Word Part	Meaning of Word Part
8. lumbosacral plexus	lumb(o)	_____
lumbosacral plexus	sacr(o)	_____
lumbosacral plexus	-al	_____
(lum′bo-sa′kral plek′sis)	Meaning of Word	_____
9. neuralgia	neur(o)	_____
neuralgia	-algia	_____
(nu-ral′je-ah)	Meaning of Word	_____
10. meningomyelitis	mening(o)	_____
meningomyelitis	myel(o)	_____
meningomyelitis	-itis	_____
(me-ning′go-mi′e-li′tis)	Meaning of Word	_____
11. epilepsy	epi-	_____
epilepsy	-lepsy	_____
(ep′i-lep′se)	Meaning of Word	_____
12. brachial plexus	brachi(o)	_____
brachial plexus	-al	_____
brachial plexus	plexus	_____
(bra′ke-al plek′sis)	Meaning of Word	_____
13. quadriplegia	quadr(i)	_____
quadriplegia	-plegia	_____
(kwod′ri- ple′je-ah)	Meaning of Word	_____
14. paraplegia	para-	_____
paraplegia	-plegia	_____
(par′ah-ple′je-ah)	Meaning of Word	_____
15. narcolepsy	narc(o)	_____
narcolepsy	-lepsy	_____
(nar′ko-lep′se)	Meaning of Word	_____

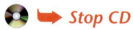 *Stop CD*

On the lines provided, write in the meanings of as many suffixes, prefixes, roots, and words as you can from memory. Check your definitions in the glossary or a medical dictionary, and make any needed corrections.

CHAPTER 12

Terminology Review

Complete this review, and turn it in to your instructor when you are finished.

Definition

Each phrase below defines one of the words you have just studied. Without looking at your previous work, write in the word that matches each definition.

Definition	Term
1. pertaining to the brain	_____
2. inflammation of the spinal cord	_____
3. any disease of the nervous system	_____
4. inflammation of the meninges	_____
5. network of nerves	_____
6. abnormal softening of the cerebrum	_____
7. membrane that surrounds the brain and the spinal cord	_____
8. roentgenogram (X-ray) of the spinal cord	_____
9. inflammation of the nerves	_____
10. paroxysmal transient disturbances of brain function with episodic impairment or loss of consciousness	_____
11. pertaining to the brain and the spinal cord	_____
12. sheath surrounding some nerves; electrical insulator	_____
13. viral inflammation of the gray matter of the spinal cord	_____
14. nerve glue	_____
15. pertaining to the loss of speech capabilities	_____
16. paralysis on one side of the body	_____
17. network of nerves in the shoulders between the neck and the armpits	_____

Definition	Term

18. paralysis in all four limbs _____

19. paralysis of the legs and lower part of the body _____

20. a network _____

Matching

Match the following definitions with the terms given. Put the letter of the correct definition to the left of the term.

Term	Definition
_____ **21.** cerebrospinal	**a.** pertaining to someone with epilepsy
_____ **22.** meningopathy	**b.** pertaining to the brain
_____ **23.** myelitis	**c.** inflammation of the cerebellum
_____ **24.** brachial plexus	**d.** any disease of the meninges
_____ **25.** epileptic	**e.** inflammation of the spinal cord and the peripheral nerves
_____ **26.** myeloneuritis	**f.** inflammation of the spinal cord
_____ **27.** encephalic	**g.** tumor of the meninges
_____ **28.** meningioma	**h.** pertaining to someone with narcolepsy
_____ **29.** narcoleptic	**i.** network of nerves in the shoulders between the neck and the armpits
_____ **30.** cerebellitis	**j.** pertaining to the brain and the spinal cord

CHAPTER 12

Terminology Review

Case Studies

Read the following brief case studies. In each case study, some terms are followed by a superscript letter. Write a brief definition for each of those terms on the corresponding lines below.

1. K.A. suffered cranial[a] trauma that resulted in encephalorrhagia[b]. Because of the swelling, ER surgeons performed a cephalocentesis[c] to relieve the pressure.

   a. _____

   b. _____

   c. _____

2. Before the development of the Salk or Sabin vaccines, poliomyelitis[a] was a terrifying and greatly feared disease in the United States. Patients who were treated for the disease had symptoms of neuritis[b], kinesalgia[c], neuralgia[d], and paralysis.

   a. _____

   b. _____

   c. _____

   d. _____

3. W.H. has chronic myalgia, which causes excruciating pain that she has difficulty coping with psychologically[a]. She is currently in psychotherapy[b] to learn how to deal with this chronic problem. Her doctor has prescribed analgesics[c] to enable her to remain mobile, and the psychotherapist has prescribed an antidepressant[d] as well as an antianxiety[e] medication to aid her in her progress.

   a. _____

   b. _____

   c. _____

   d. _____

   e. _____

4. A.Q. has epilepsy and takes an anticonvulsant[a] daily. Before he was diagnosed with this neurological[b] problem, he fell during a seizure and broke several small bones. He now visits his doctor every 6 months for an encephalogram[c] in order to monitor his progress on the medication.

a. _____

b. _____

c. _____

Labeling

Fill in the blanks with the correct terminology.

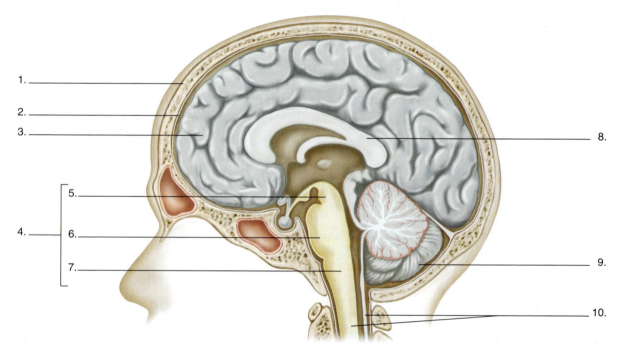

1. _____

2. _____

3. _____

4. _____

5. _____

6. _____

7. _____

8. _____

9. _____

10. _____

FIGURE 12-5   Side view of the brain.

You may now go on to Chapter Test 12.

13

Endocrine System

Objectives

After completing Chapter 13, you should be able to do the following:

1. identify the glands in the endocrine system;

2. know the names of the hormones produced by each gland;

3. understand the purpose/effect of each hormone;

4. identify terms associated with excessive/deficient amounts of sodium, potassium, and calcium in the blood; and

5. identify several types of drugs associated with endocrine disorders and treatments.

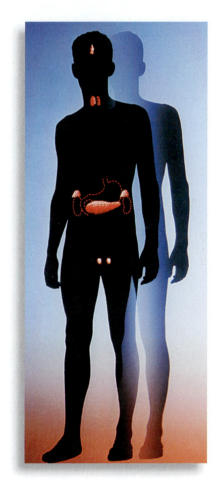

Orientation to the Endocrine System

The endocrine system is made up of ductless glands that produce hormones, which help control various body processes. Each gland produces a different hormone, and each hormone has a unique function.

The pituitary gland, also called the hypophysis cerebri, is located in the brain. The front lobe of the pituitary, the adenohypophysis cerebri, and the back lobe, the neurohypophysis cerebri, produce different hormones. Because the pituitary gland produces hormones that direct the functions of the other glands in the endocrine system, the pituitary gland is referred to as the "master gland."

The hormones produced by the endocrine system are released slowly into the circulatory system and help maintain homeostasis, a state of equilibrium within the body. The endocrine system works in conjunction with the nervous system in this process.

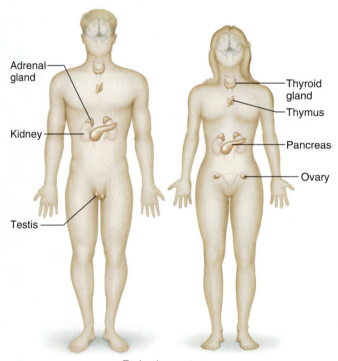

Endocrine system

Terminology Presentation

Pituitary Gland, Terms Indicating Glandular Structures, and Pineal Gland

As you listen to the CD, read the words and notice the pronunciations given.

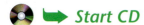 **Start CD**

Look at Figure 13-1

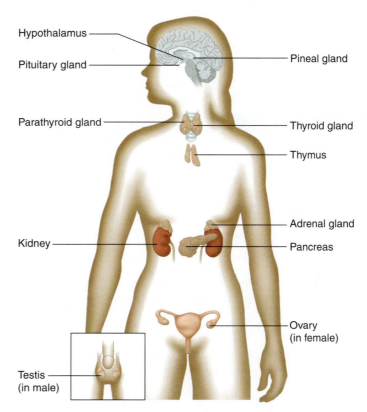

FIGURE 13-1 The glands of the endocrine system.

hypophysis a word denoting the pituitary gland			
Word	**Word Part**	**Definition**	**Answer**
1. hypophysis cerebri (hi-pof'i-sis se-re'bree)	hypo- -physis cerebri	under growing brain	1. _____
2. hypophysitis (hi-pof'i-si'tis)	hypo- -physis -itis	under growing inflammation	2. _____
3. hypophysectomy (hi-pof'i-sek'to-me)	hypo- -physis -ectomy	under growing excision, removal	3. _____

aden(o)	a word element denoting a gland		
Word	**Word Part**	**Definition**	**Answer**
4. adenitis (ad'e-ni'tis)	-itis	inflammation	4. _____
5. adenoma (ad'e-no'mah)	-oma	tumor	5. _____
6. adenomegaly (ad'e-no-meg'ah-le)	-megaly	enlargement	6. _____
7. adenomalacia (ad'e-no-mah-la'she-ah)	-malacia	softening	7. _____
8. adenocarcinoma (ad'e-no-kar'si-no'mah)	carcin(o) -oma	cancer tumor	8. _____

pineal	a word denoting the pineal body		
Word	**Word Part**	**Definition**	**Answer**
9. pinealectomy (pin'e al ek'to-me)	-ectomy	excision, removal	9. _____
10. pinealopathy (pin'e-ah-lop'ah-the)	-pathy	disease	10. _____

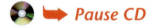 *Pause CD*

After practicing each word several times, use a sheet of paper to cover all columns except the Answer column. As each word is pronounced again on the CD, write it in the space provided.

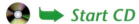 *Start CD*

Check the words you have written against the words in the left-hand column. If you have misspelled any words, practice writing them correctly.

Practice

_____

_____

_____

_____

_____

_____

_____

_____

LESSON
13-1

Terminology Application

Without looking at your previous work, write the word that matches each definition.

Definition	Term
1. abnormal softening of a gland	_____
2. glandular tumor	_____
3. the anterior lobe of the pituitary gland	_____
4. inflammation of a gland	_____
5. abnormal enlargement of a gland	_____
6. inflammation of the pituitary gland	_____
7. excision of the pineal gland	_____
8. cancer of a gland	_____
9. any disease of the pineal gland	_____
10. the posterior lobe of the pituitary gland	_____

Check your answers against the information given in this lesson's terminology presentation. If you have any errors, count them and write the number in the blank at the top of the page. Sign your work and give it to your instructor.

Practice

13-2 Terminology Presentation

Thyroid and Parathyroid Glands

As you listen to the CD, read the words and notice the pronunciations given.

 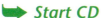 **Start CD**

Look at Figures 13-2 and 13-3

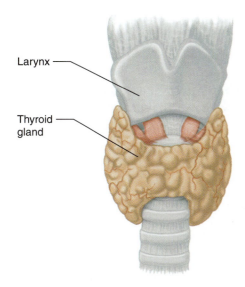

FIGURE 13-2 The thyroid gland.

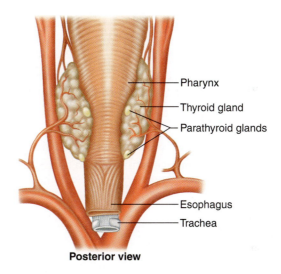

Posterior view

FIGURE 13-3 The four parathyroid glands.

thyr(o) a combining form denoting relationship to the thyroid gland			
Word	**Word Part**	**Definition**	**Answer**
1. thyrocele (thi′ro-sel)	-cele	tumor	**1.** _____
2. thyrotoxic (thi′to-tok′sik)	-toxic	pertaining to a toxin or poison	**2.** _____
3. thyroidectomy (thi′roi-dek′to-me)	-ectomy	excision, removal	**3.** _____
4. thyropathy (thi-rop′ah-the)	-pathy	disease	**4.** _____
5. thyroidotomy (thi′roi-dot′o-me)	-tomy	incision into	**5.** _____

continued

	parathyroid	a word denoting the endocrine glands located dorsal to the thyroid	

Word	Word Part	Definition	Answer
6. parathormone (par'ah-thor'mon)	-hormone	endocrine secretion	6. _____
7. parathyropathy (par'ah-thi-rop'ah-the)	-pathy	disease	7. _____
8. parathyroidal (par'ah-thi-roi'dal)	-al	pertaining to	8. _____
9. parathyroidectomy (par'ah-thi'roi-dek'to-me)	-ectomy	excision, removal	9. _____
10. parathyroidoma (par'ah-thi'roi-do'mah)	-oma	tumor	10. _____

 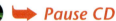 *Pause CD*

After practicing each word several times, use a sheet of paper to cover all columns except the Answer column. As each word is pronounced again on the CD, write it in the space provided.

 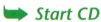 *Start CD*

Check the words you have written against the words in the left-hand column. If you have misspelled any words, practice writing them correctly.

Practice

_____

_____

_____

_____

_____

_____

_____

_____

_____

_____

_____

_____

LESSON
13-2

Terminology Application

Without looking at your previous work, write the word that matches each definition.

Definition	Term
1. parathyroid hormone	_____
2. pertaining to toxic levels of thyroid hormones	_____
3. tumor or cancer of the parathyroid gland	_____
4. any disease of the parathyroid glands	_____
5. any disease of the thyroid gland	_____
6. thyroid tumor; goiter	_____
7. excision of the parathyroid glands	_____
8. incision into the thyroid gland	_____
9. pertaining to the parathyroid glands	_____
10. excision of the thyroid gland	_____

Check your answers against the information given in this lesson's terminology presentation. If you have any errors, count them and write the number in the blank at the top of the page. Sign your work and give it to your instructor.

Practice

Terminology Presentation

Pancreas, Thymus, and Adrenal Glands

As you listen to the CD, read the words and notice the pronunciations given.

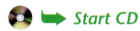 **Start CD**

Look at Figure 13-1 on page 355

pancreat(o) a combining form denoting relationship to the pancreas			
Word	**Word Part**	**Definition**	**Answer**
1. pancreatic (pan′kre-at′ik)	-ic	pertaining to	1. _____
2. pancreatitis (pan′kre-ah-ti′tis)	-itis	inflammation	2. _____
3. pancreatopathy (pan′kre-ah-top′ah-the)	-pathy	disease	3. _____
4. pancreatectomy (pan′kre-ah-tek′to-me)	-ectomy	excision, removal	4. _____
5. pancreatolith (pan′kre-at′o-lith)	-lith(o)	stone, calculus	5. _____
6. pancreatolithectomy (pan′kre-ah-to-li-thek′to-me)	-lith(o) -ectomy	stone, calculus excision, removal	6. _____

thym(o) a combining form denoting relationship to the thymus			
Word	**Word Part**	**Definition**	**Answer**
7. thymopathy (thi-mop′ah-the)	-pathy	disease	7. _____
8. thymitis (thi-mi′tis)	-itis	inflammation	8. _____
9. thymic (thi′mik)	-ic	pertaining to	9. _____
10. thymectomy (thi-mek′to-me)	-ectomy	excision, removal	10. _____

continued

	adren(o)	a combining form denoting the adrenal glands, which secrete the hormone epinephrine
		(adrenalin, ad = near + renal = kidney)

	Word	Word Part	Definition	Answer
11.	adrenomegaly (ad-ren′o-meg′ah-le)	-megaly	enlargement	11._____
12.	adrenal (ah-dre′nal)	-al	pertaining to	12._____
13.	adrenaline (ah-dren′ah-len)	-ine	pertaining to an organic base	13._____
14.	adrenalectomy (ah-dre′nal-ek′to-me)	-ectomy	excision, removal	14._____
15.	adrenalitis (ah-dre′nal-i′tis)	-itis	inflammation	15._____
16.	adrenalopathy (ah-dre′nal-op′ah-the)	-pathy	disease	16._____

 Pause CD

After practicing each word several times, use a sheet of paper to cover all columns except the Answer column. As each word is pronounced again on the CD, write it in the space provided.

 Start CD

Check the words you have written against the words in the left-hand column. If you have misspelled any words, practice writing them correctly.

Practice

_____

_____

_____

_____

_____

_____

_____

_____

_____

_____

LESSON
13-3

Terminology Application

Without looking at your previous work, write the word that matches each definition.

Definition	Term
1. pertaining to the thymus gland	_____
2. inflammation of the pancreas	_____
3. enlargement of an adrenal gland	_____
4. a pancreatic calculus	_____
5. inflammation of the thymus gland	_____
6. pertaining to the adrenal glands	_____
7. excision of the pancreas	_____
8. excision of an adrenal gland	_____
9. any disease of the thymus gland	_____
10. any disease of the adrenal glands	_____
11. pertaining to the pancreas	_____
12. inflammation of the adrenal gland	_____
13. excision of the thymus gland	_____
14. epinephrine	_____
15. any disease of the pancreas	_____
16. excision of a pancreatic calculus	_____

Check your answers against the information given in this lesson's terminology presentation. If you have any errors, count them and write the number in the blank at the top of the page. Sign your work and give it to your instructor.

Practice

LESSON

13-4 Terminology Presentation

Blood Glucose, Sodium, Potassium, and Calcium

As you listen to the CD, read the words and notice the pronunciations given.

 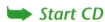 *Start CD*

	glyc(o), gluc(o) combining forms denoting a relationship to sugar or glucose		
Word	**Word Part**	**Definition**	**Answer**
1. hypoglycemia (hi'po-gli-se'me-ah)	hypo- -emia	under, deficiency condition of the blood	1. _____
2. hyperglycemia (hi'per-gli-se'me-ah)	hyper- -emia	excessive condition of the blood	2. _____
3. glycosuria (gli'ko-su're-ah)	-uria	urine	3. _____
4. glucogenic (gloo'ko-jen'ik)	-genic	producing	4. _____

	natrium a word denoting sodium		
Word	**Word Part**	**Definition**	**Answer**
5. hyponatremia (hi'po-nah-tre'me-ah)	hypo- -emia	under, deficiency condition of the blood	5. _____
6. hypernatremia (hi'per-ni-tre'me-ah)	hyper- -emia	excessive condition of the blood	6. _____

	kalium a word denoting potassium		
Word	**Word Part**	**Definition**	**Answer**
7. hypokalemia (hi'po-ka-le'me-ah)	hypo- -emia	under, deficiency condition of the blood	7. _____
8. hyperkalemia (hi'per-kah-le'me-ah)	hyper- -emia	excessive condition of the blood	8. _____

continued

calci, calc(o)	combining forms denoting a relationship to calcium		
Word	**Word Part**	**Definition**	**Answer**
9. hypocalcemia (hi'po-kal-se'me-ah)	hypo- -emia	under, deficiency condition of the blood	9. _____
10. hypercalcemia (hi'per-kal-se'me-ah)	hyper- -emia	excessive condition of the blood	10. _____

-dipsia	a suffix that denotes thirst		
Word	**Word Part**	**Definition**	**Answer**
11. polydipsia (pol'e-dip'se-ah)	poly-	many, much	11. _____

➡ *Pause CD*

After practicing each word several times, use a sheet of paper to cover all columns except the Answer column. As each word is pronounced again on the CD, write it in the space provided.

➡ *Start CD*

Check the words you have written against the words in the left-hand column. If you have misspelled any words, practice writing them correctly.

Practice

_____

_____

_____

_____

_____

_____

_____

_____

_____

_____

_____

_____

LESSON 13-4

Terminology Application

Without looking at your previous work, write the word that matches each definition.

Definition	Term
1. excessive sodium in the blood	_____
2. excessive calcium in the blood	_____
3. presence of sugar in the urine	_____
4. deficiency of sodium in the blood	_____
5. deficiency of potassium in the blood	_____
6. producing glucose	_____
7. excessive thirst	_____
8. excessive sugar in the blood	_____
9. deficiency of calcium in the blood	_____
10. excessive potassium in the blood	_____
11. deficiency of sugar in the blood	_____

Check your answers against the information given in this lesson's terminology presentation. If you have any errors, count them and write the number in the blank at the top of the page. Sign your work and give it to your instructor.

Practice

As you listen to the CD, read the words and notice the pronunciations given.

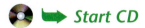 **Start CD**

Gland	Hormone	Purpose	Answer
1. adenohypophysis cerebri (ad'e-no-hi-pof'i-sis) (se-re'bree)			1. _____
adenohypophysis cerebri (anterior portion of the pituitary)	a. thyroid-stimulating hormone (TSH)	stimulates thyroid secretion	a. _____
	b. adrenocorticotropic hormone (ACTH)	stimulates adrenal cortex secretion	b. _____
	c. follicle-stimulating hormone (FSH)	stimulates growth of ovarian follicle; also stimulates secretion of estrogen (in females) and testosterone (in males)	c. _____
	d. luteinizing hormone (LH)	causes ovulation; stimulates progesterone (in females) and testosterone (in males)	d. _____
	e. melanocyte-stimulating hormone (MSH)	for skin pigmentation	e. _____
	f. somatotropin	affects growth	f. _____
	g. prolactin	stimulates the development of the breast and stimulates the production of milk during pregnancy	g. _____
2. neurohypophysis cerebri (nu'ro-hi-pof'i-sis) (se-re'bree)			2. _____
neurohypophysis cerebri (posterior portion of the pituitary)	a. antidiuretic hormone (ADH)	aids in kidney absorption of water	a. _____
	b. oxytocin	stimulates uterine contractions	b. _____

continued

Gland	Hormone	Purpose	Answer
3. pineal gland (pin′e-al)			3._____
pineal gland	a. serotonin	function unclear; thought to be a precursor to melatonin	a. _____
	b. melatonin	related to the day/night cycle; increases before sleep	b. _____
4. thyroid gland (thi′roid)			4._____
thyroid gland	a. thyroxine— tetraiodothyronine (T_4)	regulates metabolism	a. _____
	b. triiodothyronine (T_3)	regulates metabolism	b. _____
	c. calcitonin	regulates calcium and phosphorous metabolism	c. _____
5. parathyroid glands (par′ah-thi′roid)			5._____
parathyroid glands	a. parathyroid hormone (PTH) (also called parathormone)	regulates calcium and phosphorous metabolism	a. _____
6. pancreas (pan′kre-as)			6._____
pancreas	a. insulin	regulates sugar and carbohydrate metabolism	a. _____
	b. glucagon	regulates sugar and carbohydrate metabolism	b. _____
7. thymus (thi′mus)			7._____
thymus	a. thymosin	regulates immune response	a. _____
8. adrenal (ah-dre′nal)			8._____
adrenal	a. cortical hormones (steroid hormones)	regulate carbohydrate metabolism and salt and water balance; affects sexual characteristics	a. _____
	b. medullary hormones		b. _____
	i. epinephrine	increases cardiac activity, increases fat usage for energy, causes vasoconstriction in skeletal muscles	i. _____
	ii. norepinephrine	raises blood pressure, constricts vessels	ii. _____

Gland	Hormone	Purpose	Answer
9. ovaries (o'vah-rez)			9._____
ovaries	a. estrogen	increases development of female sexual characteristics; regulate reproduction	a._____
	b. progesterone	increases development of female sexual characteristics; regulate reproduction	b._____
10. testes (tes'tez)			10._____
testes	a. testosterone	increases development of male sexual characteristics; affects reproduction	a._____

  Pause CD

After practicing each word several times, use a sheet of paper to cover all columns except the Answer column. As each word is pronounced again on the CD, write it in the space provided.

  Start CD

Check the words you have written against the words in the left-hand column. If you have misspelled any words, practice writing them correctly.

Practice

_____

_____

_____

_____

_____

_____

_____

_____

_____

_____

_____

_____

_____

_____

Practice

LESSON 13-5

Hormone Terminology Application

Without looking at your previous work, write the name of the gland that matches each definition.

Definition	Term
1. produces estrogen and progesterone	_____
2. produces calcitonin	_____
3. produces steroid hormones	_____
4. produces oxytocin	_____
5. produces ACTH	_____
6. produces thymosin	_____
7. produces testosterone	_____
8. produces melatonin and serotonin	_____
9. produces insulin	_____
10. produces parathyroid hormone (PTH) (also called parathormone)	_____

Check your answers against the information given in this lesson's terminology presentation. If you have any errors, count them and write the number in the blank at the top of the page. Sign your work and give it to your instructor.

  Pause CD

After practicing each word several times, use a sheet of paper to cover all columns except the Answer column. As each word is pronounced again on the CD, write it in the space provided.

  Start CD

Check the words you have written against the words in the left-hand column. If you have misspelled any words, practice writing them correctly.

Practice

Drug Terminology Presentation

As you listen to the CD, read the words and notice the pronunciations given.

 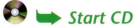 **Start CD**

Word	Definition	Example: Generic Name	Example: Brand/Trade Name	Answer
antidiabetics	agents used to decrease blood sugar or to improve the body's use of insulin	rosiglitazone (improves insulin resistance) insulin	Avandia (various)	1. _____
antilipidemics	agents that counteract high levels of lipids (fats) in the blood	simvastatin atorvastatin lovastatin	Zocor Lipitor Mevacor	2. _____
corticosteroids	any adrenal cortex steroid used to alleviate or decrease inflammation; for immunosuppression or for allergies	cortisone prednisone hydrocortisone	(various) (various) Cortef, Hydrocortone	3. _____
thyroid hormones	agents used for thyroid replacement therapy	levothyroxine (T_4) liothyronine (T_3)	Synthroid Cytomel	4. _____

 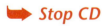 **Stop CD**

After practicing each word several times, use a sheet of paper to cover all columns except the Answer column. As each word is pronounced again on the CD, write it in the space provided.

 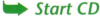 **Start CD**

Check the words you have written against the words in the left-hand column. If you have misspelled any words, practice writing them correctly.

Practice

LESSON
13-6

Drug Terminology Application

Without looking at your previous work, write the word that matches each definition.

Definition	Term
1. any adrenal cortex steroid used to alleviate or decrease inflammation	_____
2. agents used to decrease blood sugar or to improve the body's use of insulin	_____
3. agents used for thyroid replacement therapy	_____
4. agents used to counteract high levels of lipids in the blood	_____

Check your answers against the information given in this lesson's terminology presentation. If you have any errors, count them and write the number in the blank at the top of the page. Sign your work and give it to your instructor.

Practice

CHAPTER 13

Terminology Review

This is a review of the word parts and words you have learned in the preceding lessons. Some of the medical terms listed below may be new, but they are composed of the word parts and word roots that you have already learned. Read the words below as they are pronounced on the CD.

 Start CD

Word Element Review

Word	Word Part	Meaning of Word Part
1. parathyroidal parathyroidal (par'ah-thi-roi'dal)	parathyroid -al Meaning of Word	_____ _____ _____
2. pancreatolithectomy pancreatolithectomy pancreatolithectomy (pan'kre-ah-to-li-thek'to-me)	pancreat(o) -lith(o) -ectomy Meaning of Word	_____ _____ _____ _____
3. thryoidectomy thryoidectomy (thi'roi-dek'to-me)	thyr(o) -ectomy Meaning of Word	_____ _____ _____
4. adenomegaly adenomegaly (ad'e-no-meg'ah-le)	aden(o) -megaly Meaning of Word	_____ _____ _____
5. thyrocele thyrocele (thi'ro-sel)	thyr(o) -cele Meaning of Word	_____ _____ _____
6. pinealectomy pinealectomy (pin'e-al-ek'to-me)	pineal -ectomy Meaning of Word	_____ _____ _____
7. hypophysitis hypophysitis hypophysitis (hi-pof'i-si'tis)	hypo- -physis -itis Meaning of Word	_____ _____ _____ _____

Word	Word Part	Meaning of Word Part
8. pancreatitis	pancreat(o)	_____
pancreatitis	-itis	_____
(pan′kre-ah-ti′tis)	Meaning of Word	_____
9. hypophysectomy	hypo-	_____
hypophysectomy	-physis	_____
hypophysectomy	-ectomy	_____
(hi-pof′i-sek′to-me)	Meaning of Word	_____
10. thymectomy	thym(o)	_____
thymectomy	-ectomy	_____
(thi-mek′to-me)	Meaning of Word	_____
11. adrenalitis	adren(o)	_____
adrenalitis	-itis	_____
(ah-dre′nal-i′tis)	Meaning of Word	_____
12. hyponatremia	hypo-	_____
hyponatremia	natrium	_____
hyponatremia	-emia	_____
(hi′po-nah-tre′me-ah)	Meaning of Word	_____
13. adrenomegaly	adren(o)	_____
adrenomegaly	-megaly	_____
(ad-ren′o-meg′ah-le)	Meaning of Word	_____
14. thymopathy	thym(o)	_____
thymopathy	-pathy	_____
(thi-mop′ah-the)	Meaning of Word	_____
15. hypercalcemia	hyper-	_____
hypercalcemia	calc(o)	_____
hypercalcemia	-emia	_____
(hi′per-kal-se′me-ah)	Meaning of Word	_____

  Stop CD

On the lines provided, write in the meanings of as many suffixes, prefixes, roots, and words as you can from memory. Check your definitions in the glossary or a medical dictionary, and make any needed corrections.

CHAPTER 13

Terminology Review

Complete this review, and turn it in to your instructor when you are finished.

Definition

Each phrase below defines one of the words you have just studied. Without looking at your previous work, write in the word that matches each definition.

Definition	Term
1. pertaining to toxic levels of thyroid hormones	_____
2. enlargement of an adrenal gland	_____
3. inflammation of a gland	_____
4. excision of the parathyroid glands	_____
5. presence of sugar in the urine	_____
6. inflammation of the thymus gland	_____
7. the posterior lobe of the pituitary gland	_____
8. excessive sodium in the blood	_____
9. inflammation of the pituitary gland	_____
10. excessive potassium in the blood	_____
11. any disease of the pineal gland	_____
12. any disease of the parathyroid glands	_____
13. the anterior lobe of the pituitary gland	_____
14. thyroid tumor; goiter	_____
15. excessive sugar in the blood	_____
16. excision of the pancreas	_____
17. excessive calcium in the blood	_____
18. excessive thirst	_____
19. excision of an adrenal gland	_____
20. producing glucose	_____

Matching

Match the following definitions with the terms given. Put the letter of the correct definition to the left of the term.

Term	Definition
_____ 21. adenocarcinoma	**a.** blood sugar deficiency
_____ 22. pinealectomy	**b.** pertaining to the thymus gland
	c. any disease of the adrenal glands
_____ 23. hypocalcemia	**d.** excision of the pineal gland
_____ 24. thymic	**e.** pertaining to toxic levels of thyroid hormones
_____ 25. hypoglycemia	**f.** deficiency of potassium in the blood
_____ 26. parathyroidoma	**g.** cancer of a gland
_____ 27. thyrotoxic	**h.** deficiency of calcium in the blood
_____ 28. pancreatolith	**i.** a stone/calculus in the pancreas
_____ 29. hypokalemia	**j.** tumor or cancer of the parathyroid glands
_____ 30. adrenalopathy	

CHAPTER 13   Terminology Review

Case Studies

Read the following brief case studies. In each case study, some terms are followed by a superscript letter. Write a brief definition for each of those terms on the corresponding lines below.

1. L. has a history of hypophysitis[a]. He was recently diagnosed with a pituitary[b] tumor, and his doctor has scheduled him for a hypophysectomy[c].

    a. _____

    b. _____

    c. _____

2. Y.D. sustained pancreatic[a] injuries in a car accident and thought that she might have to undergo a pancreatectomy[b]. However, during exploratory surgery her doctor found only mild pancreatitis[c] and decided not to pursue the other surgery.

    a. _____

    b. _____

    c. _____

3. T.E. has arthritis and has been treated with a corticosteroid[a] to relieve some of the pain she has been experiencing. She also suffers from hypothyroidism[b] and has had a complete thyroidectomy[c]. Now she must take specific medications for thyroid replacement therapy.

    a. _____

    b. _____

    c. _____

4. A.G. has a pituitary[a] deficiency, and her body does not produce the ACTH[b] it needs. She has been to an endocrinologist[c] who is going to provide a medical regimen for her to follow.

    a. _____

    b. _____

    c. _____

5. L. is a diabetic whose body does not use the insulin[a] it produces. In addition, his body reacts as though it does not have enough insulin and thus overproduces it. His doctor has given him a prescription for an antidiabetic[b] and has suggested that he monitor his blood sugar.

   a. _____

   b. _____

6. A patient whose andenohypophysis cerebri[a] produces too much growth hormone[b] can suffer from acromegaly[c] or from giantism. A patient with a deficient amount of the growth hormone could suffer from dwarfism.

   a. _____

   b. _____

   c. _____

Labeling

Fill in the blanks with the correct terminology.

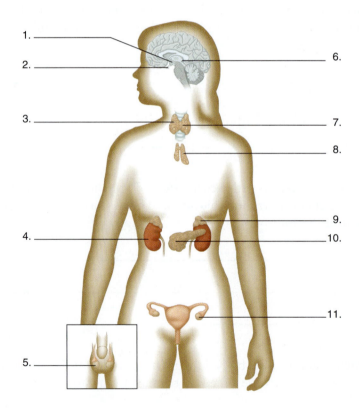

1. _____
2. _____
3. _____
4. _____
5. _____
6. _____
7. _____
8. _____
9. _____
10. _____
11. _____

FIGURE 13-4 The glands of the endocrine system.

You may now go on to Chapter Test 13.

14

Musculoskeletal System

Objectives

After completing Chapter 14, you should be able to do the following:

1. know the difference between the axial and the appendicular skeletons;

2. identify the various bones and their locations in both the axial and appendicular skeletons;

3. identify word roots pertaining to bones, the skull, the spine, joints, cartilage, and bone marrow;

4. identify various muscles;

5. identify the locations and functions of various muscles;

6. identify word roots pertaining to muscles, tendons, and fascia; and

7. identify several types of drugs associated with musculoskeletal disorders and treatments.

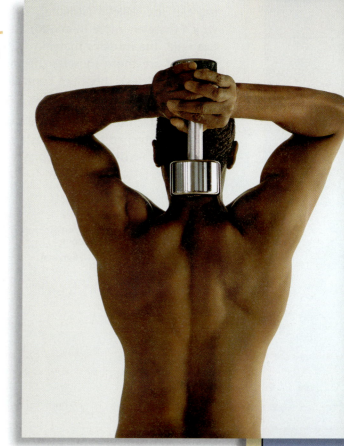

Orientation to the Musculoskeletal System

The musculoskeletal system—made up of bones, muscles, and joints—provides a supporting framework for the body and protects delicate internal structures. Bones also provide areas to which muscles, tendons, and ligaments attach to aid in movement, and they provide a storage area for minerals such as calcium and phosphorus. Inside the larger bones is bone marrow, which produces blood cells (in the process of hemopoiesis).

Most bones are covered by a connective tissue called the periosteum, which contains nerve fibers and lymphocytes. At places where bones are connected (the joints), the bone ends are lined with cartilage, and the ligaments help hold the bones in place.

The skeleton is divided into two basic structures, the axial skeleton and the appendicular skeleton. Muscles work in conjunction with the skeletal structure to provide movement. The three types of muscles are skeletal (striated), smooth, and cardiac. Skeletal muscles (the voluntary muscles, of which there are more than 600) are those muscles that the individual controls and moves at will (for example, the muscles that move the hands, the arms, the tongue). Smooth muscles (involuntary muscles) are those muscles the individual does not control (for example, the lung muscles and arterial muscles); these are controlled by the autonomic nervous system. Cardiac muscle (another type of striated muscle), another kind of involuntary muscle, composes most of the heart wall.

Muscles attach to bones several ways. In some parts of the body, the connective tissue within the muscle is attached to the periosteum of the bone. These attachments are called tendons. Ligaments are connective tissues that connect one bone to another.

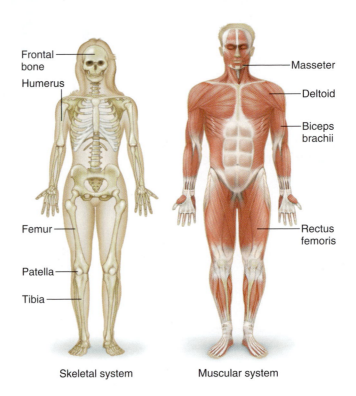

Skeletal system — Frontal bone, Humerus, Femur, Patella, Tibia

Muscular system — Masseter, Deltoid, Biceps brachii, Rectus femoris

14-1 Terminology Presentation

Axial Skeleton Bones

As you listen to the CD, read the words and notice the pronunciations given.

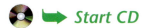 **Start CD**

Look at Figures 14-1 and 14-2

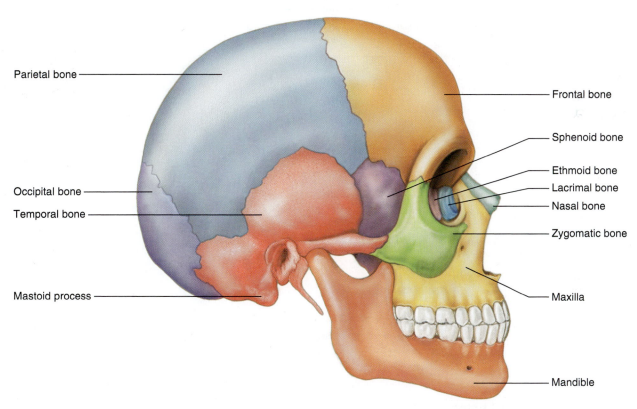

Parietal bone

Occipital bone

Temporal bone

Mastoid process

Frontal bone

Sphenoid bone

Ethmoid bone

Lacrimal bone

Nasal bone

Zygomatic bone

Maxilla

Mandible

FIGURE 14-1 The skull bones.

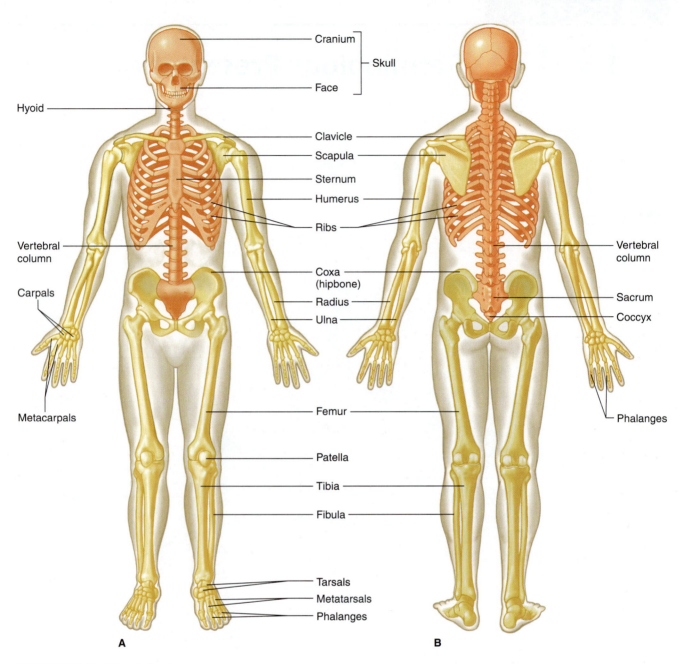

FIGURE 14-2 The skeletal system.

Skull bones		
Axial Skeleton	**Location**	**Answer**
1. frontal (frun'tal)	front of skull above the eyes	1. _____
2. parietal (pah-ri'e-tal)	sides of skull behind the frontal bone; fused at the midline	2. _____

Axial Skeleton	Location	Answer
3. temporal (tem′po-ral)	connected to the parietal bone and the base of the skull	3. _____
4. occipital (ok-sip′i-tal)	back of the skull forming the base	4. _____
5. nasal (na′zal)	forms the bridge of the nose	5. _____
6. zygomatic (zi′go-mat′ik)	cheek bone	6. _____
7. maxilla (mak-sil′ah)	the upper jaw bone	7. _____
8. mandible (man′di-b′l)	the lower jaw bone	8. _____
9. sphenoid (sfe′noid)	winglike structure wedged in the front portion of the cranium	9. _____
10. ethmoid (eth′moid)	in front of the sphenoid bone	10. _____

Vertebral bones

Axial Skeleton	Location	Answer
11. cervical (ser′vi-kal)	seven bones that form the neck	11. _____
12. atlas (at′las)	first cervical vertebra that supports the head	12. _____
13. axis (ak′sis)	second cervical vertebra inside the atlas	13. _____
14. thoracic (tho′ras′ik)	twelve bones that are inferior to the cervical vertebrae	14. _____
15. lumbar (lum′bar)	five bones that are inferior to the thoracic vertebrae	15. _____
16. sacrum (sa′krum)	five fused vertebrae superior to the tailbone	16. _____
17. coccyx (kok′sik)	four (usually) fused bones that form the tailbone	17. _____

Thoracic bones

Axial Skeleton	Location	Answer
18. sternum (ster′num)	breastbone located in the front midline of the chest	18. _____
19. ribs (ribz′)	one pair attached to each of the twelve thoracic vertebrae	19. _____

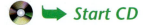

Pause CD

After practicing each word several times, use a sheet of paper to cover all columns except the Answer column. As each word is pronounced again on the CD, write it in the space provided.

Start CD

Check the words you have written against the words in the left-hand column. If you have misspelled any words, practice writing them correctly.

Practice

_____

_____

_____

_____

_____

_____

_____

_____

_____

_____

_____

_____

_____

_____

_____

_____

_____

_____

_____

_____

_____

_____

Terminology Application

Without looking at your previous work, write the word that matches each definition.

Definition	Term
1. lower jaw bone	_____
2. connected to the parietal bone and the base of the skull	_____
3. first cervical vertebra that supports the head	_____
4. twelve bones inferior to the cervical vertebrae	_____
5. sides of skull behind the frontal bone	_____
6. forms the bridge of the nose	_____
7. upper jaw bone	_____
8. seven bones that form the neck	_____
9. tailbone	_____
10. second cervical vertebra inside the atlas	_____
11. back of the skull forming the base	_____
12. front of the skull above the eyes	_____
13. five bones inferior to the thoracic vertebrae	_____
14. in front of the sphenoid	_____
15. cheek bone	_____
16. five fused bones superior to the tailbone	_____
17. one pair attached to each of the twelve thoracic vertebrae	_____
18. breastbone	_____
19. winglike structure wedged in the front portion of the cranium	_____

Check your answers against the information given in this lesson's terminology presentation. If you have any errors, count them and write the number in the blank at the top of the page. Sign your work and give it to your instructor.

Practice

14-2   Terminology Presentation

Appendicular Skeleton Bones

As you listen to the CD, read the words and notice the pronunciations given.

  Start CD

Look at Figure 14-2 on page 390

Appendicular Skeleton	Location	Answer
1. clavicle (klav′i-k′l)	collarbone	1. _____
2. scapula (skap′u-lah)	shoulderblade	2. _____
3. humerus (hu′mer-us)	upper arm bone connected to the elbow	3. _____
4. radius (ra′de-us)	forearm bone connected to the thumb side	4. _____
5. ulna (ul′nah)	the longer of the two forearm bones	5. _____
6. carpals (kar′palz)	wrist bones	6. _____
7. metacarpals (met′ah-kar′palz)	hand bones that extend from the wrist	7. _____
8. phalanx (fa′lanks)	finger (and toe) bones (also called digits and dactyls) (pl. *phalanges*)	8. _____
9. pelvic bones	hip bones	9. _____
10. ilium (il′e-um)	the superior portion of the hip bone	10. _____
11. ischium (is′ke-um)	the inferior portion of the hip bone	11. _____
12. pubis (pu′bis)	one of two bones that connect at the midline of the base of the pelvis	12. _____
13. femur (fe′mur)	thigh bone	13. _____
14. patella (pah-tel′ah)	kneecap	14. _____

continued

Appendicular Skeleton	Location	Answer
15. tibia (tib'e-ah)	shin bone	15._____
16. fibula (fib'u-lah)	lateral to the tibia	16._____
17. tarsals (tahr'salz)	ankle bones	17._____
18. metatarsals (met'ah-tahr'salz)	foot bones that extend from the ankle	18._____
19. phalanx (fa'lanks)	finger (and toe) bones (also called digits and dactyls) (pl. *phalanges*)	19._____
20. calcaneous (kal-ka'ne-us)	heel bone	20._____

 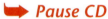 *Pause CD*

After practicing each word several times, use a sheet of paper to cover all columns except the Answer column. As each word is pronounced again on the CD, write it in the space provided.

  Start CD

Check the words you have written against the words in the left-hand column. If you have misspelled any words, practice writing them correctly.

Practice

_____

_____

_____

_____

_____

_____

_____

_____

_____

_____

_____

LESSON 14-2 Terminology Application

Without looking at your previous work, write the word that matches each definition.

Definition	Term
1. wrist bones	_____
2. foot bones that extend from the ankle	_____
3. longer of the two forearm bones	_____
4. heel bone	_____
5. upper arm connected to the elbow	_____
6. hip bones	_____
7. thigh bone	_____
8. collarbone	_____
9. hand bones that extend from the wrist	_____
10. the superior portion of the hip bone	_____
11. kneecap	_____
12. shoulderblade	_____
13. bone lateral to the tibia	_____
14. finger bones	_____
15. forearm connected to the thumb side	_____
16. ankle bones	_____
17. the inferior portion of the hip bone	_____
18. shin bone	_____
19. one of two bones that connect at the midline of the base of the pelvis	_____
20. toe bones	_____

Check your answers against the information given in this lesson's terminology presentation. If you have any errors, count them and write the number in the blank at the top of the page. Sign your work and give it to your instructor.

Practice

Terminology Presentation

Skull, Spine, Joints, Cartilage, and Bone Marrow

As you listen to the CD, read the words and notice the pronunciations given.

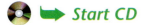 **Start CD**

Look at Figure 14-1, on page 389, and Figure 14-3

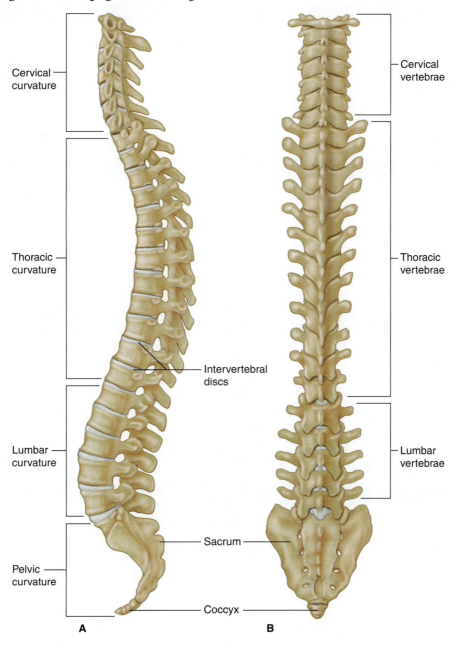

Cervical curvature

Thoracic curvature

Lumbar curvature

Pelvic curvature

Intervertebral discs

Sacrum

Coccyx

Cervical vertebrae

Thoracic vertebrae

Lumbar vertebrae

A   B

FIGURE 14-3   The spinal column.

crani(o) a combining form denoting relationship to the skull

	Word	Word Part	Definition	Answer
1.	craniotomy (kra'ne-ot'o-me)	-tomy	incision into	1. _____
2.	cranial (kra'ne-al)	-al	pertaining to	2. _____
3.	craniectomy (kra'ne-ek'to-me)	-ectomy	excision, removal	3. _____

vertebr(o) a combining form denoting relationship to a vertebra or to the spinal column

	Word	Word Part	Definition	Answer
4.	vertebral (ver'te-bral)	-al	pertaining to	4. _____
5.	vertebrocostal (ver'te-bro-kos'tal)	cost(o) -al	rib pertaining to	5. _____

spondyl(o) a combining form denoting relationship to a vertebra or to the spinal column

	Word	Word Part	Definition	Answer
6.	spondylitis (spon'di-li'tis)	-itis	inflammation	6. _____
7.	spondylosis (spon'di-lo'sis)	-osis	disease	7. _____

rachi(o) a combining form denoting relation to the spine

	Word	Word Part	Definition	Answer
8.	rachialgia (ra'ke-al'je-ah)	-algia	pain	8. _____
9.	rachitis (ra-ki'tis)	-itis	inflammation	9. _____

sacr(o) a combining form denoting relationship to the sacrum, the fused triangular bone just above the tailbone

	Word	Word Part	Definition	Answer
10.	sacral (sa'kral)	-al	pertaining to	10. _____

coccyx	a term referring to the fused vertebrae called the tailbone		
Word	**Word Part**	**Definition**	**Answer**
11. coccygeal (kok-sij′e-al)	-eal	pertaining to	11. _____

oste(o)	a combining form denoting relationship to bone or the bones		
Word	**Word Part**	**Definition**	**Answer**
12. osteitis (os′te-i′tis)	-itis	inflammation	12. _____
13. osteomalacia (os′te-o-mah-la′she-ah)	-malacia	softening	13. _____
14. osteoporosis (os′te-o-po-ro′sis)	-porosis	callosity	14. _____

arthr(o)	a combining form denoting some relationship to a joint or joints		
Word	**Word Part**	**Definition**	**Answer**
15. arthrocentesis (ar′thro-sen-te′sis)	-centesis	surgical puncture	15. _____
16. arthritis (ar′thri′tis)	-itis	inflammation	16. _____

chondr(o)	a combining form denoting relationship to cartilage		
Word	**Word Part**	**Definition**	**Answer**
17. chondrolysis (kon-drol′i-sis)	-lysis	dissolution	17. _____
18. chondritis (kon-dri′tis)	-itis	inflammation	18. _____

myel(o)	a combining form denoting relationship to bone marrow, to the spinal cord, or to myelin		
Word	**Word Part**	**Definition**	**Answer**
19. osteomyelitis (os′te-o-mi′e-li′tis)	oste(o) -itis	bone inflammation	19. _____

 ➡ *Pause CD*

After practicing each word several times, use a sheet of paper to cover all columns except the Answer column. As each word is pronounced again on the CD, write it in the space provided.

 ➡ *Start CD*

Check the words you have written against the words in the left-hand column. If you have misspelled any words, practice writing them correctly.

continued

Practice

LESSON 14-3

Terminology Application

Without looking at your previous work, write the word that matches each definition.

Definition	Term
1. inflammation of a joint	_____
2. excision of part of the skull	_____
3. any disease of the vertebrae	_____
4. incision into the skull	_____
5. callosity of bones	_____
6. pain in the spinal column	_____
7. pertaining to the skull	_____
8. a form of osteomalacia; rickets	_____
9. pertaining to the vertebrae and a rib	_____
10. softening of bone	_____
11. inflammation of bone marrow	_____
12. inflammation of the vertebrae	_____
13. inflammation of cartilage	_____
14. pertaining to the sacrum	_____
15. degeneration of cartilage	_____
16. pertaining to the vertebrae	_____
17. inflammation of a bone	_____
18. pertaining to the coccyx	_____
19. surgical puncture of a joint	_____

Check your answers against the information given in this lesson's terminology presentation. If you have any errors, count them and write the number in the blank at the top of the page. Sign your work and give it to your instructor.

Practice

14-4 Terminology Presentation

Muscles, Tendons, and Fascia

As you listen to the CD, read the words and notice the pronunciations given.

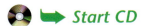 **Start CD**

Look at Figures 14-4 and 14-5

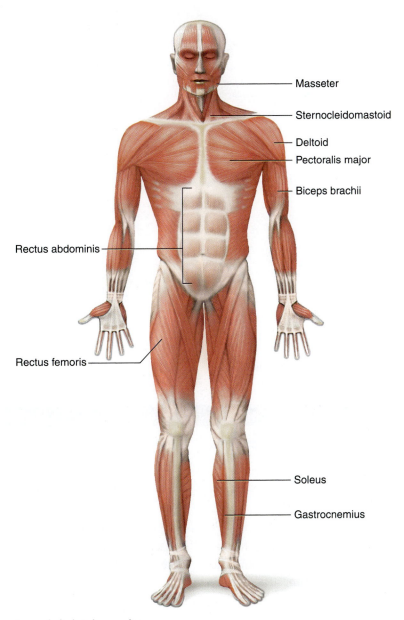

FIGURE 14-4 Anterior view of skeletal muscles.

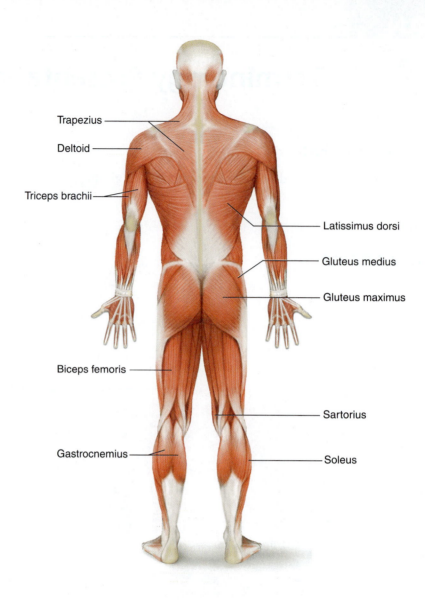

FIGURE 14-5 Posterior view of skeletal muscles.

	Name of Muscle	Location	Function	Answer
1.	masseter (mas-se′ ter)	side of mandible	chewing and closes jaw	**1.** _____
2.	trapezius (trah-pe′ze-us)	shoulder region	raises shoulder and arm	**2.** _____
3.	sternocleidomastoid (ster′no-kli′do-mas′toid)	connects the sternum to the clavicle and the mastoid process	pulls head laterally and toward the chest; raises breastbone	**3.** _____

Name of Muscle	Location	Function	Answer
4. deltoid (del'toid)	spine of scapula and clavicle	extends arm	4. _____
5. biceps (bi'seps)	two-headed muscle at front of forearm above elbow	flexes the arm, supinates hand	5. _____
6. triceps (tri'seps)	three-headed muscle at side and middle of forearm	extends the forearm, extends arm	6. _____
7. brachialis (bra'ke-al'is)	front of humerus	flexes the forearm at the elbow	7. _____
8. pectoralis (pek'to-ra'lis)	chest / chest	major—flexes and rotates arm medially / minor—draws shoulder downward	8. _____
9. rectus abdominus (rek'tus ab dom'e-nis)	straight abdominal muscle	supports abdomen, flexes lumbar vertebrae	9. _____
10. latissimus dorsi (lah-tis'i-mus dor'si)	largest back muscle	extends, rotates humerus medially	10. _____
11. gluteus maximus (gloo'te-us mak'si-mus)	largest muscle of buttocks	extends, rotates thigh laterally	11. _____
12. sartorius (sar-to're-us)	side of proximal end of tibia	flexes thigh and leg	12. _____
13. rectus femoris (rek'tus fem'or-is)	from iliac spine to patella	flexes thigh	13. _____
14. soleus (so'le-us)	fibula, fascia at back of knee, tibia	flexes ankle joint	14. _____
15. gastrocnemius (gas'trok-ne'me-us)	calf muscle	flexes ankle joint and knee joint	15. _____

my(o)	a combining form denoting relationship to muscle		
Word	**Word Part**	**Definition**	**Answer**
16. myocele (mi'o-sel)	-cele	herniation	16. _____
17. myopathy (mi-op'ah-the)	-pathy	disease	17. _____

continued

tendon	a fibrous cord by which a muscle is attached to a bone or other structure		
Word	**Word Part**	**Definition**	**Answer**
18. tendinitis (ten'di-ni'tis)	-itis	inflammation	18. _____
19. tenalgia (te-nal'je-ah)	-algia	pain	19. _____

fascia	sheet of fibrous tissue that forms an investment for muscles and other organs of the body		
Word	**Word Part**	**Definition**	**Answer**
20. fasciitis (fas'e-i'tis)	-itis	inflammation	20. _____

➡️ *Pause CD*

After practicing each word several times, use a sheet of paper to cover all columns except the Answer column. As each word is pronounced again on the CD, write it in the space provided.

➡️ *Start CD*

Check the words you have written against the words in the left-hand column. If you have misspelled any words, practice writing them correctly.

Practice

_____

_____

_____

_____

_____

_____

_____

_____

_____

_____

_____

_____

_____

LESSON 14-4

Terminology Application

Without looking at your previous work, write the word that matches each definition.

Definition	Term
1. straight abdominal muscle	_____
2. muscle herniation	_____
3. inflammation of a tendon	_____
4. chest muscle that draws shoulder downward	_____
5. any disease of the muscles	_____
6. raises the shoulder and arm	_____
7. three-headed muscle	_____
8. connects the sternum to the clavicle and the mastoid process	_____
9. largest back muscle	_____
10. from iliac spine to patella; flexes thigh	_____
11. calf muscle	_____
12. chewing muscle; closes jaw	_____
13. connects spine of scapula and clavicle; extends arm	_____
14. inflammation of fascia	_____
15. located at front of humerus; flexes forearm at elbow	_____
16. flexes ankle joint	_____
17. two-headed muscle	_____
18. pain in a tendon	_____
19. located at the side of the proximal end of the tibia; flexes thigh	_____

Definition	Term

20. largest muscle of the buttocks _____

21. chest muscle that flexes and rotates arm medially _____

Check your answers against the information given in this lesson's terminology presentation. If you have any errors, count them and write the number in the blank at the top of the page. Sign your work and give it to your instructor.

14-5 Drug Terminology Presentation

As you listen to the CD, read the words and notice the pronunciations given.

  Start CD

Word	Definition	Example: Generic Name	Example: Brand/Trade Name	Answer
analgesics	agents that relieve pain	hydrocodone meperidine acetaminophen oxycodone codeine morphine	Vicodin Demerol Tylenol (various) (various) (various)	1. _____
anti-inflammatories	agents that counteract or suppress inflammation	celecoxib indomethacin ibuprofen naproxen sodium acetaminophen aspirin	Celebrex Indocin Motrin Anaprox, Aleve Datril, Tylenol (various)	2. _____
corticosteroids	any adrenal cortex steroid used to alleviate or to decrease inflammation; for immunosuppression, or for allergies	cortisone prednisone hydrocortisone	(various) (various) Cortef, Hydrocortone	3. _____
muscle relaxants	agents that lessen muscle tension	cyclobenzaprine diazepam chlorzoxazone	Flexeril Valium Paraflex, Remular	4. _____

  PauseCD

After practicing each word several times, use a sheet of paper to cover all columns except the Answer column. As each word is pronounced again on the CD, write it in the space provided.

  Start CD

Check the words you have written against the words in the left-hand column. If you have misspelled any words, practice writing them correctly.

Practice

LESSON
14-5
Drug Terminology Application

Without looking at your previous work, write the word that matches each definition.

Definition	Term
1. any adrenal cortex steroid used to alleviate or to decrease inflammation	_____
2. agents that counteract or suppress inflammation	_____
3. agents that lessen muscle tension	_____
4. agents that relieve pain	_____

Check your answers against the information given in this lesson's terminology presentation. If you have any errors, count them and write the number in the blank at the top of the page. Sign your work and give it to your instructor.

Practice

CHAPTER 14

Terminology Review

This is a review of the word parts and words you have learned in the preceding lessons. Some of the medical terms listed below may be new, but they are composed of the word parts and word roots that you have already learned. Read the words below as they are pronounced on the CD.

 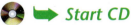 **Start CD**

Word Element Review

Word	Word Part	Meaning of Word Part
1. sacral sacral (sa′kral)	sacr(o) -al Meaning of Word	_____ _____ _____
2. arthrocentesis arthrocentesis (ar′thro-sen-te′sis)	arthr(o) -centesis Meaning of Word	_____ _____ _____
3. osteomyelitis osteomyelitis osteomyelitis (os′te-o-mi′e-li′tis)	oste(o) myel(o) -itis Meaning of Word	_____ _____ _____ _____
4. chondrolysis chondrolysis (kon-drol′i-sis)	chrondr(o) -lysis Meaning of Word	_____ _____ _____
5. cranial cranial (kra′ne-al)	crani(o) -al Meaning of Word	_____ _____ _____
6. myocele myocele (mi′o-sel)	my(o) -cele Meaning of Word	_____ _____ _____
7. spondylitis spondylitis (spon′di-li′tis)	spondyl(o) -itis Meaning of Word	_____ _____ _____

continued

Word	Word Part	Meaning of Word Part
8. fasciitis	fascia	_____
fasciitis	-itis	_____
(fas'e-i'tis)	Meaning of Word	_____
9. vertebral	vertebr(o)	_____
vertebral	-al	_____
(ver'te-bral)	Meaning of Word	_____
10. rachitis	rachi(o)	_____
rachitis	-itis	_____
(ra-ki'tis)	Meaning of Word	_____
11. tendinitis	tendon	_____
tendinitis	-itis	_____
(ten'di-ni'tis)	Meaning of Word	_____
12. craniectomy	crani(o)	_____
craniectomy	-ectomy	_____
(kra'ne-ek'to-me)	Meaning of Word	_____
13. rachialgia	rachi(o)	_____
rachialgia	-algia	_____
(ra'ke-al'je-ah)	Meaning of Word	_____
14. osteitis	oste(o)	_____
osteitis	-itis	_____
(os'te-i'tis)	Meaning of Word	_____
15. coccygeal	coccyx	_____
coccygeal	-eal	_____
(kok-sij'e-al)	Meaning of Word	_____

 Stop CD

On the lines provided, write in the meanings of as many suffixes, prefixes, roots, and words as you can from memory. Check your definitions in the glossary or a medical dictionary, and make any needed corrections.

CHAPTER 14

Terminology Review

Complete this review, and turn it in to your instructor when you are finished.

Definition

Each phrase below defines one of the words you have just studied. Without looking at your previous work, write in the word that matches each definition.

Definition	Term
1. chewing muscle	_____
2. seven bones that form the neck	_____
3. chest muscle that draws shoulder downward	_____
4. shoulderblade	_____
5. two-headed muscle that extends the arm	_____
6. bone located at the back of the skull forming the base	_____
7. largest back muscle	_____
8. flexes ankle joint and knee joint	_____
9. the lower jaw bone	_____
10. winglike bone wedged in the front portion of the cranium	_____
11. second cervical vertebra inside the atlas	_____
12. bone connected to the parietal bone and the base of the skull	_____
13. superior portion of the hip bone	_____
14. largest muscle of the buttocks	_____
15. first cervical vertebra that supports the head	_____
16. chest muscle that flexes and rotates arm medially	_____
17. one pair attached to each of the twelve thoracic vertebrae	_____

continued

Definition	Term

18. three-headed muscle _____

19. flexes the forearm at the elbow _____

20. straight abdominal muscle _____

Matching

Match the following definitions with the terms given. Put the letter of the correct definition to the left of the term.

Term	Definition
_____ **21.** craniotomy	**a.** a form of osteomalacia; rickets
_____ **22.** vertebrocostal	**b.** disease of the spine
_____ **23.** rachitis	**c.** inflammation of cartilage
_____ **24.** osteoporosis	**d.** inflammation of bone marrow
_____ **25.** chondritis	**e.** incision into the skull
_____ **26.** myopathy	**f.** herniation of a muscle
_____ **27.** myocele	**g.** inflammation of the fascia
_____ **28.** spondylosis	**h.** any disease of muscles
_____ **29.** fasciitis	**i.** callosity of the bones
_____ **30.** osteomyelitis	**j.** pertaining to the vertebrae and the ribs

CHAPTER 14

Terminology Review

Read the following brief case studies. In each case study, some terms are followed by a superscript letter. Write a brief definition for each of those terms on the corresponding lines below.

Case Studies

1. S. suffers from osteoporosis[a], which causes her considerable pain. She takes an anti-inflammatory[b] drug on a daily basis and has a corticosteroid[c] injection, which seems to relieve her arthritis[d]. S. must be careful not to fall because she is at risk for bone fractures.

   a. _____

   b. _____

   c. _____

   d. _____

2. H.D. was injured in a car accident and had to have several surgeries to repair damaged and broken bones. His first surgery was to repair a fractured tibia[a]. That was followed by a reconstruction of the humerus[b] in his right arm. Two months later he had a repair of his thoracic vertebrae[c], which helped alleviate some of his post-trauma pain.

   a. _____

   b. _____

   c. _____

3. R.D. is an athlete who has had a right gastrocnemius[a] reattachment to repair damage he sustained while playing soccer. His doctor has him scheduled for physical therapy three times a week to help him to regain his strength and to help alleviate the persistent pain. In addition, he will eventually need to have a right soleus[b] repair.

   a. _____

   b. _____

4. C.R. has arthritis[a] and has a family history of osteomalacia[b]. This past year she has had surgery to remove a vertebra[c] and an arthrocentesis[d] to remove fluid from her shoulder.

   a. _____

   b. _____

   c. _____

   d. _____

Labeling

Fill in the blanks with the correct terminology.

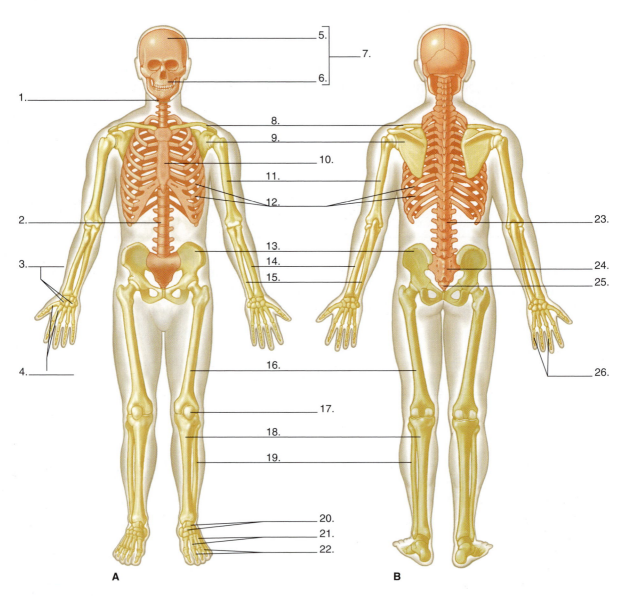

FIGURE 14-6   The skeletal system.

You may now go on to Chapter Test 14.

15

Special Senses

Objectives

After completing Chapter 15, you should be able to do the following:

1. identify word roots pertaining to the eyes and parts of the eye;

2. identify word roots associated with the tear sacs and tear glands;

3. identify word roots associated with the ear and hearing;

4. identify word roots associated with the eardrum and inner ear; and

5. identify several types of drugs associated with visual and hearing disorders and treatments.

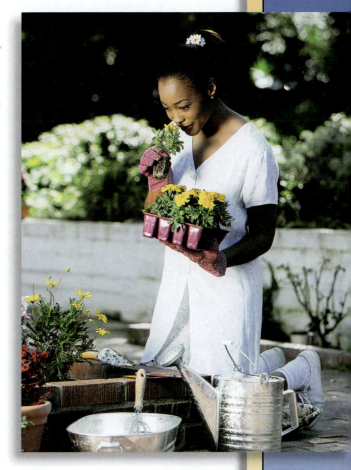

Orientation to Special Senses

The special senses (the sensory system) give us information about the environment. These senses allow us to see, hear, smell, taste, and feel. The sensory system includes the eyes, the ears, the nose, the taste buds of the tongue, and the sense receptors in the skin (see Chapter 12 for information regarding nerve receptors). This chapter focuses specifically on the eye and the ear.

The eye is a spherical organ that has a tough, protective outer covering, the sclera (the white portion). The conjunctiva lines the eyelid and covers the exposed portion of the eyeball. The middle layer, the choroid, is a vascular layer that provides blood to the eye. Inflammation of the conjunctiva is called conjunctivitis. The cornea is a section of the sclera that is situated in front of the optical lens and allows light to pass into the eye. The lens is held in place by ligaments and is situated between the two chambers of the eye. The anterior chamber contains a fluid called aqueous humor that nourishes the lens and the cornea. The posterior chamber contains a gelatinous fluid called vitreous humor that works in conjunction with the lens and the aqueous humor to refract light as it enters the eye.

The iris is a colored, contractile membrane that expands and contracts based on the amount of light present; the opening in the center of the iris is called the pupil. Inside the eye is a membrane called the retina that connects to the optic nerve, which transmits light impulses to the brain. The retina includes cells called rods and cones, which are the photoreceptors in the eye.

The tear glands, called lacrimal glands, are located above and near the outer edge of each eye; these glands produce fluid that cleanses and lubricates the eyes. Tears flow to the inner edges of the eyes and pass through lacrimal ducts into the nose (via the nasolacrimal ducts).

The ear has three divisions: the outer ear, the tympanic cavity (the middle section), and the labyrinth (the inner ear). The outer ear includes the auricle and the external auditory meatus (the ear canal). The middle ear includes the tympanic membrane (eardrum), which responds to vibrations and transmits these vibrations to the tiny bones in the middle ear (the malleus, incus, and stapes), which in turn transmit the vibrations to the cochlea in the inner ear. The eustachian tube connects the middle ear to the nasopharynx.

The cochlea contains fluid and has small nerve endings called hairs of Corti. Sound vibrations cause the fluid to move and to stimulate the hairs of Corti, which transmit impulses to the brain via the auditory nerve. The inner ear also contains the semicircular canals and the vestibule that connect to the cochlea and function to maintain equilibrium during movement.

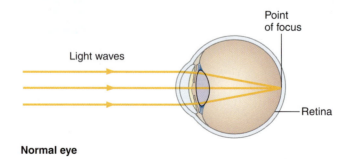

Normal eye

Terminology Presentation

Eye, Iris, and Cornea

As you listen to the CD, read the words and notice the pronunciations given.

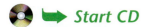

➡ Start CD

Look at Figure 15-1

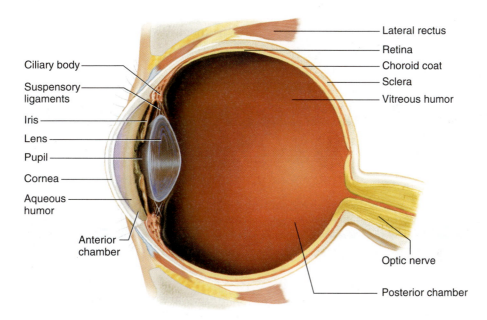

FIGURE 15-1   Side view of the eye.

ophthalm(o) a combining form denoting the eye			
Word	**Word Part**	**Definition**	**Answer**
1. ophthalmic (of-thal′mik)	-ic	pertaining to	1. _____
2. ophthalmology (of′thal-mol′o-je)	-logy	science of, study of	2. _____
3. ophthalmomycosis (of-thal′mo-mi-ko′sis)	myc(o) -osis	fungus abnormal condition	3. _____

continued

ocul(o)   a combining form denoting relationship to the eye

Word	Word Part	Definition	Answer
4. ocular (ok′u-lar)	-ar	pertaining to	4. _____
5. oculus (ok′u-lus)	-us	singular spelling	5. _____

opt(o)   a combining form denoting relationship to vision and sight

Word	Word Part	Definition	Answer
6. optical (op′ti-kal)	-al	pertaining to	6. _____
7. optometer (op-tom′e-ter)	-meter	instrument used for measurement	7. _____

-opia   a suffix denoting a condition or defect of the eye or of vision

Word	Word Part	Definition	Answer
8. presbyopia (pres′be-o′pe-ah)	presby-	old age	8. _____

irid(o)   a combining form denoting a relationship to the iris of the eye

Word	Word Part	Definition	Answer
9. iridectomy (ir′i-dek′to-me)	-ectomy	excision, removal	9. _____
10. iridectasis (ir′i-dek′tah-sis)	-ectasis	dilation, expansion	10. _____
11. iritis (i-ri′tis)	-itis	inflammation	11. _____
12. iridoplegia (ir′i-do-ple′je-ah)	-plegia	paralysis	12. _____

kerat(o), corne(o)   combining forms denoting relationship to the cornea or to horny tissue

Word	Word Part	Definition	Answer
13. keratocele (ker′ah-to-sel′)	-cele	herniation	13. _____
14. keratoplasty (ker′ah-to-plas′te)	-plasty	plastic surgery	14. _____

Word	Word Part	Definition	Answer
15. keratoscleritis (ker'ah-to-skle-ri'tis)	sclera -itis	white portion of eyeball inflammation	15. _____
16. radial keratotomy (ra'de-al) (ker'ah-tot'o-me)	radial -tomy	spoke-like incision into	16. _____
17. corneal (kor'ne-al)	-al	pertaining to	17. _____

 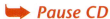 *Pause CD*

After practicing each word several times, use a sheet of paper to cover all columns except the Answer column. As each word is pronounced again on the CD, write it in the space provided.

 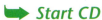 *Start CD*

Check the words you have written against the words in the left-hand column. If you have misspelled any words, practice writing them correctly.

Practice

_____

_____

_____

_____

_____

_____

_____

_____

_____

_____

_____

_____

_____

_____

_____

Practice

LESSON
15-1
Terminology Application

Without looking at your previous work, write the word that matches each definition.

Definition	Term
1. excision of all or part of the iris	_____
2. herniation of the cornea	_____
3. inflammation of the iris	_____
4. plastic surgery of the cornea; corneal graft	_____
5. the study of the science of the eye	_____
6. the eye	_____
7. fungal condition of the eye	_____
8. hardening of the lens due to old age	_____
9. pertaining to the eye	a. _____
	b. _____
10. paralysis of the iris	_____
11. pertaining to the cornea	_____
12. abnormal dilation of the iris	_____
13. pertaining to sight	_____
14. inflammation of the cornea and the sclera	_____
15. instrument used for measuring sight	_____
16. spoke-like incisions that flatten the cornea and correct myopia	_____

Check your answers against the information given in this lesson's terminology presentation. If you have any errors, count them and write the number in the blank at the top of the page. Sign your work and give it to your instructor.

Practice

Terminology Presentation

Lens, Pupil, Retina, Tear Sacs, Tear Glands, and Eyelids

As you listen to the CD, read the words and notice the pronunciations given.

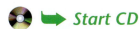 **Start CD**

See Figure 15-1, on page 423, and Figure 15-2

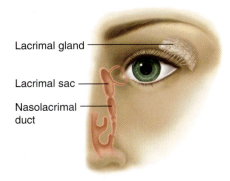

Lacrimal gland

Lacrimal sac

Nasolacrimal duct

FIGURE 15-2 The lacrimal gland and the lacrimal sac.

phac(o), phak(o) combining forms denoting relationship to the lens			
Word	**Word Part**	**Definition**	**Answer**
1. phacocele (fak′o-sel)	-cele	herniation	**1.** _____
2. phakitis (fak′i-tis)	-itis	inflammation	**2.** _____
3. phacomalacia (fak′o-mah-la′she-ah)	-malacia	softening	**3.** _____

pupill(o) a combining form denoting the pupil			
Word	**Word Part**	**Definition**	**Answer**
4. pupillary (pu′pi-ler-e)	-ary	pertaining to	**4.** _____

retin(o) a combining form denoting the retina			
Word	**Word Part**	**Definition**	**Answer**
5. retinal (ret′i-nal)	-al	pertaining to	**5.** _____

Word	Word Part	Definition	Answer
6. retinitis (ret′i-ni′tis)	-itis	inflammation	6. _____
7. retinopathy (ret′i-nop′ah-the)	-pathy	disease	7. _____
8. retinoscopy (ret′i-nos′ko-pe)	-scopy	visual examination	8. _____

lacrim(o), dacry(o)   combining forms denoting tears

Word	Word Part	Definition	Answer
9. lacrimal (lak′ri-mal)	-al	pertaining to	9. _____
10. dacryocyst (dak′re-o-sist′)	cyst(o)	sac	10. _____
11. dacryocystitis (dak′re-o-sis-ti′tis)	cyst(o) -itis	sac inflammation	11. _____
12. dacryoadenitis (dak′re-o-ad′e-ni′tis)	aden(o) -itis	gland inflammation	12. _____

blephar(o)   a combining form denoting the eyelid

Word	Word Part	Definition	Answer
13. blepharal (blef′ah-ral)	-al	pertaining to	13. _____
14. blepharoplasty (blef′ah-ro-plas′te)	-plasty	plastic surgery	14. _____
15. blepharoptosis (blef′ah-rop-to′sis)	-ptosis	falling	15. _____
16. blepharoplegia (blef′ah-ro-ple′je-ah)	-plegia	paralysis	16. _____
17. blepharitis (blef′ah-ri′tis)	-itis	inflammation	17. _____

  ➡ *Pause CD*

After practicing each word several times, use a sheet of paper to cover all columns except the Answer column. As each word is pronounced again on the CD, write in the space provided.

  ➡ *Start CD*

Check the words you have written against the words in the left-hand column. If you have misspelled any words, practice writing them correctly.

Practice

_____

_____

LESSON
15-2

Terminology Application

Without looking at your previous work, write the word that matches each definition.

Definition	Term
1. pertaining to tears	_____
2. pertaining to the eyelid	_____
3. pertaining to the retina	_____
4. the tear sac	_____
5. herniated lens	_____
6. paralysis of the eyelid	_____
7. inflammation of the tear sac	_____
8. plastic surgery of the eyelid	_____
9. inflammation of the retina	_____
10. drooping eyelid	_____
11. visual examination of the retina to detect refractive errors	_____
12. inflammation of the lens	_____
13. inflammation of the tear gland	_____
14. softening of the lens; a soft cataract	_____
15. inflammation of the eyelid	_____
16. pertaining to the pupil	_____
17. any disease of the retina	_____

Check your answers against the information given in this lesson's terminology presentation. If you have any errors, count them and write the number in the blank at the top of the page. Sign your work and give it to your instructor.

Practice

15-3   Terminology Presentation

The Ear and Hearing

As you listen to the CD, read the words and notice the pronunciations given.

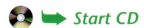 **Start CD**

Look at Figure 15-3

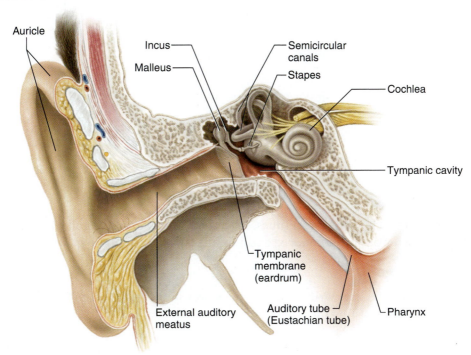

FIGURE 15-3   The parts of the ear.

auricle a word denoting the ear			
Word	**WordPart**	**Definition**	**Answer**
1. auricular (aw-rik′u-lar)	-ar	pertaining to	**1.** _____

ot(o) a combining form denoting relationship to the ear			
Word	**WordPart**	**Definition**	**Answer**
2. otitis (o-ti′tis)	-itis	inflammation	**2.** _____
3. otalgia (o-tal′je-ah)	-algia	pain	**3.** _____

continued

Word	WordPart	Definition	Answer
4. otoscope (o′to-skop)	-scope	instrument for viewing	**4.** _____
5. otomycosis (o′to-mi-ko′sis)	-mycosis	fungus	**5.** _____

audi(o), acou-	combining forms denoting relationship to hearing

Word	WordPart	Definition	Answer
6. audiologist (aw′de-ol′o-jist)	-ist	specialist	**6.** _____
7. auditory (aw′di-to′re)	-ory	pertaining to	**7.** _____
8. audiometry (aw′de-om′e-tre)	-metry	measurement	**8.** _____
9. acoustic (ah′koos′tik)	-ic	pertaining to	**9.** _____
10. presbycusis (pres′be-ku′sis)	presby-	old age	**10.** _____

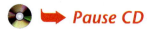 ➡ *Pause CD*

After practicing each word several times, use a sheet of paper to cover all columns except the Answer column. As each word is pronounced again on the CD, write it in the space provided.

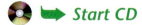 ➡ *Start CD*

Check the words you have written against the words in the left-hand column. If you have misspelled any words, practice writing them correctly.

Practice

_____

_____

_____

_____

_____

_____

_____

_____

_____

LESSON 15-3

Terminology Application

Without looking at your previous work, write the word that matches each definition.

Definition	Term
1. inflammation of the ear	_____
2. instrument used for viewing the ear	_____
3. pertaining to hearing	a. _____
	b. _____
4. pertaining to the ear	_____
5. loss of hearing due to old age	_____
6. pain in the ear	_____
7. a hearing specialist	_____
8. fungal infection of the ear	_____
9. measurement of hearing	_____

Check your answers against the information given in this lesson's terminology presentation. If you have any errors, count them and write the number in the blank at the top of the page. Sign your work and give it to your instructor.

Practice

LESSON

15-4 Terminology Presentation

Eardrum and Inner Ear

As you listen to the CD, read the words and notice the pronunciations given.

 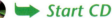 **Start CD**

Look at Figure 15-3 on page 433

tympan(o), myring(o)	combining forms denoting relationship to the tympanic cavity or the tympanic membrane; the eardrum		
Word	**Word Part**	**Definition**	**Answer**
1. tympanic (tim-pan′ik)	-ic	pertaining to	1. _____
2. tympanotomy (tim′pah-not′o-me)	-tomy	incision into	2. _____
3. myringectomy (mir′in-jek′to-me)	-ectomy	excision, removal	3. _____
4. myringomycosis (mi-ring′go-mi-ko′sis)	-myc(o) -osis	fungus abnormal condition	4. _____
5. myringitis (mir′in-ji′tis)	-itis	inflammation	5. _____

labyrinth	a word denoting the inner ear		
Word	**Word Part**	**Definition**	**Answer**
6. labyrinthitis (lab′i-rin-thi′tis)	-itis	inflammation	6. _____
7. labyrinthotomy (lab′i-rin-thot′o-me)	-tomy	incision into	7. _____

cochlea	a word denoting the organ of hearing in the inner ear		
Word	**Word Part**	**Definition**	**Answer**
8. cochlear (kok′le-ar)	-ar	pertaining to	8. _____
9. cochleitis (kok′le-i′tis)	-itis	inflammation	9. _____

continued

salping(o)	a combining form denoting relationship to a tube: specifically the auditory (eustachian) tube or the uterine (fallopian) tube			

	Word	Word Part	Definition	Answer
10.	salpingoscopy (sal′ping-gos′ko-pe)	-scopy	visual examination	10. _____
11.	auditory salpingitis (aw′di-to′re sal′pin-ji′tis)	auditory -itis	pertaining to hearing inflammation	11. _____

  Pause CD

After practicing each word several times, use a sheet of paper to cover all columns except the Answer column. As each word is pronounced again on the CD, write it in the space provided.

  Start CD

Check the words you have written against the words in the left-hand column. If you have misspelled any words, practice writing them correctly.

Practice

_____

_____

_____

_____

_____

_____

_____

_____

_____

_____

_____

_____

_____

_____

_____

_____

LESSON
15-4

Terminology Application

Without looking at your previous work, write the word that matches each definition.

Definition	Term
1. visual examination of the auditory tube	_____
2. pertaining to the cochlea	_____
3. incision into the labyrinth	_____
4. inflammation of the eardrum	_____
5. pertaining to the eardrum	_____
6. inflammation of the cochlea	_____
7. incision into the eardrum	_____
8. inflammation of the labyrinth	_____
9. fungal infection of the eardrum	_____
10. pertaining to an inflammation of the auditory tube	_____
11. excision of the eardrum	_____

Check your answers against the information given in this lesson's terminology presentation. If you have any errors, count them and write the number in the blank at the top of the page. Sign your work and give it to your instructor.

Practice

As you listen to the CD, read the words and notice the pronunciations given.

 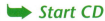 **Start CD**

Word	Definition	Example: Generic Name	Example: Brand/ Trade Name	Answer
ophthalmics	agents used in the treatment of disorders/diseases of the eye			1._____
a. conjunctivitis drugs		azelastine erythromycin levofloxacin	Astelin (various) Levaquin	2._____
b. glaucoma drugs		apraclonidine hydrochloride betaxolol hydrochloride	Iopidine Betoptic	3._____
c. mydriatics; pupil-dilating drugs		atropine sulfate	Atropair, Atropen, Atropinol	4._____
otics	agents used to treat ear disorders	benzocaine chloramphenicol	Americaine Chloromycetin	5._____

 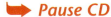 **Pause CD**

After practicing each word several times, use a sheet of paper to cover all columns except the Answer column. As each word is pronounced again on the CD, write it in the space provided.

  Start CD

Check the words you have written against the words in the left-hand column. If you have misspelled any words, practice writing them correctly.

Practice

LESSON
15-5

Terminology Application

Without looking at your previous work, write the word that matches each definition.

Definition	Term
1. agents used to treat conjunctivitis	_____
2. agents used to treat any disorder/disease of the eye	_____
3. agents used to treat glaucoma	_____
4. agents used to treat ear disorders	_____
5. agents used to dilate the pupil of the eye	_____

Check your answers against the information given in this lesson's terminology presentation. If you have any errors, count them and write the number in the blank at the top of the page. Sign your work and give it to your instructor.

Practice

CHAPTER 15 Terminology Review

This is a review of the word parts and words you have learned in the preceding lessons. Some of the medical terms listed below may be new, but they are composed of the word parts and word roots that you have already learned. Read the words below as they are pronounced on the CD.

  Start CD

Word Element Review

Word	Word Part	Meaning of Word Part
1. audiometry	audi(o)	_____
audiometry	-metry	_____
(aw'de-om'e-tre)	Meaning of Word	_____
2. cochlear	cochlea	_____
cochlear	-ar	_____
(kok'le-ar)	Meaning of Word	_____
3. myringectomy	myring(o)	_____
myringectomy	-ectomy	_____
(mir'in-jek'to-me)	Meaning of Word	_____
4. iridoplegia	irid(o)	_____
iridoplegia	plegia	_____
(ir'i-do-ple'je-ah)	Meaning of Word	_____
5. presbycusis	presby-	_____
presbycusis	acou-	_____
(pres'be-ku'sis)	Meaning of Word	_____
6. otoscope	ot(o)	_____
otoscope	-scope	_____
(o'to-skop)	Meaning of Word	_____
7. ophthalmic	ophthalm(o)	_____
ophthalmic	-ic	_____
(of-thal'mik)	Meaning of Word	_____

Word	Word Part	Meaning of Word Part
8. phakitis	phak(o)	_____
phakitis	-itis	_____
(fak'i-tis)	Meaning of Word	_____
9. presbyopia	presby-	_____
presbyopia	-opia	_____
(pres'be-o'pe-ah)	Meaning of Word	_____
10. pupillary	pupill(o)	_____
pupillary	-ary	_____
(pu'pi-ler-e)	Meaning of Word	_____
11. corneal	corne(o)	_____
corneal	-al	_____
(kor'ne-al)	Meaning of Word	_____
12. retinitis	retin(o)	_____
retinitis	-itis	_____
(ret'i-ni'tis)	Meaning of Word	_____
13. keratocele	kerat(o)	_____
keratocele	-cele	_____
(ker'ah-to-sel')	Meaning of Word	_____
14. dacryocystitis	dacry(o)	_____
dacryocystitis	cyst(o)	_____
dacryocystitis	-itis	_____
(dak're-o-sis-ti'tis)	Meaning of Word	_____
15. radial keratotomy	radial	_____
radial keratotomy	kerat(o)	_____
radial keratotomy	-tomy	_____
(ra'de-al ker'ah-tot'o-me)	Meaning of Word	_____

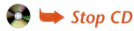 ➡ *Stop CD*

On the lines provided, write in the meanings of as many suffixes, prefixes, roots, and words as you can from memory. Check your definitions in the glossary or a medical dictionary, and make any needed corrections.

CHAPTER 15
Terminology Review

Complete this review, and turn it in to your instructor when you are finished.

Definition

Each phrase below defines one of the words you have just studied. Without looking at your previous work, write in the word that matches each definition.

Definition	Term
1. pertaining to an inflammation of the auditory tube	_____
2. hardening of the lens of the eye due to old age	_____
3. cornea grafting	_____
4. expansion of the iris	_____
5. pertaining to the eardrum	_____
6. instrument used to measure sight	_____
7. inflammation of the cornea and the sclera	_____
8. fungal infection of the eardrum	_____
9. instrument used for viewing the ear	_____
10. inflammation of a tear sac	_____
11. incision into the labyrinth	_____
12. paralysis of an eyelid	_____
13. fungal infection of the eye	_____
14. visual examination of retina to look for refractive errors	_____
15. visual examination of the auditory tube	_____
16. inflammation of the cochlea	_____
17. the lacrimal sac	_____
18. inflammation of a tear gland	_____

Definition	Term
19. drooping eyelid	_____
20. hearing specialist	_____

Matching

Match the following definitions with the terms given. Put the letter of the correct definition to the left of the term.

Term	Definition
_____ **21.** acoustic	**a.** excision of the eardrum
_____ **22.** labyrinthitis	**b.** pertaining to inflammation of the auditory tube
_____ **23.** tympanotomy	**c.** loss of hearing due to old age
_____ **24.** oculus	**d.** paralysis of the iris
_____ **25.** iridoplegia	**e.** any disease of the retina
_____ **26.** phacocele	**f.** herniation of the lens
_____ **27.** myringectomy	**g.** pertaining to hearing
_____ **28.** retinopathy	**h.** the eye
_____ **29.** presbycusis	**i.** incision into the eardrum
_____ **30.** auditory salpingitis	**j.** inflammation of the labyrinth

CHAPTER 15

Terminology Review

Case Studies

Read the following brief case studies. In each case study, some terms are followed by a superscript letter. Write a brief definition for each of those terms on the corresponding lines below.

1. G.Z. contracted ophthalmomycosis[a] and has visited her ophthalmologist[b] several times for examination and treatment. She has developed mild conjunctivitis[c] and blepharitis[d], which will require continued treatment.

   a. _____

   b. _____

   c. _____

   d. _____

2. Y.J. has chronic sinus problems, which often cause her to have swollen nasal[a] passages, otitis[b], and pharyngitis[c]. Her goal is to buy a home in the western United States where the climate will not exacerbate her condition.

   a. _____

   b. _____

   c. _____

3. D.R. was hit in the eye while he was playing baseball and developed severe iritis[a], which necessitated his having a partial iridectomy[b]. The surgery was successful, and he has not had much pain during his recovery.

   a. _____

   b. _____

4. E. has a swollen right dacryocyst[a] in addition to dacryoadenitis[b]. His symptoms have included painful dacryocystitis[c] and phakitis[d].

   a. _____

   b. _____

   c. _____

   d. _____

5. When B. goes to her ophthalmologist[a], a nurse administers a mydriatic[b] as a prep for the ophthalmoscopy[c]. The doctor examines the internal structure of the eyes, checks the internal blood vessels, and checks the pressure of the aqueous chamber to determine whether or not glaucoma[d] is present.

a. _____

b. _____

c. _____

d. _____

Labeling

Fill in the blanks with the correct terminology.

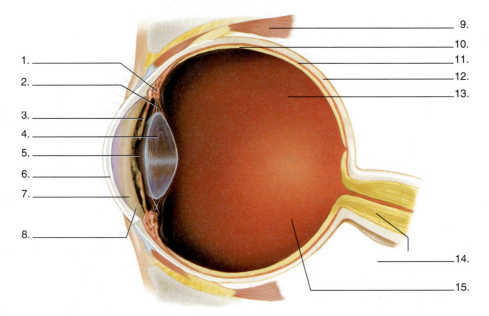

FIGURE 15-4 Side view of the eye.

You may now go on to Chapter Test 15.

PART
3

Medical Specialties and Psychiatric Terminology

16

Medical Specialties

Objectives

After completing Chapter 16, you should be able to do the following:

1. identify the terms associated with various medical specialties;

2. identify the terms used to denote specialists in specific medical fields; and

3. understand the terms used to denote combined medical specialties such as gastroenterology (stomach and intestines specialty).

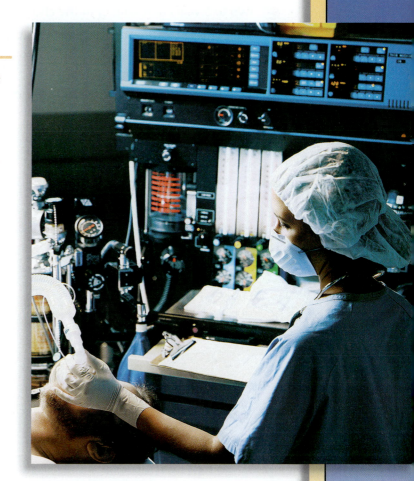

Orientation to Medical Specialties

The lessons in this chapter provide general information regarding a sampling of medical specialties. Students working in any area of health care will come into contact with specialists in many of these areas, so you need to familiarize yourself with many of the terms presented in this chapter.

It is also important to understand the process an individual must follow to become a physician or a specialist. The chronological sequence of this process includes the successful completion of the following steps:

▶ A 4-year pre-med undergraduate program.

▶ A 4-year term in medical school.

▶ Two to 5 years of residency in the chosen specialty internal medicine, radiology, etc.

▶ Sometimes a post-residency fellowship in a subspecialty (for example, an internist might choose cardiology or gastroenterology as a subspecialty; a general surgeon might choose thoracic surgery or proctology).

A clear knowledge of various specialties and their functions is essential for anyone working in the medical field.

16-1 Terminology Presentation

Medical Specialties, Part 1

As you listen to the CD, read the words and notice the pronunciations given.

 Start CD

Specialty	Specialist	Answer
1. anesthesiology (an'es-the'ze-ol'o-je)	anesthesiologist (an'es-the'ze-ol'o-jist)	1. _____

Anesthesiology is the study and practice of administering anesthetic agents.

2. dermatology (der'mah-tol'o-je)	dermatologist (der'mah-tol'o-jist)	2. _____

Dermatology deals with the diagnosis and treatment of diseases of the skin.

3. family practice (family medicine) (fam'i-le prak'tis)	family practitioner (fam'i-le prak-tish'un-er)	3. _____

Family medicine concerns the diagnosis and treatment of disorders of all members of the family, regardless of age or sex, on a continuing basis.

4. obstetrics and gynecology (ob-stet'riks) (gi'ne-kol'o-je)	obstetrician and gynecologist (ob'ste-trish'un) (gi'ne-kol'o-jist)	4. _____

Obstetrics deals with pregnancy, prenatal care, and childbirth and its aftermath; gynecology deals with disorders of women.

5. ophthalmology (of'thal-mol'o-je)	ophthalmologist (of'thal-mol'o-jist)	5. _____

This specialty deals with diseases of the eye. The ophthalmologist is a physician who deals with all areas involving the eye, as distinct from the optometrist who examines and tests eyes and treats visual defects with corrective lenses but is not a physician.

6. physical medicine and rehabilitation (fiz'e-kal med'i-sin)	physiatrist (fiz'e-at'rist)	6. _____

Physical medicine and rehabilitation deal with the diagnosis and treatment of diseases with the aid of physical agents such as heat, light, water, or mechanical apparatus. Exercise therapy and the use of braces are involved. The nonphysician in this area is known as a physical therapist.

7. psychiatry and neurology (si-ki'ah-tre) (nu-rol'o-je)	psychiatrist and neurologist (si-ki'ah-trist) (nu-rol'o-jist)	7. _____

Psychiatry deals with functional disorders of the mind. Neurology deals with disorders of the nervous system caused by organic disease or injury.

continued

Specialty	Specialist	Answer
8. otolaryngology (o′to-lar′in-gol′o-je)	otolaryngologist (o′to-lar′in-gol′o-jist)	8. _____

Otolaryngology involves the diagnosis and treatment of diseases of the ear, nose, and throat. Both surgical and nonsurgical techniques are employed.

Specialty	Specialist	Answer
9. pathology (pah-thol′o-je)	pathologist (pah-thol′o-jist)	9. _____

The pathologist deals primarily with the diagnosis of disease. By studying the structural changes that have taken place, the pathologist can also determine the cause of death.

Specialty	Specialist	Answer
10. pediatrics (pe′de-at′riks)	pediatrician (pe′de-ah′trish′un)	10. _____

Pediatrics involves the diagnosis and treatment of diseases of children.

➥*Pause CD*

After practicing each word several times, use a sheet of paper to cover everything except the Answer column. As each word is pronounced again on the CD, write it in the space provided.

➥ *Start CD*

Check the words you have written against the words in presented. If you have misspelled any words, practice writing them correctly.

Practice

_____

_____

_____

_____

_____

_____

_____

_____

_____

_____

_____

_____

_____

Terminology Application

Complete the sentences below with the names of the specialties and specialists.

1. _____ is the branch of medicine that treats disorders of the skin. The specialist

   is known as a(n) _____.

2. The division of medicine that studies and administers anesthetic agents is known as

   _____. The specialist is called a(n) _____.

3. A _____ deals with the diagnosis of diseases by studying structural changes in

   the body. This branch of medicine is called _____.

4. _____ is the branch of medicine treating disorders and diseases of children. The

   specialist is known as a(n) _____.

5. _____ and _____ are branches of medicine
   dealing with female disorders and pregnancy and childbirth. The specialists are known as

   _____ and _____.

6. The _____ is the specialist who treats disorders of the ear, nose, and throat. The

   specialty is called _____.

7. The _____ treats disorders of the eye. The specialty is known

   as _____.

8. The specialist who uses natural elements, such as heat and light, for treatment is known as a(n)

   _____. The branch of medicine is called _____.

continued

9. The _____ and _____ deal with disorders of the

nervous system and the mind. These branches of medicine are called _____ and

_____.

10. The _____ _____ specializes in the diagnosis and
treatment of all family members, regardless of age or sex, on a continuing basis. The specialty is known as

_____ _____.

Check your answers against the information given in this lesson's terminology presentation. If you have any errors, count them and write the number in the blank at the top of the page. Sign your work and give it to your instructor.

16-2 Terminology Presentation

Medical Specialties, Part 2

As you listen to the CD, read the words and notice the pronunciations given.

  Start CD

Specialty	Specialist	Answer
1. surgery (general surgery) (sur′jer-e)	surgeon (general surgeon) (sur′jun)	1. _____

Surgery is the branch of medicine that treats pathologic or traumatic conditions by operative procedures. The general surgeon operates for a variety of conditions, but some surgeons limit their work to just one.

2. thoracic surgery (tho-ras′ik)	thoracic surgeon (tho-ras′ik)	2. _____

The thoracic surgeon deals with the diagnosis and treatment (mainly surgical) of disorders of the organs of the thoracic cavity, generally the heart and lungs.

3. urology (u-rol′o-je)	urologist (u-rol′o-jist)	3. _____

Urology deals with the diagnosis and treatment of disorders and diseases of the urogenital system. Disorders of the urinary system of both men and women are treated by the urologist. Treatment of male genital disorders are common in this practice.

4. proctology (colon and rectal surgery) (prok-tol′o-je)	proctologist (prok-tol′o-jist)	4. _____

Diseases and disorders of the rectum and sigmoid colon are included under this heading. Treatment often involves surgery for such disorders as cancer, hemorrhoids, and anal fissures.

5. plastic surgery (plas′tik sur′jer-e)	plastic surgeon (plas′tik sur′jun)	5. _____

Plastic surgery deals with the restoration or repair of defects of the human body. This repair often is accomplished by means of tissue grafting.

6. orthopedic surgery (or′tho-pe′dik)	orthopedic surgeon or orthopedist (or′tho-pe′dist)	6. _____

Orthopedic surgery is concerned with the treatment of musculoskeletal disorders. Surgery is often done to alleviate these conditions, but nonsurgical techniques utilizing casts, braces, or strappings are sometimes used. *Orthopedic* is also spelled *orthopaedic*, but the pronunciation remains the same.

7. neurological surgery (nu′ro-loj′ ik-al)	neurosurgeon (nu′ro-sur′jun)	7. _____

This branch of medicine deals with the diagnosis and mainly surgical treatment of diseases and disorders of the central nervous system (brain and spinal cord).

continued

Specialty	Specialist	Answer
8. radiology (ra′de-ol′o-je)	radiologist (ra′de-ol′o-jist)	8. _____

Radiology involves the diagnostic and therapeutic use of radiant energy. Roentgen rays, commonly called X-rays, are a major tool in diagnosing disease. Cobalt and other types of energy are used in treating diseases such as cancer.

9. nuclear medicine (nu′kle-ar)		9. _____

This branch of medicine is concerned with the use of radionuclides in the diagnosis and treatment of disease.

10. preventive medicine (pre-ven′tiv)		10. _____

This branch of study and practice aims at the prevention of disease.

➡️ *Pause CD*

After practicing each word several times, use a sheet of paper to cover everything except the Answer column. As each word is pronounced again on the CD, write it in the space provided.

➡️ *Start CD*

Check the words you have written against the words presented. If you have misspelled any words, practice writing them correctly.

Practice

_____

_____

_____

_____

_____

_____

_____

_____

_____

_____

_____

_____

_____

Terminology Application

Complete the sentences below with the names of the specialties and specialists.

1. _____ is the branch of medicine dealing with the restoration or repair of injuries or defects of the human body. The specialist in this field is called a(n)

   _____ _____.

2. The _____ is the specialist in using X-ray or roentgenography. This branch of

   medicine is called _____.

3. _____ deals with the diagnosis and treatment of disorders of the urinary tract.

   The specialist is called a(n) _____.

4. A(n) _____ treats, mainly with surgery, disorders of the central nervous system.

   This specialty is known as _____ _____.

5. A(n) _____ _____ diagnoses and surgically treats

   disorders of the organs of the thoracic cavity. The specialty is known as _____

   _____.

6. _____ is that branch of medicine dealing with disorders of the rectum and

   colon. The specialist is a(n) _____.

7. The _____ treats pathological conditions by operative procedures. This practice

   is known as _____.

8. _____ _____ is the branch of medicine that aims at
   the prevention of disease.

continued

9. The branch of medicine concerned with the use of radionuclides in the diagnosis and treatment of disease

is known as _____ _____.

10. _____ _____ is the branch of medicine dealing with

the treatment of bones, muscles, etc. The specialist is known as a(n) _____

_____ or a(n) _____.

Check your answers against the information given in this lesson's terminology presentation. If you have any errors, count them and write the number in the blank at the top of the page. Sign your work and give it to your instructor.

Medical Specialties, Part 3

As you listen to the CD, read the words and notice the pronunciations given.

 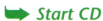 **Start CD**

Specialty	Specialist	Answer
1. internal medicine (in-ter′nal med′i-sin)	internist (in-ter′nist)	1. _____

The internist diagnoses and treats disorders and diseases of the internal structures of the body.

2. allergy and immunology (al′er-je) (im′u-nol′o-je)	allergist and immunologist (al′er-jist) (im′u-nol′o-jist)	2. _____

These specialties are concerned with the diagnosis and treatment of allergies and the body's resistance to disease.

3. cardiology (kar-de-ol′o-je)	cardiologist (kar-de-ol′o-jist)	3. _____

The diagnosis and treatment of heart disorders is the cardiologist's area of specialization.

4. gastroenterology (gas′tro-en′ter-ol′o-je)	gastroenterologist (gas′tro-en′ter-ol′o-jist)	4. _____

The gastroenterologist deals with the diagnosis and treatment of diseases of the stomach and intestines.

5. pulmonary disease (pul′mo-ner′e)	chest specialist	5. _____

The diagnosis and treatment of diseases of the chest or thorax is the concern of this specialist.

6. endocrinology and metabolism (en′do-kri-nol′o-je) (me-tab′o-lizm)	endocrinologist (en′do-kri-nol′o-jist)	6. _____

The endocrinologist studies the internally secreting glands and their effect on the body and its metabolism.

7. hematology-oncology (hem′ah-tol′o-je) (ong-kol′o-je)	hematologist-oncologist (hem′ah-tol′o-jist) (ong-kol′o-jist)	7. _____

Hematology is the branch of medicine that treats the blood and blood-forming elements, and oncology deals with tumors, primarily cancer.

8. infectious disease (epidemiology) (in-fek′shus)	epidemiologist (ep′i-de′me-ol′o-jist)	8. _____

Epidemiology is the diagnosis and treatment of diseases capable of being communicated from one host to another.

Specialty	Specialist	Answer
9. nephrology (ne-frol′o-je)	nephrologist (ne-frol′o-jist)	9. _____

The nephrologist diagnoses and treats diseases and disorders that involve the kidneys.

| 10. rheumatology
(roo′mah-tol′o-je) | rheumatologist
(roo′mah-tol′o-jist) | 10. _____ |

The science of rheumatism, a variety of disorders involving connective tissues (joints and related structures), is the area of this specialist.

➡ *Pause CD*

After practicing each word several times, use a sheet of paper to cover everything except the Answer column. As each word is pronounced again on the CD, write it in the space provided.

➡ *Start CD*

Check the words you have written against the words presented. If you have misspelled any words, practice writing them correctly.

Practice

_____

_____

_____

_____

_____

_____

_____

_____

_____

_____

_____

_____

_____

_____

_____

_____

LESSON
16-3

Terminology Application

Complete the sentences below with the names of the specialties and specialists.

1. The _____ and _____ deal with the diagnosis and

   treatment of allergies and the body's resistance to disease. The specialties are known as

   _____ and _____.

2. A(n) _____ deals with the diagnosis and treatment of diseases capable of being
   communicated from one host to another.

3. _____ _____ is the branch of medicine that deals
   with the diagnosis and treatment of the internal structures of the body. This specialist is known as a(n)

   _____.

4. The _____ specializes in the diagnosis and treatment of kidney disorders. The

   specialty is known as _____.

5. _____ and _____ are the branches of medicine
   dealing with blood and blood-forming elements and cancer. The specialists in these areas are

   _____ and _____.

6. A(n) _____ treats heart disorders. Her or his specialty is known as

   _____.

7. A(n) _____ treats a variety of disorders of connective tissue (rheumatism).

   The specialty is _____.

8. _____ is the science of the diagnosis and treatment of diseases of the stomach

   and intestines. This specialist is known as a(n) _____.

continued

9. The specialty involved with the study of internally secreting glands is known as

_____ and _____. The specialist is called

a(n) _____.

10. _____ _____ is the branch of medicine that deals
with the diagnosis and treatment of diseases of the chest or thorax. The specialist is called

a(n) _____ _____.

Check your answers against the information given in this lesson's terminology presentation. If you have any errors, count them and write the number in the blank at the top of the page. Sign your work and give it to your instructor.

CHAPTER
16

Terminology Review

This is a review of the specialties and specialists you have learned about in the preceding lessons. Read the words below as they are pronounced on the CD.

 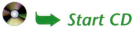 **Start CD**

Word Review

Word	Definition
1. radiologist	_____
	_____
	_____
2. ophthalmology	_____
	_____
	_____
3. pharmacology	_____
	_____
	_____
4. urology	_____
	_____
	_____
5. nephrologist	_____
	_____
	_____
6. pathology	_____
	_____
	_____
7. internal medicine	_____
	_____
	_____

Word	Definition

8. hematology _____

_____

_____

9. pathologist _____

_____

_____

10. orthopedic surgery _____

_____

_____

11. pediatrics _____

_____

_____

12. rheumatology _____

_____

_____

13. proctologist _____

_____

_____

14. gastroenterologist _____

_____

_____

15. otolaryngology _____

_____

_____

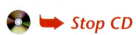 *Stop CD*

On the lines provided, write in the definitions of as many words as you can from memory. Check your definitions in the glossary or a medical dictionary, and make any needed corrections.

CHAPTER 16   Terminology Review

Complete this review, and turn it in to your instructor when you are finished.

Definition

Write the definition for each of the following terms to the right of the term.

Term	Definition
1. dermatology	_____
2. anesthesiology	_____
3. ophthalmologist	_____
4. urology	_____
5. plastic surgeon	_____
6. preventive medicine	_____
7. otolaryngologist	_____
8. pathology	_____
9. nephrology	_____
10. rheumatology	_____
11. ophthalmology	_____
12. neurosurgeon	_____
13. internal medicine	_____
14. pediatrician	_____
15. orthopedic surgery	_____
16. anesthesiologist	_____
17. radiologist	_____
18. obstetrician	_____
19. thoracic surgeon	_____
20. psychiatry	_____

continued

Matching

Match the following definitions with the terms given. Place the letter of the correct definition to the left of the term.

Term	Definition
_____ 21. gynecology	**a.** diagnosis and treatment of diseases and disorders of the rectum and sigmoid colon
_____ 22. epidemiology	**b.** diagnosis and treatment of diseases and disorders of the urogenital system
_____ 23. thoracic surgery	**c.** diagnosis and treatment of diseases of the stomach and intestines
_____ 24. proctology	**d.** diagnosis and treatment of tumors and cancers
_____ 25. nephrology	**e.** diagnosis and treatment of disorders of women
_____ 26. endocrinology	**f.** diagnosis and treatment of diseases and disorders of the kidneys
_____ 27. urology	**g.** diagnosis and treatment of diseases capable of being communicated from one host to another
_____ 28. hematology	**h.** diagnosis and treatment of diseases of the internally secreting glands
_____ 29. gastroenterology	**i.** diagnosis and treatment of diseases of the blood
_____ 30. oncology	**j.** diagnosis and treatment of disorders of the thoracic (chest) cavity

You may now go on to Chapter Test 16.

17

Psychiatric Terminology

Objectives

After completing Chapter 17, you should be able to do the following:

1. identify general terms used to describe psychiatric disorders;

2. know the difference between an organic disorder and a functional disorder;

3. understand the terms used to describe organic disorders;

4. understand the terms used to describe functional disorders; and

5. identify several types of drugs associated with psychiatric disorders and treatments.

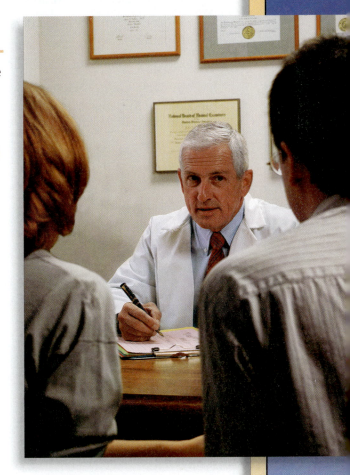

Orientation to Psychiatric Terminology

Unlike the other chapters in this textbook, this chapter does not, by the nature of its content, follow anatomic categories. For centuries the function of the mind has intrigued people, and many theories abound regarding its complexities.

When discussing psychiatric terminology, we use terms such as *personality disorders, behavior disorders, mental illness, psychosis, eating disorders, and mental health*. There are two primary categorizations of personality, mental, and behavior disorders:

▶ Organic disorders—disorders in which an organic cause (i.e., originating in a body organ) can be identified

   Examples: alcoholism, drug-induced disorder, brain disease

▶ Functional disorders—disorders without an organic basis (i.e., not originating in a body organ; idiopathic)

   Examples: feelings of inadequacy, antisocial behavior, phobias

In both cases, these disorders cause significant distress, disability, or impairment in areas of social functioning. In general, good mental health is indicated in our society by success in working and loving and by the ability to resolve conflicts maturely.

Terminology Presentation

Personality Disorders

As you listen to the CD, read the terms and notice the pronunciations given.

 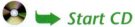 *Start CD*

Term	Definition	Answer
1. personality disorders	Mental disorders characterized by an inflexible and poorly adaptive personality. These traits result in definite impairment in social functioning. Because of these impairments, the patient's actions may have a generally adverse effect on society.	1. _____
2. affective type (cyclothymia) (si-klo-thi′me-ah)	Cyclic personality disorder characterized by symptoms of manic (excited or violent) and depressive (sad or despairing) episodes of behavior.	2. _____
3. antisocial type	Personality disorder marked by continuous and chronic antisocial behavior in which the rights of others are often violated.	3. _____
4. avoidant type	Personality disorder characterized by hypersensitivity to criticism, anxiety, an exaggeration of difficulties, and general timidity.	4. _____
5. borderline type	Personality disorder marked by instability of mood. Impulsive and self-damaging acts are common.	5. _____
6. dependent type	Personality disorder characterized by an excessive need to be taken care of, resulting in submissive and clinging behavior.	6. _____
7. histrionic type (his-tre-on′ik)	Personality disorder marked by excessive attention-seeking behavior.	7. _____
8. inadequate type	Personality disorder marked by general ineptness or social, intellectual, and physical awkwardness.	8. _____

continued

Term	Definition	Answer
9. introverted type	Form of schizoidal personality in which there is a defect in forming interpersonal relationships.	9. _____
10. masochistic type (mas-o-kis′tik)	Personality disorder in which the person seems to derive pleasure from physical or psychological pain inflicted on oneself either by the self or by others.	10. _____
11. narcissistic type (self-love) (nahr-si-sis′tik)	Personality disorder in which interpersonal problems arise because of an inflated sense of self-worth.	11. _____
12. obsessive-compulsive type	Personality disorder characterized by a preoccupation with orderliness, perfection, and control.	12. _____ _____
13. paranoid type (par′ah-noid)	Personality disorder characterized by a pattern of distrust and suspiciousness of others without reason.	13. _____
14. passive-aggressive type	Personality disorder marked by aggressive behavior manifested in a passive way, such as pouting, procrastination, or stubborness.	14. _____
15. schizoid type (skiz′oid) (skit′soid)	Personality disorder in which there is withdrawal from affectional and social contacts.	15. _____
16. schizotypal type (skiz′o-ti-pal) (skit-so-ti′pal)	Personality disorder that appears to be a form of schizoid personality. Individuals with this disorder manifest oddities of thinking, perception, communication, and behavior.	16. _____

  Pause CD

After practicing each term several times, use a sheet of paper to cover all columns except the Answer column. As each term is pronounced again on the CD, write it in the space provided.

  Start CD

Check the terms you have written against the terms in the left-hand column. If you have misspelled any terms, practice writing them correctly.

Practice

_____

_____

_____

Terminology Application

Without looking at your previous work, write the term that matches each definition.

Definition	Term
1. Personality disorder marked by continuous and chronic antisocial behavior in which the rights of others are often violated.	_____
2. Cyclic personality disorder characterized by symptoms of manic (excited or violent) and depressive (sad or despairing) episodes of behavior.	_____
3. Personality disorder in which interpersonal problems arise because of an inflated sense of self-worth.	_____
4. Personality disorder characterized by an excessive need to be taken care of, resulting in submissive and clinging behavior.	_____
5. Personality disorder characterized by hypersensitivity to criticism, anxiety, an exaggeration of difficulties, and general timidity.	_____
6. A form of schizoidal personality in which there is a defect in forming interpersonal relationships.	_____
7. Personality disorder marked by excessive attention-seeking behavior.	_____
8. Personality disorder marked by instability of mood. Impulsive and self-damaging acts are common.	_____
9. Personality disorder characterized by a pattern of distrust and suspiciousness of others without reason.	_____
10. Personality disorder characterized by a preoccupation with orderliness, perfection, and control.	_____
11. Mental disorders characterized by an inflexible and poorly adaptive personality. These traits result in definite impairment in social functioning. Because of these impairments, the patient's actions may have a generally adverse effect on society.	_____

continued

Definition	Term
12. Personality disorder in which the person seems to derive pleasure from physical or psychological pain inflicted on oneself either by the self or by others.	_____
13. Personality disorder marked by general ineptness or social, intellectual, and physical awkwardness.	_____
14. Personality disorder in which there is withdrawal from affectional and social contacts.	_____
15. Personality disorder that appears to be a form of schizoid personality. Individuals with this disorder manifest oddities of thinking, perception, communication, and behavior.	_____
16. Personality disorder marked by aggressive behavior manifested in a passive way, such as pouting, procrastination, or stubbornness.	_____

Check your answers against the information given in this lesson's terminology presentation. If you have any errors, count them and write the number in the blank at the top of the page. Sign your work and give it to your instructor.

LESSON
17-2 Terminology Presentation

Anxiety, Somatoform, Factitious, and Dissociative Disorders

As you listen to the CD, read the terms and notice the pronunciations given.

  Start CD

Term	Definition	Answer
1. anxiety disorders	A group of mental disorders in which apprehension, tension, or uneasiness from anticipation of danger predominate.	1. _____
2. panic attack	A period of intense fear or discomfort, with fears of dying or losing control. Some physical symptoms include smothering sensations and trembling.	2. _____
3. agoraphobia (ag-o-ra-fo′be-ah)	Anxiety about being in places where help may not be available should a panic attack occur.	3. _____
4. specific phobia	Intense fear caused by a specific object or situation. Examples: *claustrophobia*—fear of closed places; *acrophobia*—fear of heights; *ailurophobia*—fear of cats; *xenophobia*—fear of strangers.	4. _____
5. social phobia	Characterized by an anxiety provoked by exposure to types of social or performance situations. Example: performing in front of others.	5. _____
6. obsessive-compulsive disorders	Disorders marked by recurrent compulsions (repetitive behaviors) and obsessions (persistent ideas, thoughts, and impulses). Compulsions may involve repetitive washing of hands, checking constantly to see if a door is locked, etc. Obsessions may involve repeated thoughts such as thoughts of becoming contaminated by shaking hands.	6. _____
7. somatoform disorders (so-mat′o-form)	A group of disorders with symptoms suggesting physical ailments but without organic findings evident.	7. _____

continued

Term	Definition	Answer
8. somatization disorder (so-mah-ti-za′shun)	Disorder marked by multiple physical complaints not fully explained by any known medical condition.	8. _____
9. conversion disorder	Disorder characterized by a symptom suggestive of a neurologic impairment that affects the senses (for example, blindness) or motor function (for example, paralysis).	9. _____
10. pain disorder	Somatoform disorder characterized by pain, for which there is no physical finding, in one or more parts of the body; causes distress or impairs work or social functioning.	10. _____
11. hypochondriasis (hi-po-kon-dri′ah-sis)	Mental disorder marked by a morbid preoccupation with one's health or a fear of having some disease, despite a lack of identification of disease on examination.	11. _____
12. body dysmorphic disorder (dis-mor′fik)	Disorder in which the patient imagines a defect in his or her appearance, even though he or she appears normal to others.	12. _____
13. factitious disorder (Münchausen's syndrome) (fak-tish′as)	Disorder in which there is intentional feigning of physical or psychological symptoms to obtain medical treatment.	13. _____
14. dissociative disorders (dis-so-she′ah-tiv)	A group of mental disorders in which the patient is unable to recall important personal information.	14. _____

  ➡ *Pause CD*

After practicing each term several times, use a sheet of paper to cover all columns except the Answer column. As each term is pronounced again on the CD, write it in the space provided.

  ➡ *Start CD*

Check the terms you have written against the terms in the left-hand column. If you have misspelled any terms, practice writing them correctly.

Practice

_____

_____

_____

LESSON 17-2

Terminology Application

Without looking at your previous work, write the term that matches each definition.

Definition	Term
1. Disorder marked by multiple physical complaints not fully explained by any known medical condition.	_____
2. Disorder in which there is intentional feigning of physical or psychological symptoms to obtain medical treatment.	_____
3. A group of disorders with symptoms suggesting physical ailments but *without* organic findings evident.	_____
4. A group of mental disorders in which apprehension, tension, or uneasiness from anticipation of danger predominate.	_____
5. Somatoform disorder characterized by pain, for which there is no physical finding, in one or more parts of the body; causes distress or impairs work or social functioning.	_____
6. Disorder in which the patient imagines a defect in his or her appearance, even though he or she appears normal to others.	_____
7. Period of intense fear or discomfort with fears of dying or losing control. Some physical symptoms include smothering sensations and trembling.	_____
8. A group of mental disorders in which the patient is unable to recall important personal information.	_____
9. Anxiety about being in places where help may not be available should a panic attack occur.	_____
10. Disorders marked by recurrent compulsions (repetitive behaviors) and obsessions (persistent ideas, thoughts, and impulses). Compulsions may involve repetitive washing of hands, checking constantly to see if a door is locked, etc. Obsessions may involve repeated thoughts such as thoughts of becoming contaminated by shaking hands.	_____

continued

Definition	Term

11. Intense fear caused by a specific object or situation. Examples: *claustrophobia*—fear of closed places; *acrophobia*—fear of heights; *ailurophobia*—fear of cats; *xenophobia*—fear of strangers.

                    _____

12. Disorder characterized by a symptom suggestive of a neurologic impairment that affects the senses (for example, blindness) or motor function (for example, paralysis).

                    _____

13. Characterized by an anxiety provoked by exposure to types of social or performance situations. Example: performing in front of others.

                    _____

14. Mental disorder marked by a morbid preoccupation with one's health or a fear of having some disease, despite a lack of identification of disease on examination.

                    _____

Check your answers against the information given in this lesson's terminology presentation. If you have any errors, count them and write the number in the blank at the top of the page. Sign your work and give it to your instructor.

Terminology Presentation

Psychoses

As you listen to the CD, read the terms and notice the pronunciations given.

 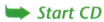 **Start CD**

Term	Definition	Answer
1. psychoses (si-ko′ses)	Group of severe mental disorders marked by gross impairment in reality testing, typically shown by delusions, hallucinations, incoherent speech, or disorganized or agitated behavior.	1. _____
2. bipolar psychosis (manic depressive) (bi-po′lar)	Mood disorder characterized by the occurrence of one or more manic episodes of behavior along with one or more depressive episodes.	2. _____
3. alcoholic psychoses	A group of major mental disorders associated with organic brain dysfunction due to long-term ingestion of large amounts of alcohol.	3. _____
4. depressive psychosis	Major depressive disorder characterized by significant lowering of mood tone, loss of interest in daily activities, feelings of worthlessness, and recurrent thoughts of death or suicide.	4. _____
5. schizophrenia (skiz-o-fre′ne-ah) (skit-so-fre′ne-ah)	A group of major mental disorders characterized by distortion in thinking, bizarre delusions, and hallucinations.	5. _____
6. drug psychoses	Organic mental syndromes caused by the consumption of drugs; some commonly used drugs are amphetamines, barbiturates, opiates, LSD groups, and solvents (inhalants).	6. _____

continued

Term	Definition	Answer
7. Alzheimer's disease (altz'hi-merz) (presenile dementia) (pre-se'nil de-men'she-ah)	Organic mental syndrome characterized by a general loss of intellectual abilities involving impairment of memory, judgment, and abstract thinking.	7. _____
8. symbiotic psychosis (sim-bi-ot'ik)	A condition found in 2- to 4-year-old children with an abnormal relationship to a mothering figure, marked by autism and regression.	8. _____

➡ *Pause CD*

After practicing each term several times, use a sheet of paper to cover all columns except the Answer column. As each term is pronounced again on the CD, write it in the space provided.

➡ *Start CD*

Check the terms you have written against the terms in the left-hand column. If you have misspelled any terms, practice writing them correctly.

Practice

_____

_____

_____

_____

_____

_____

_____

_____

_____

_____

_____

_____

_____

_____

_____

LESSON 17-3

Terminology Application

Without looking at your previous work, write the term that matches each definition.

Definition	Term
1. A group of major mental disorders characterized by distortion in thinking, bizarre delusions, and hallucinations.	_____
2. Major depressive disorder characterized by significant lowering of mood tone, loss of interest in daily activities, feelings of worthlessness, and recurrent thoughts of death or suicide.	_____
3. Condition found in 2- to 4-year-old children with an abnormal relationship to a mothering figure, marked by autism and regression.	_____
4. Organic mental syndrome characterized by a general loss of intellectual abilities involving impairment of memory, judgment, and abstract thinking.	_____
5. Mood disorder characterized by the occurrence of one or more manic episodes of behavior along with one or more depressive episodes.	_____
6. A group of severe mental disorders marked by gross impairment in reality testing, typically shown by delusions, hallucinations, incoherent speech, or disorganized or agitated behavior.	_____
7. A group of major mental disorders associated with organic brain dysfunction due to long-term ingestion of large amounts of alcohol.	_____
8. Organic mental syndromes caused by the consumption of drugs; some commonly used drugs are amphetamines, barbiturates, opiates, LSD groups, and solvents (inhalants).	_____

Check your answers against the information given in this lesson's terminology presentation. If you have any errors, count them and write the number in the blank at the top of the page. Sign your work and give it to your instructor.

Practice

Disorders of Gender and Sexual Identity, Sleep, Impulse Control, Eating, and Post-Traumatic Stress

As you listen to the CD, read the terms and notice the pronunciations given.

  Start CD

Term	Definition	Answer
1. psychosexual gender identity disorders (si-ko-seks′u-al)	Repeated desire to be of the opposite sex; a belief that one was born the wrong sex.	1. _____
2. sexual deviation	Paraphilia—abnormal sexual inclination or behavior.	2. _____
3. fetishism (fet′ish-izm)	Sexual urges involving the use of inanimate objects (fetishes), such as clothing, shoes, and underwear.	3. _____
4. nymphomania (nim-fo-ma′ne-ah)	Abnormal, excessive sexual desire in the female.	4. _____
5. pedophilia (pe-do-fil′e-ah)	Sexual thoughts about or sexual activity with children by an adult.	5. _____
6. satyriasis (sat-i-ri′ah-sis)	Abnormal, excessive sexual desire in the male.	6. _____
7. sexual masochism (mas′o-kizm)	Paraphilia in which sexual gratification is derived from being humiliated or hurt by another.	7. _____
8. sexual sadism (sad′izm)	Paraphilia in which sexual gratification is derived from humiliating or hurting another.	8. _____
9. transvestism (trans-ves′tizm)	"Cross-dressing"; the practice of wearing articles of clothing of the opposite sex.	9. _____
10. voyeurism (voi′yer-izm)	Disorder marked by recurrent sexual urges to watch unsuspecting people who are naked, disrobing, or engaging in sexual activities ("peeping Tom").	10. _____

continued

Term	Definition	Answer
11. zoophilia (zo-o-fil′e-ah)	Disorder involving sexual activity with animals.	11. _____
12. dyssomnias (dis-som′ne-ahs)	Sleep disturbances involving the amount,quality, or timing of sleep.	12. _____
13. insomnia (in-som′ne-ah)	Inability to sleep.	13. _____
14. hypersomnia (hi-per-som′ne-ah)	Sleep disorder consisting of the need for excessive sleep.	14. _____
15. narcolepsy (nar′ko-lep-se)	Recurrent, uncontrolled, brief episodes of sleep.	15. _____
16. breathing-related sleep disorder	Sleep disruption due to a sleep-related breathing condition (sleep apnea).	16. _____
17. parasomnias (par-ah-som′ne-ahs)	Category of sleep disorder in which abnormal events occur during sleep.	17. _____
18. nightmare disorder	Repeated awakenings from sleep due to extremely frightening dreams.	18. _____
19. sleep terror disorder	Parasomnia marked by panic and confusion when abruptly awakening from sleep.	19. _____
20. sleepwalking	Recurrent episodes of arising from bed during sleep and walking about.	20. _____
21. impulse control disorder	Failure to resist a temptation to perform an act that is harmful to oneself or others.	21. _____
22. pathological gambling	Morbid preoccupation with gambling; a need to gamble.	22. _____
23. kleptomania (klep-to-ma′ne-ah)	Disorder consisting of episodes of stealing objects that are not needed for personal use or for their monetary value.	23. _____
24. pyromania (pi-ro-ma′ne-ah)	Deliberate and purposeful firesetting; the completion of this act brings a sense of gratification. Not to be confused with arson, which is usually done for a profit motive.	24. _____
25. anorexia nervosa (an-o-rek′se-ah ner-vo′sa)	Eating disorder characterized by refusal or inability to maintain minimum normal weight, with an intense fear of gaining weight.	25. _____

Term	Definition	Answer
26. bulimia nervosa (bu-lim′e-ah)	Binge eating, followed by compensatory behavior such as self-induced vomiting or the use of diuretics and laxatives.	26. _____
27. post-traumatic stress disorder (PTSD) (traw-mat′ik)	Various psychological symptoms occurring after a traumatic event, such as military combat, flood, fire, or an automobile accident.	27. _____

➡ Pause CD

After practicing each term several times, use a sheet of paper to cover all columns except the Answer column. As each term is pronounced again on the CD, write it in the space provided.

➡ Start CD

Check the terms you have written against the terms in the left-hand column. If you have misspelled any terms, practice writing them correctly.

Practice

_____

_____

_____

_____

_____

_____

_____

_____

_____

_____

_____

_____

_____

_____

_____

Practice

LESSON
17-4

Terminology Application

Without looking at your previous work, write the term that matches each definition.

Definition	Term
1. Failure to resist a temptation to perform an act that is harmful to oneself or others.	_____
2. Abnormal sexual inclinations or behavior (paraphilia).	_____
3. Various psychological symptoms occurring after a traumatic event, such as military combat, flood, fire, an automobile accident.	_____
4. Sleep disruption due to a sleep-related breathing condition (sleep apnea).	_____
5. Paraphilia in which sexual gratification is derived from humiliating or hurting another.	_____
6. Disorder consisting of episodes of stealing objects that are not needed for personal use or for their monetary value.	_____
7. Eating disorder characterized by refusal or inability to maintain minimum normal weight, with an intense fear of gaining weight.	_____
8. Sexual thoughts or sexual activity of adults with children.	_____
9. Repeated awakenings from sleep due to extremely frightening dreams.	_____
10. Deliberate and purposeful firesetting; the completion of this act brings a sense of gratification. Not to be confused with arson, which is usually done for a profit motive.	_____
11. Repeated desire to be of the opposite sex; a belief that one was born the wrong sex.	_____
12. Binge eating, followed by compensatory behavior such as self-induced vomiting or the use of diuretics and laxatives.	_____
13. Paraphilia in which sexual gratification is derived from being humiliated or hurt by another.	_____
14. Recurrent episodes of arising from bed during sleep and walking about.	_____

continued

Definition	Term

15. Disorder marked by recurrent sexual urges to watch unsuspecting people who are naked, disrobing, or engaging in sexual activities ("peeping Tom").   _____

16. Inability to sleep.   _____

17. Morbid preoccupation with gambling; a need to gamble.   _____

18. Abnormal, excessive sexual desire in the female.   _____

19. Recurrent, uncontrolled, brief episodes of sleep.   _____

20. "Cross-dressing"; the practice of wearing articles of clothing of the opposite sex.   _____

21. Category of sleep disorders in which abnormal events occur during sleep.   _____

22. Sexual urges involving the use of inanimate objects (fetishes), such as clothing, shoes, or underwear.   _____

23. Sleep disturbances involving the amount, quality, or timing of sleep.   _____

24. Abnormal, excessive sexual desire in the male.   _____

25. Parasomnia marked by panic and confusion when abruptly awakening from sleep.   _____

26. Sleep disorder consisting of the need for excessive sleep.   _____

27. Disorder involving sexual activity with animals.   _____

Check your answers against the information given in this lesson's terminology presentation. If you have any errors, count them and write the number in the blank at the top of the page. Sign your work and give it to your instructor.

As you listen to the CD, read the words and notice the pronunciations given.

  Start CD

Word	Definition	Example: Generic Name	Example:Brand/ Trade Name	Answer
antianxiety drugs (psychotropics)	agents that reduce or eliminate anxiety	diazepam alprazolam lorazepam	Valium Xanax Ativan	1._____
anticonvulsants	agents that prevent or relieve convulsions	diazepam phenobarbital primidone phenytoin	Valium Solfoton, Luminal Sertan Dilantin	2._____
antidepressants	agents that prevent or relieve depression	venlafaxine sertraline fluoxetine paroxetine	Effexor Zoloft Prozac Paxil	3._____
antipsychotics	agents that are effective in the treatment of psychoses	lithium haloperidol chlorpromazine	Lithotabs Haldol Thorazine	4._____
sedatives (hypnotics)	agents that allay activity and excitement; used for short-term treatment of insomnia	zolpidem diphenhydramine chloral hydrate lorazepam pentobarbital secobarbital	Ambien Benadryl, Sominex 2, Nytol, Allerdryl Aquachloral Ativan Nembutal Seconal	5._____
tranquilizers (major)	agents that have a calming, soothing effect; antipsychotic agents	lithium haloperidol chlorpromazine	Lithotabs Haldol Thorazine	6._____
tranquilizers (minor)	agents that have a calming, soothing effect; antianxiety drugs	diazepam alprazolam lorazepam	Valium Xanax Ativan	7._____

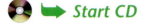 *Pause CD*

After practicing each word several times, use a sheet of paper to cover all columns except the Answer column. As each word is pronounced again on the CD, write it in the space provided.

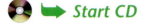 *Start CD*

Check the words you have written against the words in the left-hand column. If you have misspelled any words, practice writing them correctly.

Practice

_____

_____

_____

_____

_____

_____

_____

_____

_____

_____

_____

_____

_____

_____

_____

_____

_____

_____

_____

_____

_____

_____

_____

Terminology Application

Without looking at your previous work, write the word that matches each definition.

Definition	Term
1. agents that have a calming, soothing effect; antianxiety drugs	_____
2. agents that allay activity and excitement; used for the short-term treatment of insomnia	_____
3. agents that prevent or relieve depression	_____
4. agents that are effective in the treatment of psychoses	_____
5. agents that have a calming, soothing effect; antipsychotic agents	_____
6. agents that prevent or relieve convulsions	_____

Check your answers against the information given in this lesson's terminology presentation. If you have any errors, count them and write the number in the blank at the top of the page. Sign your work and give it to your instructor.

Practice

CHAPTER
17

Terminology Review

This is a review of the terms you have learned in the preceding four lessons. As each term is pronounced on the CD, write the appropriate definition in the space to the right.

 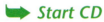 *Start CD*

Word Review

Term	Definition
1. personality disorder—dependent type	
2. social phobia	
3. voyeurism	
4. post-traumatic stress disorder (PTSD)	
5. personality disorder—masochistic type	
6. bipolar psychosis (manic depressive)	
7. conversion disorder	
8. pyromania	
9. Alzheimer's disease	

Term	Definition

10. anorexia nervosa _____

_____

11. personality disorder—schizoid type _____

_____

12. hypochondriasis _____

_____

13. satyriasis _____

_____

14. personality disorder—paranoid type _____

_____

15. transvestism _____

_____

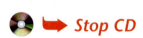 *Stop CD*

On the lines provided, fill in the meanings of as many definitions as you can from memory. Check your definitions in the glossary or a medical dictionary, and make any needed corrections.

CHAPTER 17
Terminology Review

Complete this review, and return it to your instructor when you are finished.

Definition

Write the definition for each of the following terms to the right of the term.

Term	Definition
1. somatization disorder	_____
2. pedophilia	_____
3. factitious disorder (Münchausen's syndrome)	_____
4. personality disorder-narcissistic type	_____
5. psychosexual gender identity disorder	_____
6. dissociative disorder	_____
7. alcoholic psychoses	_____
8. parasomnias	_____
9. pathological gambling	_____
10. body dysmorphic disorder	_____
11. personality disorder-introverted type	_____
12. zoophilia	_____
13. symbiotic psychosis	_____
14. fetishism	_____
15. agoraphobia	_____

Matching

Match the following definitions with the terms given. Place the letter of the correct definition to the left of the term.

Term	Definition
_____ 16. pain disorder	**a.** a group of major mental disorders characterized by distortion in thinking, bizarre delusions, and hallucinations
_____ 17. bulimia nervosa	**b.** abnormal, excessive sexual desire in the female
_____ 18. kleptomania	
_____ 19. depressive psychosis	**c.** personality disorder marked by instability of mood; impulsive and self-damaging acts are common
_____ 20. sexual deviations	
_____ 21. schizophrenia	**d.** personality disorder marked by excessive attention-seeking behavior
_____ 22. personality disorder—histrionic	
_____ 23. personality disorder—borderline type	**e.** somatoform disorder characterized by pain, for which there is no physical finding, in one or more parts of the body; causes distress or impairs work or social functioning
_____ 24. sleepwalking	
_____ 25. nymphomania	

You may now go on to Chapter Test 17.

f. disorder consisting of episodes of stealing objects that are not needed for personal use or for their monetary value

g. major depressive disorder characterized by significant lowering of mood tone, loss of interest in daily activities, feelings of worthlessness, and recurrent thoughts of death or suicide

h. recurrent episodes of arising from bed during sleep and walking about

i. abnormal sexual inclinations or behavior (paraphilia)

j. binge eating, followed by compensatory behavior such as self-induced vomiting or the use of diuretics and laxatives

APPENDIX

Selected Medical and Chemical Abbreviations

AB	abort
ACG	angiocardiography
ACTH	adrenocorticotropic hormone
AG	atrial gallop
AIDS	acquired immunodeficiency syndrome
AMA	American Medical Association
AMI	acute myocardial infarction
ANA	American Nurses' Association; antinuclear antibodies
anat.	anatomy; anatomical
ant.	anterior
AOA	American Optometric Association; American Orthopsychiatric Association; American Osteopathic Association
AP	acid phosphatase; action potential; alkaline phosphatase; aminopeptidase; angina pectoris; antepartum; anterior pituitary; anteroposterior; aortic pressure; appendix; arterial pressure
ASA	argininosuccinic acid; acetylsalicylic acid
AT	atrial tachycardia
Au	gold
AV	atrioventricular; arteriovenous
ax.	axis
BMR	basal metabolic rate
BP	blood pressure
BUN	blood urea nitrogen
c̄	with

C1	first cervical vertebra (C1–C7)
°C	degrees Celsius
C.	Celsius
ca., CA.	carcinoma
CA	cardiac arrest; coronary artery; chronological age
CAD	coronary artery disease
cal	calorie
CAT (scan)	computerized axial tomography
cbc	complete blood count
CC	chief complaint
CCU	coronary care unit
CDC	Centers for Disease Control and Prevention
CEA	carcinoembryonic antigen
CHD	coronary heart disease
CHF	congestive heart failure
CI	color index
CK	creatine kinase
cm.	centimeter
CNS	central nervous system
Co	cobalt
CO_2	carbon dioxide
CPC	clinicopathological conference
CPK	creatine phosphokinase
CPR	cardiopulmonary resuscitation
CRNA	Certified Registered Nurse Anesthetist
CSF	cerebrospinal fluid
CT	computerized tomography
CVA	cerebrovascular accident; cardiovascular accident
D1	first dorsal vertebra (D1–D12)
dB	decibel
↓	decrease
D & C	dilation and curettage
DNA	deoxyribonucleic acid
DNR	do not resuscitate
DOA	dead on arrival

DTR	deep tendon reflex
Dx	diagnosis
ECG	electrocardiogram
ECT	electroconvulsive therapy
EEG	electroencephalogram
EKG	electrocardiogram
ENA	extractable nuclear antigens
ENT	ear, nose, and throat
EOM	extraocular movement; extraocular muscle
ER	emergency room
°F	degrees Fahrenheit
F.	Fahrenheit
GI	gastrointestinal
GU	genitourinary
Hb	hemoglobin
HDL	high-density lipoprotein
HEENT	head, eyes, ears, nose, and throat
Hgb	hemoglobin
HMO	health maintenance organization
Hz	hertz
↑	increase
ICP	intracranial pressure
ICU	intensive care unit
Ig	immunoglobulin
IM	intramuscularly; by intramuscular injection
IOP	intraocular pressure
IQ	intelligence quotient
IUD	intrauterine contraceptive device
IV	intravenously; by intravenous injection
IVP	intravenous pyelogram
K	potassium
kg	kilogram
KUB	kidney, ureter, and bladder
kV	kilovolt
L1	first lumbar vertebra (L1–L5)

L&A	light and accommodation (reaction of pupils of eyes)
LDH	lactate dehydrogenase
LDL	low-density lipoprotein
LPN	licensed practical nurse
m	median; meter; milli-
mEq	milliequivalent
MI	myocardial infarction
MRI	magnetic resonance imaging
MS	multiple sclerosis
Na	sodium
NG	nasogastric
NPN	nonprotein nitrogen
NPO	nothing by mouth
NSR	normal sinus rhythm
O	oxygen
O_2	diatomic form of oxygen
OB	obstetrics
O.D.	right eye
O.L.	left eye
O.P.D.	outpatient department
OR	operating room
PBI	protein-bound iodine
PCO_2	carbon dioxide partial pressure
PERRLA	pupils equal, round, reactive to light and accomodation
PET	positron emission tomography
pH	hydrogen ion concentration
PMI	point of maximal impulse
PO_2	oxygen partial pressure
PT	prothrombin time
PTA	plasma thromboplastin antecedent
RBC	red blood (cell) count
REM	rapid eye movements
RNP	ribonucleoprotein
R_x	drug, prescription

s̄	without
S1	first sacral vertebra (S1–S5)
segs	segmented neutrophils
SGOT	serum glutamic-oxaloacetic transaminase
SGPT	serum glutamate pyruvate transaminase
SIDS	sudden infant death syndrome
sp. gr.	specific gravity
ST	sinus tachycardia
stat.	immediately
T&A	tonsils and adenoids
TAT	thematic apperception test
T1	first thoracic vertebra (T1–T12)
TB	tuberculosis
TIA	transient ischemic attack
TSH	thyroid-stimulating hormone
UV	ultraviolet
V	volt
var.	variety
VD	venereal disease
W	watt; work
WBC	white blood (cell) count
wt	weight

B

Selected Abbreviations Used in Pharmacy and Prescription Writing

aa	equal parts of each
a.c.	before meals
ad lib.	at pleasure
Alt. dieb.	every other day
b.i.d.	twice a day
c̄	with
cc.	cubic centimeter
d.d.	let it be given to
dil.	dilute or dissolve
dr.	dram
extr.	extract
female ♀	female
Fl.	fluid
Fl.oz.	fluid ounce
g.	gram
gr.	grain
gt.	drop
gtt.	drops
>	greater than
h.s.	at bedtime
<	less than
l	liter

male ♂	male
mg.	milligram
min.	minim
ml	milliliter
mm	millimeter
Noct.	at night
n.p.o.	nothing by mouth
o.h.	every hour
o.m.	every morning
o.n.	every night
oz.	ounce
p.a.	in equal parts
p.c.	after food, after meals
P.O.	by mouth; orally
p.r.n.	as needed; as required
pt.	patient
q	every; quart
q.a.m.	every morning
q.d.	every day
q.h.	every hour (q.2h.: every second hour; q.3h.: every third hour)
q.i.d.	four times a day
q.p.m.	every night
Rx	drug; prescription
s̄	without
Sig.	let it be labeled
Stat	immediately
subq.	subcutaneous
Syr.	syrup
t.i.d.	three times a day
tr.	tincture
wt	weight

Common Latin and Greek Singular and Plural Endings

Singular	Example	Plural	Example
-a	vertebra fascia sclera gingiva	-ae	vertebrae fasciae sclerae gingivae
-em	lumen foramen	-ina	lumina foramina
-is	naris diagnosis anastomosis stenosis	-es	nares diagnoses anastomoses stenoses
-ix, -ax	varix calix appendix thorax	-ices	varices calices appendices thoraces
-nx	pharynx larynx phalanx	-nges	pharynges larynges phalanges
-oma	adenoma carcinoma stoma keratoma	-omata	adenomata carcinomata stomata keratomata
-um	diverticulum cranium ovum septum	-a	diverticula crania ova septa
-us	bronchus glomerulus thrombus enterococcus	-i	bronchi glomeruli thrombi enterococci

D

Common Prefixes

PREFIX	MEANING
a-, an-	without, negative
ab-	away from
ad-	toward
alb-	white
all-	other
ambi-	both
amphi-	around, both sides
ana-	up
andro-	man
ankylo-	bent, crooked
ante(ro)	before
anti-	against
apo-	from, apposed
auto-	self
baso-	basic
bi-	two, double
bio-	life, living
brachy-	short
brady-	slow
cata-	down
caud-	tail
centi-	one-hundredth (1/100)

chloro-	green
chrom-	color
circum-	around
cirrho-	yellow
co-, con-, com-	together
conio-	dust
contra-	against
cryo-	cold
cyano-	blue
de-	from, not, down
deca-	ten (10)
deci-	tenth (1/10)
demi-	half
dextro-	right
di-	double
dia-	through
diplo-	double
dipso-	thirst
dis-	negative, apart
dorsa-	back
dys-	difficult, bad, painful
ec-, ecto-	out, outside
en-	into
endo-	within
eosin-	rose-colored
epi-	above, upon
erythro-	red
eu-	well, normal
ex-	away from
exo-	out
extra-	outside of
fibro-	fibrous
flexed-	bent
fore-	before, front
glauco-	bluish-green

glyco-	sugar
hecto-	hundred (100)
hemi-	half (1/2)
holo-	all
homo-	same
hydro-	water
hyper-	above, excess
hypo-	under, deficient
idio-	self
im-	not
in-	in, not
infra-	below
inter-	between
intra-	below, within
iso-	equal
juxta-	near
kilo-	thousand
kines-	motion
lat(ero)	side
lepto-	small, soft
leuko-	white
lipo-	fat
macro-	large
mal-	bad
med-	middle
mega-	large
melan-	black
meso-	middle
meta-	beyond, change
micro-	small
milli-	one-thousandth (1/1000)
mono-	one (1)
morph-	shape, form
multi-	many
myco-	fungus

neo-	new
neutro-	neither
noct-	night, dark
non-	not
nyct-	night, dark
oligo-	few
ortho-	straight, normal
pachy-	thick
pan-	all
para-	beside, near
path-	disease
per-	through
peri-	around
pharm(aco)-	drug
photo-	light
pleo-	more, many
polio-	gray
poly-	many
post-	after
pre-	before, in front of
primi-	one
pro-	before
proto-	first
pseudo-	false
quadri-	four (4)
quinqui-	five (5)
re-	back
retro-	backward
rube-	red
sclero-	hard
semi-	half (1/2)
sinistro-	left
somat-	body
steno-	narrow
sub-	under

supra-	above
syn-	with, together
tachy-	fast
tele-	distant, far
ter-	three (3)
tetra-	four (4)
trans-	across
tri-	three (3)
ultra-	beyond
uni-	one
xantho-	yellow
xero-	dry
zoo-	animal

Common Suffixes

SUFFIX	MEANING
-ac	pertaining to
-al	pertaining to
-algesia	pain
-algia	pain
-ant	denotes a noun
-ar, -ary	pertaining to
-ase	enzyme
-asthenia	lack of strength
-ate	denotes a verb
-blast	immature cell
-cele	tumor, swelling, hernia
-centesis	surgical puncture
-cide, -cidal	death, killer
-clasis, -clast	break, fracture
-cleisis	closure
-cylsis	wash out
-coccus, -cocci (pl.)	bacteria
-crit	separate
-cyesis	pregnancy
-cyte	cell
-cytosis	cellular content (increase)

-desis	binding
-duct	to draw
-dynia	pain
-ectasis	dilatation (dilation)
-ectomy	excision, removal
-edema	swelling
-emesis	vomit
-emia	blood
-esthesia	feeling, sensation
-fuge	to drive away
-gen(ous)	produce
-genic	produce
-genesis	produce, origin
-gnosis	knowledge
-gram	tracing, chart
-graphy	recording
-ia	condition, process
-iasis	diseased condition
-iatrics	treatment
-ic, -iac	pertaining to
-iferous	bear, produce
-ion	denotes a noun
-ism	condition
-itis	inflammation
-kinesia, kinesis	motion
-listhesis	to slip
-lith	stone
-(o)logist	specialist
-(o)logy	science of
-(o)lysis, lytic	dissolve, break down
-malacia	soft
-mania	compulsion
-megaly	enlargement

-meter	measure
-motor	mover
-mycosis	fungus
-oid	resembling
-oma	tumor
-ose	pertaining to
-osis	condition
-ous	pertaining to
-oxia	oxygen
-palpation	feeling
-pathy	disease
-penia	lack of
-pexy	fix, fasten
-phagia	to eat
-phasia	speech
-philia	desire, attraction
-phobia	fear
-phonia	voice, sound
-phylaxis	protection
-phyll	leaf
-phyte	plant, organism
-plasia	formation
-plasm	to mold
-plastic	mold, form
-plasty	plastic surgery
-plegia	paralyis, stroke
-pnea	breathing, air
-poiesis	making, producing
-ptosis	falling, prolapse
-ptysis	cough up, spit up
-rrhagia	flow (of blood)
-rrhaphy	suture, sew up
-rrhea	flow

-rrhexis	rupture, break
-schesis	to check
-schisis	splitting
-scirrhus	hardening
-sclerosis	hardening
-scope	viewing instrument
-scopy	visual examination
-sect	cut
-sepsis	poison
-spasm	contraction
-stasis	stop
-stat	stop
-stenosis	narrowing
-sthenia	strength
-stomy	connection, opening
-therapy	treatment
-tomy	incision, cut
-toxic	poison
-tractor	to draw back
-tripsy	crush
-trophy	nourishment
-uria	urine

Sexually Transmitted Diseases for Men and Women

Types of STDs	Common Name	Symptoms/Effects in Men	Symptoms/Effects in Women
Bacteria/Protozoa			
Chlamydia trachomatis	chlamydia (klah-mid′e-ah)	urethritis and white discharge from the penis	uterine cervicitis and mucopurulent discharge
Neisseria gonorrhoeae	gonorrhea (gon′o-re′ah)	urethritis, dysuria, and cystitis	green-yellow cervical discharge, oophoritis, salpingitis, and infant blindness
Treponema pallidum	syphilis (sif′i-lis)	stage 1—external lesions (chancre) stage 2—sytemic infection stage 3—destructive lesions in organs and tissues	stage 1—external lesions (chancre) stage 2—systemic infection stage 3—destructive lesions in organs and tissues
Trichomonas vaginalis	trichomonas (trik′o-mo′nas)	urethritis, prostate enlargement, and epididymitis	green vaginal discharge, burning, pruritis, and chafing
Virus			
herpes simplex (HSV-2)	genital herpes (jen′i-tal her′pez)	blisters/lesions on the glans penis, the prepuce, and the penis	blisters on external genitalia; can result in cervical cancer or miscarriage
human immunodeficiency virus (HIV)	acquired immunodeficiency syndrome (AIDS)	the virus attacks the T-cells and breaks down the immune system	the virus attacks the T-cells and breaks down the immune system

Glossary

A

aberrant Wandering or deviating from the norm.

abnormal Not normal.

aboral Situated away, or remote, from the mouth.

acetaminophen A generic agent that relieves pain and suppresses inflammation.

acoustic Pertaining to hearing; auditory.

ACTH Adrenocorticotropic hormone; stimulates adrenal cortex secretions.

adduct To draw toward.

aden(o) A combining form denoting the glands.

adenitis Inflammation of a gland or glands.

adenocarcinoma Glandular cancer or carcinoma.

adenohypophysis The anterior (front) lobe of the pituitary gland; also called adenohypophysis cerebri.

adenohypophysis cerebri The anterior lobe of the pituitary gland.

adenoid Like or resembling a gland or the glands.

adenoma A benign tumor of a gland.

adenomalacia Abnormal softening of a gland.

adenomegaly Abnormal enlargement of a gland.

adipoid Resembling fat; lipoid.

adipoma A fatty tumor; lipoma.

adipose Fatty tissue.

adiposis Obesity or corpulence; excessive accumulation of fat in the body.

adiposuria Fat in the urine; lipuria.

adren(o) A combining form denoting the adrenal glands, which secrete the hormone epinephrine (adrenaline, ad = near + renal = kidney).

adrenal cortex The outer layer of adrenal gland; produces cortical (steroid) hormones.

adrenal glands Glands located above each kidney that produce cortical hormones and medullary hormones; also called suprarenals.

adrenal medulla The middle layer of adrenal gland; produces medullary (nonsteroid) hormones.

adrenalectomy Excision of an adrenal gland.

adrenaline A hormone that increases cardiac activity, increases fat usage for energy, and causes vasoconstriction in skeletal muscles.

adrenalitis Inflammation of the adrenal glands.

adrenocorticotropic hormone A hormone that stimulates adrenal cortex secretion; ACTH.

adrenokinetic Stimulating the adrenal glands.

adrenomegaly Enlargement of the adrenal glands.

adrenopathy Any disease of the adrenal glands.

adrenotoxin Toxic or poisonous to the adrenal glands.

Aerobid The brand name for flunisolide (a corticosteroid); used to expand the air passages in the lungs.

affective type (cyclothymia) Cyclic personality disorder characterized by symptoms of manic (excited or violent) and depressive (sad or despairing) episodes of behavior.

afferent nerves Nerves that note changes within the body and in the environment and send electrical impulses to the brain.

agoraphobia Anxiety about being in places where help may not be available should a panic attack occur.

AIDS A disease caused by the sexually transmitted human immunodeficiency virus (HIV); acquired immunodeficiency syndrome.

albuminuria Presence of serum albumin in the urine.

alcoholic psychoses A group of major mental disorders associated with organic brain dysfunction due to long-term ingestion of large amounts of alcohol.

algia or algesia A word element (suffix, usually) denoting pain or ache.

Allegra Brand name for fexofenadine; used to treat allergies.

Allerdryl Brand name for diphenhydramine; used for short-term treatment of insomnia.

allergist (allergy)   Specialist concerned with the diagnosis and treatment of allergies.

Alloprim   Brand name for allopurinol; used in the treatment of gout.

allopurinol   Generic name for Zyloprim, prescribed for the treatment of gout.

alveolus, alveoli   Singular and plural terms referring to the air sacs in the lungs where gaseous exchange occurs.

Alzheimer's disease   Organic mental syndrome characterized by a general loss of intellectual abilities involving impairment of memory, judgment, and abstract thinking.

Ambien   Brand name for zolpidem; used for short-term treatment of insomnia.

Amicar   Brand name for aminocaproic acid; used to arrest the flow of blood.

ammonium chloride   A generic agent used to promote the ejection of mucus from the lower respiratory tract.

amniocentesis   Surgical puncture of the amnion to remove fluid.

amnion   The thin extra-embryonic membrane that contains the fetus.

amyl nitrite   A generic agent used to dilate blood vessels.

anal   Pertaining to the anus.

analgesics   Agents that relieve pain.

anastomosis   An opening or connection between two vessels or organs.

androcyte   A male sex cell.

androgen   Any substance that conduces to masculinization.

androgenic   Producing masculine characteristics.

andrology   The scientific study of the masculine constitution and diseases in males.

andropathy   Any disease peculiar to men.

anemia   Reduction in the number of red blood cells in the blood.

anesthesiologist   Specialist who studies and administers anesthetic agents.

anesthesiology   The study and practice of administering anesthetic agents.

anesthetics   Agents that reduce or eliminate the perception of sensation.

angi(o)   A combining form indicating relationship to a vessel, usually a blood vessel.

angiectasis   Dilatation (dilation) of a blood vessel.

angiocarditis   Inflammation of the heart and major blood vessels.

angiogram   X-ray picture (roentgenogram) of a blood vessel.

angiomegaly   Enlarged blood vessels.

angiomyolipoma   A tumor of blood vessels, muscle, or fat.

angioplasty   Dilatation (dilation) of a blood vessel by means of a balloon catheter inserted through the skin to the site of the narrowing; the balloon flattens plaque in the vessel.

angiorrhaphy   The suturing of vessels, especially blood vessels.

angiospasm   Contraction of a blood vessel.

angiostenosis   Narrowing of the lumen (inside) of a blood vessel.

angiostomy   Making an opening into the blood vessel.

anorexia nervosa   An eating disorder characterized by refusal or inability to maintain minimum normal weight, with an intense fear of gaining weight.

antacids   Agents that counteract or neutralize acidity, usually in the stomach.

antianginals   Agents that alleviate angina pectoris by dilating coronary arteries to improve blood flow.

antianxiety drugs   Agents that reduce or eliminate anxiety.

anticoagulants   Agents that prevent blood clotting.

anticonvulsants   Agents that prevent or relieve convulsions.

antidepressants   Agents that prevent or relieve depression.

antidiabetics   Agents used to decrease blood sugar or to improve the body's use of Insulin.

antidiarrheals   Agents that counteract diarrhea.

antidiuretic hormone (ADH)   A hormone that helps the kidneys absorb water.

antiemetics   Agents that prevent or alleviate nausea and vomiting.

anti-fungals   Agents that destroy fungus or suppress its growth.

antihistamines   Agents that counter the effects of histamines; used to treat allergies.

antihypertensives   Agents that counteract high blood pressure.

antihypotensives   Agents that counteract low blood pressure by causing contraction of blood vessels.

anti-infectives   Agents that can kill infectious agents or prevent them from spreading.

anti-inflammatories   Agents that counteract or suppress inflammation.

antilipidemics   Agents that counteract high levels of lipids (fats) in the blood.

antipruritics   Agents that relieve or prevent itching.

antipsychotics   Agents that are effective in the treatment of psychoses.

antisocial type   A personality disorder marked by continuous and chronic antisocial behavior, often involving violation of others' rights.

antitussives   Agents that relieve or prevent coughs.

Anturane   Brand name for sulfinpyrazone; used in the treatment of gout.

anuria   Absence of the secretion of urine.

anus   The distal (terminal) orifice of the alimentary canal.

anusitis   Inflammation of the anus.

Anusol-HC   Brand name for hydrocortisone; used to relieve or prevent itching.

anxiety disorders   A group of mental disorders in which apprehension, tension, or uneasiness from anticipation of danger predominate.

aorta   The main trunk from which the systemic arterial system proceeds.

aortic   Pertaining to the aorta.

aortitis   Inflammation of the aorta.

aortosclerosis   Hardening of the aorta.

aphasia   Without speech; loss of speech.

aphasic   Pertaining to the loss of speech.

aphasiologist   A specialist in the treatment of aphasia.

apnea   Temporary absence of breathing.

apocrine glands   Sweat glands found in the pubic, anal, and mammary regions.

appendices   Plural spelling of *appendix*.

appendicular skeleton   The shoulder, upper extremities, hips, and lower extremities.

Aquachloral   Brand name for chloral hydrate; used for short-term treatment of insomnia.

aqueous humor   The fluid in the anterior cavity of the eyeball; nourishes the lens and the cornea.

arachnoid   The weblike middle layer of the meninges.

art, arteri(o)   Combining forms denoting the arteries.

arterial   Of or pertaining to an artery.

arteriectasis   Expansion of an artery.

arteries   Blood vessels that carry blood away from the heart.

arteriole   A minute arterial branch.

arteriopathy   Any disease of the arteries.

arteriorrhexis   Rupture of an artery.

arteriosclerosis   Hardening of the arteries.

arteriostenosis   Narrowing of an artery.

arteritis   Inflammation of an artery.

arthr(o)   A combining form denoting the joints.

arthralgia   Pain in a joint; painful joints.

arthrectomy   Excision of a joint.

arthritis   Inflammation of a joint.

arthrocentesis   Surgical puncture of a joint to remove fluid.

arthropathy   Any disease affecting a joint.

aspirin   An agent that counteracts or suppresses inflammation.

astrocytes   A type of neuroglial cells that cover the brain capillaries.

Atarax   Brand name for hydroxyzine; used to relieve or prevent itching.

Ativan   Brand name for lorazepam; used to reduce or eliminate anxiety; a minor tranquilizer.

atlas   First cervical vertebra that supports the head.

atrium, atria   Singular and plural spelling for the two heart chambers that collect blood.

Atrovent   Brand name for ipratropium; used to expand the air passages in the lungs.

audiologist   A hearing specialist.

audiometry   Measurement of hearing.

auditory   Pertaining to hearing; acoustic.

auditory salpingitis   Inflammation of the eustachian tube.

Augmentin   Brand name for amoxicillin/clavulanate potassium; used to kill infectious agents or prevent them from spreading.

auricle   The visible part of the outer ear.

auricular   Pertaining to the auricle.

auscultation   Listening to sounds made by body structures.

autograft   A graft of tissue from the patient's body.

autonomic nervous system   The part of the peripheral nervous system responsible for involuntary activities.

autopsy   Postmortem examination of a body.

Avalox   Brand name for moxifloxacin; used to kill infectious agents or prevent them from spreading.

avoidant type   A personality disorder characterized by hypersensitivity to criticism, anxiety, an exaggeration of difficulties, and general timidity.

axial skeleton   The skull, thoracic, and vertebral bones.

axis   The second cervical vertebra inside the atlas.

Azmacort   Brand name for triamcinolone (acorticosteroid); used to expand the air passages in the lungs.

azoturia   Excessive urea or other nitrogen compounds in the urine.

B

bacteriuria   Presence of bacteria in the urine.

balanitis   Inflammation of the glans penis.

balanoplasty   Plastic surgery of the glans penis.

balanorrhagia   Balanitis with free discharge of pus.

Baridium   Brand name for phenazopyridine; used to eliminate urinary spasms.

Bartholin's glands   Glands lateral to the vagina; produce secretions for the vagina.

Benadryl   Brand name for diphenhydramine; used to treat allergies; used for short-term treatment of insomnia.

Benemid   Brand name for probenecid; used in the treatment of gout.

biceps muscle   A two-headed muscle at the front of the forearm above the elbow; flexes the arm, supinates the hand.

bicuspid valve   A heart valve with two leaflets; also called a mitral valve.

bifurcate   Divide into two (2) branches.

Biosaren   Brand name for tranexamic acid; used to arrest the flow of blood.

bipolar psychosis (manic depressive)   A mood disorder characterized by the occurrence of one or more manic episodes of behavior along with one or more depressive episodes.

blephar(o)   A combining form denoting the eyelid.

blepharal   Pertaining to the eyelid.

blepharitis   Inflammation of the eyelid.

blepharoplasty   Plastic surgery on the eyelid.

blepharoplegia   Paralysis of the eyelid.

blepharoptosis   Drooping of the eyelid.

body dysmorphic disorder   A disorder in which the patient imagines a defect in his or her appearance, even though he or she appears normal to others.

bone marrow   A substance located in the larger bones; produces blood cells.

borderline type   A personality disorder marked by instability of mood. Impulsive and self-damaging acts are common.

brachial plexus   The network of nerves in the shoulders between the neck and armpits.

brachialis muscle   The muscle located in front of the humerus that flexes the forearm at the elbow.

bradycardia   Abnormally slow heartbeat.

bradypnea   Abnormally slow breathing.

brain stem   The part of the brain made up of the midbrain, the medulla oblongata, and the pons.

breathing-related sleep disorder   Sleep disruption due to a sleep-related breathing condition (sleep apnea).

bronch(o)   A combining form denoting the bronchi (plural) or bronchus (singular), the air passages within the lungs.

bronchi   Plural spelling of bronchus.

bronchial   Pertaining to a bronchus.

bronchiectasis   Expansion of the bronchus.

bronchioles   Finer subdivisions of the bronchi.

bronchitis   Inflammation of the bronchi.

bronchodilators   Agents that expand the air passages in the lungs.

bronchoedema   Swelling of the mucosa of the bronchi.

bronchoplegia   Paralysis of the bronchi.

bronchopneumonitis   An inflammation of the lungs that originates in the bronchi.

bronchorrhea   Excessive secretion of mucus from the bronchial mucous membrane.

bronchoscopy   Inspection or examination of the bronchi.

bronchus   Any of the larger air passages of the lungs; the bronchi branch extends from the trachea and contains irregularly placed plates of cartilage.

bulbourethral gland   The gland located below the prostate and connected to the urethra by means of a duct; produces a fluid component of semen that promotes the viability of sperm.

bulimia nervosa   Binge eating, followed by compensatory behavior such as self-induced vomiting or the use of diuretics and laxatives.

bursa, bursae (pl.)   A fluid-filled sac (located in certain joints) that prevents friction between moving parts.

C

calcaneous   Heel bone.

calcitonin   A hormone that regulates the metabolism of calcium and phosphorous.

capillaries Thin-walled blood vessels that connect arteries and veins.

carcinomata Plural spelling of *carcinoma*.

cardi(o), cardi(a) Combining forms denoting the heart.

cardiac Pertaining to the heart.

cardiogram The recording of the heart's movements.

cardiograph An instrument for recording the heart rate.

cardiography The process of recording heart movements.

cardiologist A specialist in diagnosing and treating heart disorders.

cardiology The science or study of the heart.

cardiomegaly Abnormal enlargement of the heart.

cardiomyopathy Primary myocardial disease.

carditis Inflammation of the heart.

Cardizem Brand name for diltiazem hydrochloride; used to alleviate angina pectoris and hypertension.

carpals Wrist bones.

Casodex Brand name for bicalutamide; used to treat menopause, prostatic cancer, osteoporosis, and abnormal menses.

Ceclor Brand name for cefaclor; used to kill infectious agents or prevent them from spreading.

Celebrex Brand name for celecoxib; used to counteract or suppress inflammation.

celiac Pertaining to the abdomen.

Cenestin Brand name for estrogen; used to treat menopause, prostatic cancer, osteoporosis, and abnormal menses.

centimeter A unit of the metric system being one one-hundredth part of a meter (.01 meter).

central nervous system The brain and the spinal cord.

cephal(o) A combining form indicating the cranium (head) or the head of a body part.

cephaledema Swelling or edema of the head.

cephalic Pertaining to the head.

cephalocaudal Pertaining to the long axis of the body (head to tail).

cephalocele A hernial protrusion of part of the cranial contents.

cephalocentesis Surgical puncture of the head to remove fluid.

cephalometer An instrument used to measure the head.

cephaloplegia Paralysis of the head muscles.

cerebellar Pertaining to the cerebellum.

cerebellitis Inflammation of the cerebellum.

cerebellum A small portion of the metencephalon behind the brain stem.

cerebral Pertaining to the cerebrum.

cerebromalacia Softening of the brain.

cerebrospinal Pertaining to the cerebrum and the spinal cord.

cerebrum The main portion of brain; divided into two hemispheres.

cervical Pertaining to the neck.

cervical plexus The network of nerves in the neck of the vertebrae.

cheil(o) A combining form denoting relationship to the lip.

cheilectomy Excision of the lip as for cheilocarcinoma.

cheilitis Inflammation of the lip.

cheilocarcinoma Cancer of the lip.

cheilophagia Habitual biting of the lip.

cheilorrhaphy Suture of the lip.

cheiloschisis Cleft in the lip; harelip.

cheilostomatoplasty Plastic surgery on the lip and mouth.

cheilotomy Incision into the lip.

cheir(o) A combining form denoting the hands.

cheiroplasty Plastic surgery of the hand.

chest specialist (pulmonary disease) A specialist in the diagnosis and treatment of diseases of the chest or thorax.

chir(o) A combining form denoting the hands.

chiropractic A system of therapeutics that attempts to restore normal function of the body via manipulation of the body.

chlamydia A sexually transmitted disease caused by the bacterium *Chlamydia trachomatis*.

chlorophyll The green coloring matter of plants.

cholecyst(o) A combining form that denotes the gallbladder (a bile sac).

cholecystectomy Excision or removal of the gallbladder.

cholecystitis Inflammation of the gallbladder.

cholecystography X-ray examination of the gallbladder.

choledoch(o) A combining form denoting bile or the common bile duct.

choledochogastrostomy Surgical connection of the stomach and the common bile duct.

choledocholithotripsy The crushing of a stone in the common bile duct.

choledochotomy Incision into the bile duct.

cholelithiasis A stone in the gallbladder—gallstone.

chondr(o) A combining form denoting cartilage.

chondritis Inflammation of cartilage.

chondrolysis Degeneration of cartilage.

choroid The middle layer of the eyeball; the vascular layer that provides blood to the eye.

cirrhosis A liver disorder in which the primary symptom is jaundice (yellow skin).

Claritin Brand name for loratadine; used to treat allergies and to reduce congestion and bronchial swelling.

clavicle Collarbone.

clitoris A small elongated erectile body situated at the anterior angle of the rima pudendi in women.

coccygeal Pertaining to the coccyx, or tailbone.

coccyx Four (usually fused) vertebrae that form the tailbone.

cochlea A snail-shell shaped organ of hearing in the inner ear.

cochlear Pertaining to the cochlea.

cochleitis Inflammation of the cochlea.

codeine A generic agent used to promote the ejection of mucus from the lower respiratory tract; also used to relieve pain.

colectomy Excision of all or part of the colon.

colitis Inflammation of the colon.

colonoscopy Visual examination of the colon.

colostomy Surgical creation of a new opening into the colon.

colpitis Inflammation of the vagina; vaginitis.

colpocele Herniation of the vagina.

colporrhagia Excessive flow (bleeding) from the vagina.

colporrhaphy Suturing of the vagina.

colposcopy Visual examination of the vagina and the cervix uteri.

Compazine Brand name for prochlorperazine; used to prevent or alleviate nausea and vomiting.

cones/rods Photoreceptor cells in the retina of the eye.

conjunctiva The mucous membrane that lines the eyelid and covers the exposed portion of the eyeball.

conjunctivitis Inflammation of the conjunctiva.

contraceptives Agents that prevent conception or impregnation.

contraindication Any condition that renders a certain treatment undesirable or not indicated.

conversion disorder A disorder characterized by a symptom suggestive of a neurologic impairment that affects the senses (for example, blindness) or motor function (for example, paralysis).

Corti, hairs of Small nerve endings in the cochlea that transmit impulses to the brain via the auditory nerve; also called the organ of Corti.

Corti, organ of Small nerve endings in the cochlea that transmit impulses to the brain via the auditory nerve; also called the hairs of Corti.

cortical hormones Hormones that regulate carbohydrate metabolism and salt and water balance; they also affect sexual characteristics.

cortisone An adrenal cortex steroid used to alleviate or to decrease inflammation; for immunosuppression, or for allergies.

costalgia Rib pain.

Cowper's gland Bulbourethral gland.

crani(o) A combining form denoting the skull or cranium.

cranial Pertaining to the skull.

craniectomy Removal or excision of part of the skull.

craniocele A protrusion of part of the cranial contents through a defect in the skull.

craniomalacia Softening of the skull.

cranioplasty Plastic surgery on the cranium.

craniospinal Pertaining to the skull and spine.

craniotomy An operation on or incision into the skull.

cranium The skull.

cryosurgery Destruction of tissue by the application of extreme cold.

cryotherapy The therapeutic use of cold.

cryptorchidism A congenital failure of the testes to descend into the scrotum.

cyanemia Bluishness of the blood. (Archaic)

cyanosis A bluish discoloration of skin and mucous membranes resulting from a lack of oxygen.

cystic Pertaining to a cyst or bladder.

cystitis Inflammation of the urinary bladder.

cystoptosis Prolapse of the urinary bladder into the urethra.

cystorrhagia Excessive bleeding from the urinary bladder.

cystoscope An endoscope for visual examination of the urinary bladder.

cystoscopy Visual examination of the urinary bladder.

cystospasm A spasm of the urinary bladder.

cystostomy Surgical formation of an opening into the urinary bladder.

cyt(o) A combining form denoting relationship to a cell.

cytoma A cell tumor.

D

dacry(o) A combining form denoting tears or lacrimal (tear) glands or ducts.

dacryoadenitis Inflammation of the lacrimal (tear) gland.

dacryocyst A lacrimal or tear sac.

dacryocystitis Inflammation of the tear or lacrimal sac.

dacryorrhea Excessive flowing of tears.

dacryostenosis Narrowing of lacrimal ducts.

dactyls Finger and toe bones; also called phalanges or digits.

decagram Ten grams.

decapitate To remove the head.

deciliter One-tenth of a liter.

decongestants Agents that reduce congestion and bronchial swelling.

dehydrate To remove water from a substance, such as the body.

deltoid muscle A muscle located at the spine of the scapula and clavicle; extends the arm.

Demerol Brand name for meperidine; used to relieve pain.

demilune Half-moon or crescent shaped.

dependent type A personality disorder characterized by an excessive need to be taken care of, resulting in submissive and clinging behavior.

Depogen Brand name for estradiol cypionate; used to treat menopause, prostatic cancer, osteoporosis, and abnormal menses.

depressive psychosis A major depressive disorder characterized by significant lowering of mood tone, loss of interest in daily activities, feelings of worthlessness, and recurrent thoughts of death or suicide.

derm(o), derm(a), dermat(o) Combining forms denoting the skin.

dermal Of or pertaining to the skin.

dermatitis Inflammation of the skin.

dermatoautoplasty Autografting of skin taken from another part of the patient's own body.

dermatologist A specialist in the diagnosis and treatment of skin diseases.

dermatology The specialty that deals with the diagnosis and treatment of diseases of the skin.

dermatophobia A morbid fear of acquiring a skin disease.

dermatosis Abnormal condition of the skin.

dermatotome An instrument for cutting the skin or cutting thin transplants.

dermis The middle layer of skin; also called the cutis or corium.

dermomycosis Any fungus disease of the skin.

detoxify To remove the toxic quality of a substance.

dextral Pertaining to the right (side or direction).

dextrogastria Displacement of the stomach to the right.

diagnoses Plural spelling of *diagnosis*.

diagnosis A determination of the nature of a disease.

dialysis A process of separating elements in a solution through a semipermeable membrane.

diarrhea Abnormal frequency and liquidity of fecal discharges.

diastole The resting phase of the heart.

diastolic pressure The pressure of the resting phase (expansion) of the heart; the lower of the two pressures.

Diflucan Brand name for fluconazole; used to destroy fungus or suppress its growth.

digits Finger and toe bones; also called phalanges or dactyls.

Dilantin Brand name for phenytoin; used to prevent or relieve convulsions.

diplophonia The production of double vocal sounds.

diplopia Double vision.

Diprivan Brand name for propofol; used to reduce or eliminate the perception of sensation.

dips(o), dips(ia)   Combining forms denoting thirst.

dissociative disorders   A group of mental disorders in which the patient is unable to recall important personal information.

diuretics   Agents that promote and increase the excretion of urine.

Diuril   Brand name for chlorothiazide; used to promote the production and excretion of urine.

dorsal   Pertaining to the back of the body.

Dramamine   Brand name for dimenhydrinate; used to prevent or alleviate nausea and vomiting.

drug psychoses   Organic mental syndromes caused by the consumption of drugs; some commonly used drugs are amphetamines, barbiturates, opiates, LSD groups, and solvents (inhalants).

ductus deferens   The excretory duct of the testis which unites with the excretory duct of the seminal vesicle; vas deferens

Dulcolax   Brand name for bisacodyl; used to promote peristalsis and bowel evacuation.

duodenal   Pertaining to the duodenum.

duodenectomy   Excision of all or part of the duodenum.

duodenoctomy   Surgical creation of a new opening into the duodenum.

dura mater   The tough outer layer of the meninges.

Dyrenium   Brand name for triamterine; used to promote the production and excretion or urine.

dyskinesia   Difficult or painful movement.

dysmenorrhagia   Painful and excessive bleeding during the menses.

dysmenorrhea   Difficult, painful menses.

dyspnea   Difficult breathing.

dyssomnias   Sleep disturbances involving the amount, quality, or timing of sleep.

dysuria   Painful or difficult urination.

E

eccrine glands   Sweat glands found in most regions of the body.

ectoderm   The outermost layers of skin.

efferent nerves   Nerves that send the impulses from the brain and spinal cord to the glands and muscles throughout the body.

Effexor   Brand name for venlafaxine; used to prevent or relieve depression.

electrocardiogram   Graphic tracing of the variations in electrical potential caused by excitation of the heart muscle.

electrocardiograph   An instrument used for recording the heart's activity.

electrocardiography   The process of making a recording of the heart's activity.

emetics   Agents that cause vomiting.

emia   A word element denoting relationship to the blood, or a condition of the blood.

encephal(o)   A combining form denoting the brain (en- [inside or within], combined with *cephal* [head]).

encephalic   Pertaining to the brain.

encephalitis   Inflammation of the brain.

encephaloma   Any swelling or tumor of the brain.

encephalomalacia   Softening of the brain.

encephalorrhagia   Excessive bleeding in the brain.

endocarditis   Inflammation of the endocardium.

endocardium   The membrane that lines the inside of the heart.

endocrinologist (endocrinology)   A specialist who studies the internally secreting glands and their effect on the body and its metabolism.

endometriosis   A condition in which tissue resembling endometrial tissue occurs aberrantly within the pelvic cavity.

enter(o)   A combining form indicating the intestines.

enterocleisis   Blockage or closure of the intestine.

enteroclysis   Injection or introduction of liquid into the intestine.

enterococcus   A type of intestinal bacteria.

enterokinesis   Muscular movement of the intestinal canal—peristalsis.

enterolithiasis   Stones or calculi found in the intestine.

enterorrhagia   Hemorrhage from the intestine.

enterorrhexis   Rupture of the intestinal wall.

enterostomy   Surgical creation of a new opening into the small intestine.

ependyma   Neuroglial cells that line the cavities of the central nervous system (CNS).

epicardium   The outermost layer of the heart.

epidemiologist (epidemiology)   A specialist in the diagnosis and treatment of diseases capable of being communicated from one host to another.

epidermis   The outer layer of skin.

epididymal   Pertaining to the epididymis.

epididymectomy   Removal of all or part of the epididymis.

epididymis   An elongated cordlike structure along the posterior border of the testis; provides storage, transit, and maturation of spermatozoa.

epididymitis   Inflammation of the epididymis.

epididymotomy   Incision into the epididymis.

epidiymectomy   Excision of the epididymis.

epiglottis   The cartilaginous structure that covers the glottis during swallowing to prevent food or fluid from entering the trachea.

epilepsy   Paroxysmal transient disturbance with episodic impairment or loss of consciousness.

epileptic   Pertaining to epilepsy.

epinephrine   A hormone that increases cardiac activity, increases fat usage for energy, and causes vasoconstriction in skeletal muscles; also called adrenaline.

epiotic   Situated above or upon the ear.

erectile agents   Agents that enhance the erectile function of the penis.

erotomania   An excessive or morbid inclination to erotic thoughts or behavior.

erythr(o)   A combining form denoting the color red or red blood cells.

erythroclasis   Breaking up or splitting up of red cells.

erythrocyte   A red blood cell.

erythrocytosis   An increase in red blood cells.

erythropenia   A deficiency in the number of red blood cells.

erythropoiesis   Formation of red blood cells.

esophageal   Pertaining to the esophagus.

esophagitis   Inflammation of the esophagus.

esophagoscopy   Visual examination (endoscopy) of the esophagus.

esophagostenosis   Narrowing of the esophagus.

Estrace   Brand name for estradiol; used to treat menopause, prostatic cancer, osteoporosis, and abnormal menses.

Estragyn   Brand name for estradiol cypionate; used to treat menopause, prostatic cancer, osteoporosis, and abnormal menses.

estrogen   A hormonal agent used in the treatment of menopause, prostatic cancer, osteoporosis, and abnormal menses.

estrogen hormones   Agents used to treat menopause, prostatic cancer, osteoporosis, and abnormal menses.

Estrostep 21   Brand name for estrogen and progestin; used to prevent conception or impregnation.

ethmoid bone   A bone located in front of the sphenoid bone.

etiology   The study of the cause of disease.

Eulexin   Brand name for flutamide; used to treat menopause, prostatic cancer, osteoporosis, and abnormal menses.

eupnea   Easy, normal breathing.

eustachian tube   The auditory tube that connects the middle ear to the pharynx.

exophthalmos   Abnormal protrusion of the eyeball.

expectorants   Agents that promote the ejection of mucus or other fluids from the lower respiratory tract.

F

factitious disorder (Münchausen's syndrome)   A disorder in which there is intentional feigning of physical or psychological symptoms to obtain medical treatment.

fallopian tubes   Tubes that connect the ovaries to the uterus; also called uterine tubes, oviducts.

family practice (family medicine)   The diagnosis and treatment of disorders of all members of the family regardless of age or sex, on a continuing basis.

fascia   A sheet of fibrous tissue that envelops the muscles and other organs of the body.

fasciitis   Inflammation of fascia.

femur   Thigh bone.

fetishism   Sexual urges involving the use of inanimate objects (fetishes), such as clothing, shoes, or underwear.

fetus   An unborn offspring in the post-embryonic period.

fibrin   A protein that aids in clotting blood.

fibula   The bone that is lateral to the tibia.

fimbriae   Fringe-like projections at the end of each fallopian tube that move the ovum into the uterus.

Floxin   Brand name for ofloxacin; used to kill infectious agents or prevent them from spreading.

follicle-stimulating hormone   A hormone that stimulates growth of the ovarian follicle; also stimulates secretion of estrogen (in females) and testosterone (in males); FSH.

frontal bone   Front skull bone above the eyes.

G

galact(o)   A combining form denoting milk or a resemblance to milk.

galactogenous   Production of milk by the mammary glands.

galactorrhea   Excessive or spontaneous flow of milk.

galactostasis   Halting or stoppage of milk secretion.

ganglia   Plural spelling of *ganglion*.

gastralgia   Pain in the stomach—stomachache.

gastrectomy   Excision of all or part of the stomach.

gastritis   Inflammation of the stomach.

gastrocnemius muscle   Calf muscle; flexes ankle joint and knee joint.

gastroenterologist (gastroenterology)   A specialist who deals with the diagnosis and treatment of diseases of the stomach and intestines.

gastropathy   Any disease of the stomach.

gastroscope   Instrument used to view the inside of the stomach.

gastroscopy   Visual examination of the inside of the stomach.

gastrostomy   Surgical creation of a new opening into the stomach.

genital herpes   A sexually transmitted disease caused by the herpes simplex (HSV-2) virus.

gingiva   The tissue enveloping the tooth sockets (the gums).

glans penis   The tip of the penis.

glaucoma   Opacity of the crystalline lens of the eye resulting from an increase in intraocular pressure.

glomerular   Pertaining to a renal glomerulus.

glomerulitis   Inflammation of the renal glomeruli.

glomerulopathy   Any disease of the glomerulus.

glomerulus   A tuft of capillaries located in the renal corpuscle.

gloss(o), gloss(ia)   Combining forms that denote the tongue.

glossal   Pertaining to the tongue; lingual.

glossectomy   Excision of the tongue.

glossitis   Inflammation of the tongue.

glottal   Pertaining to the glottis.

glottis   The vocal apparatus of the larynx, consisting of the true vocal cords and the opening between them.

glucagon   A hormone that regulates sugar and carbohydrate metabolism.

glucogenic   Giving rise to or producing glucose.

gluteus maximus muscle   The largest muscle of the buttocks; extends and rotates the thigh laterally.

glycemia   Presence of glucose in the blood.

glycopenia   Deficiency of glucose in tissues.

glycosuria   Presence of sugar in the urine, especially an excessive amount.

gonorrhea   A sexually transmitted disease caused by the bacterium *Neisseria gonorrhoeae*.

gravida   A word denoting a pregnant woman.

gyn(o), gynec(o)   Combining forms that denote women or the female sex.

gynecologist   A specialist in treating female disorders.

gynecology   The branch of medicine treating diseases of women.

gynopathy   Any disease of women.

gynoplasty   Plastic surgery on the female organs.

H

hairs of Corti   Small nerve endings in the cochlea that transmit impulses to the brain via the auditory nerve; also called the organ of Corti.

Haldol   Brand name for haloperidol; used to treat psychoses; a major tranquilizer.

heart   A hollow muscle that is divided into four chambers; the two atria collect blood, and the two ventricles pump the blood.

hectogram   A unit of mass being 100 grams.

hem(o), hemat(o)   Combining forms denoting the blood.

hemangioma   A benign tumor composed of newly formed blood vessels.

hemarthrosis   Accumulation of blood in a joint cavity.

hematemesis   Vomiting of blood.

hematic   Pertaining to or contained in the blood.

hematocrit   The volume percentage of red cells in whole blood (separation of red cells for counting).

hematologist (hematology)   A specialist who treats the blood and blood-forming elements.

hematologist-oncologist (hematology-oncology) A specialist who treats cancers of the blood and blood-forming elements.

hematology Study of the science of blood.

hematopoiesis/hemopoiesis The process of developing blood cells.

hematuria Presence of blood in the urine.

hemianesthesia Anesthesia (lack of feeling) on one side of the body.

hemiplegia Paralysis on one side of the body.

hemiplegic Pertaining to hemiplegia.

hemolysis Breaking down or destroying blood cells.

hemoptysis Spitting up or coughing up blood.

hemostat An instrument or medicine for stopping bleeding.

hemostatics Agents that arrest the flow of blood.

heparin Generic agent used to dissolve blood clots or to thin the blood.

hepat(o), hepat(ico) Combining forms denoting the liver.

hepatatrophy Atrophy or wasting of the liver.

hepatic Of or pertaining to the liver.

hepatitis Inflammation of the liver.

hepatomegaly Abnormally enlarged liver.

hepatorenal Pertaining to the liver and kidneys.

hepatorrhaphy Surgical repair or suture of the liver.

hidradenitis Inflammation of a sweat gland.

hidropoiesis Formation and secretion of sweat by the sweat glands.

hist(o), histi(o) Combining forms denoting relationship to tissue.

histocyte A tissue cell.

histokinesis Movement in the tissues of the body.

histology The study of tissue.

histoneurology The histology of the nervous system.

historrhexis Breaking up of tissue.

histotoxic Being poisonous to tissue or tissues.

histrionic type A personality disorder marked by excessive attention-seeking behavior.

homogenesis Reproduction by the same process each generation.

humerus Upper arm bone connected to the elbow.

Hycodan Brand name for hydrocodone; used to relieve pain.

hydralazine Generic agent used to dilate blood vessels.

hydrocodone Generic agent that relieves pain.

hydrocortisone An adrenal cortex steroid used to alleviate or to decrease inflammation; also for immunosuppression and allergies.

hyperalgesia Increased sensitivity to pain.

hypercalcemia Excessive amount of calcium in the blood.

hyperglycemia Abnormally high level of sugar in the blood

hyperkalemia Excessive amount of potassium in the blood.

hypernatremia Excessive amount of sodium in the blood.

hyperpnea An increase in the depth and rate of breathing.

hypersomnia A sleep disorder consisting of the need for excessive sleep.

hypocalcemia Deficiency of calcium in the blood.

hypochondriasis A mental disorder marked by a morbid preoccupation with one's health or a fear of having some disease, despite a lack of identification of disease on examination.

hypodermic Administered beneath the skin.

hypogastric Pertaining to the area under the stomach.

hypoglycemia Abnormally low level of glucose in the blood

hypokalemia Deficiency of potassium in the blood.

hyponatremia Deficiency of sodium in the blood.

hypophysectomy Surgical removal or destruction of the pituitary gland.

hypophysis Another term for the pituitary gland.

hypophysis cerebri Another term for the pituitary gland.

hypophysitis Inflammation of the pituitary gland.

hypothyroidism Deficiency of thyroid secretion.

hypoxemia Deficient oxygenation of the blood.

hyster(o) A combining form denoting the uterus.

hysteralgia Pain in the uterus.

hysterectomy Removal or excision of the uterus.

hysterocleisis Surgical closure of the os uteri.

hysterolith Uterine calculus.

hysteropathy Any uterine disease; metropathy.

hysteropexy Surgical fixation or fastening of the uterus.

hysteroptosis Prolapse of the uterus; metroptosis.

hysterospasm Contraction, spasm of the uterus.

I

ibuprofen   An agent that counteracts or suppresses inflammation.

ile(o)   A combining form denoting relationship to the ileum, the third or distal portion of the small intestine.

ileectomy   Excision of all or part of the ileum.

ileitis   Inflammation of the ileum.

ileocecal   Pertaining to the ileum and cecum.

ileorrhaphy   Suture of the ileum.

ileotomy   Incision into the ileum.

ili(o)   A combining form denoting relationship to the ilium, the superior portion of the hip bone.

iliac   Pertaining to the ilium.

ilium   The superior portion of the hip bone.

Imdur   Brand name for isosorbide; used to dilate blood vessels.

immature   Not fully developed.

immunologist (immunology)   A specialist in the diagnosis and treatment of the body's resistance to disease.

Imodium   Brand name for loperamide; used to counteract diarrhea.

impulse control disorders   Failure to resist a temptation to perform an act that is harmful to oneself or others.

inadequate type   A personality disorder involving being generally inept or socially, intellectually, and physically awkward.

Inapsine   Brand name for droperidol; used to reduce or eliminate the perception of sensation.

incus   The bone shaped like an anvil, located in the middle ear, that transmits vibrations to the cochlea.

infectious diseases   Diseases that can be transmitted from one host to another.

inferior   A directional term meaning located below something.

inframammary   Situated beneath the breast.

infratracheal   Beneath the trachea.

insomnia   Inability to sleep.

insulin   A hormone that regulates the metabolism of sugar and carbohydrate.

integumentary system   Skin, nails, hair, and the glands embedded in the skin.

intercostal   Situated between the ribs.

intercostal nerves   Nerves between the ribs.

interdigital   Between the fingers or toes.

internist (internal medicine)   A specialist in the diagnosis and treatment of the disorders and diseases of the internal structures of the body.

intrabuccal   Within the cheek or mouth.

intravenous   Within a vein.

introverted type   A form of schizoidal personality in which there is a defect in forming interpersonal relationships.

intubation   The process of inserting a tube for anesthesia or pulmonary assistance.

involuntary muscles   Smooth muscles (and cardiac, or striated, muscles) that you do not control and that are controlled by the autonomic nervous system.

Ipecac Syrup   Brand name for ipecac; used to cause vomiting.

irid(o)   A combining form denoting a relationship to the iris of the eye.

iridectasis   Dilatation (dilation) of the iris.

iridectomy   Excision of the iris.

iridopathy   Any disease of the iris.

iridoplegia   Paralysis of the iris.

iris   The colored, contractile membrane that expands and contracts based on the amount of light present.

iritis   Inflammation of the iris.

ischium   The inferior portion of the hip bone.

islets of Langerhans   Small groups of insulin-producing cells in the pancreas.

J

jejunitis   Inflammation of the jejunum.

jejunorrhaphy   Suturing of the jejunum.

K

Kaopectate   Brand name for loperamide; used to counteract diarrhea.

Keflex   Brand name for cephalexin; used to kill infectious agents or prevent them from spreading.

kerat(o)   A combining form denoting the cornea of the eye or horny tissue.

keratectomy   Excision of the cornea.

keratiasis   The presence of horny warts on the skin.

keratin   A scleroprotein that is the principal component of epidermis, hair, nails, and horny tissues.

keratocele   Herniation of the cornea.

keratoderma   A horny skin or covering.

keratogenous   Producing cells that result in the formation of horny tissue such as fingernails.

keratoid   Resembling a horny skin.

keratolytics   Agents that soften the horny layer of the epidermis.

keratoma   A tumor or growth of horny tissue.

keratoplasty   Plastic surgery of the cornea; cornea grafting.

keratoscleritis   Inflammation of the cornea and the sclera.

kilounit   A quantity equaling 1000 units.

kinesalgia   Pain on motion or movement.

kleptomania   A compulsion to steal. Episodes of stealing objects that are not needed for personal use or for their monetary value.

L

labia majora   The larger lips of the external female genitalia.

labia minora   The smaller lips of the external female genitalia.

labyrinth   The inner ear.

labyrinthitis   Inflammation of the inner ear.

labyrinthotomy   Incision into the inner ear.

lacrimal   Pertaining to tears or the tear glands.

lacrimal glands   Tear glands; they produce a fluid that cleanses and lubricates the eye

lactation   Secretion of milk.

lactic   Pertaining to milk.

lactogenic   Stimulating the production of milk.

laryng(o)   A combining form denoting the larynx (voice box).

laryngeal   Of or pertaining to the larynx.

laryngectomy   Excision of the larynx.

laryngitis   Inflammation of the larynx.

laryngocentesis   Surgical puncture of the larynx.

laryngopharynx   The portion of the pharynx below the upper edge of the epiglottis; opens into the larynx and esophagus.

laryngoplegia   Paralysis of the larynx.

laryngoscope   An instrument used to examine the larynx.

laryngospasm   Spasmodic closure of the larynx.

laryngostenosis   Narrowing of the larynx.

Lasix   Brand name for furosemide; used to promote the production and excretion of urine.

latissimus dorsi muscle   The largest back muscle; extends and rotates the humerus medially.

laxatives   Agents that promote peristalsis and bowel evacuation.

leukemia   A blood disease characterized by distorted proliferation and development of leukocytes.

leukocyte   White blood cell.

leukocytology   Study of the science of white blood cells.

leukopenia   Reduction in the number of leukocytes in the blood.

leukopoiesis   Formation of white blood cells.

lidocaine   A generic agent that reduces or eliminates the perception of sensation.

ligaments   A type of connective tissue that connects one bone to another.

lingual   Pertaining to the tongue; glossal.

lipedema   Excess fat and fluid in the subcutaneous tissue.

lipemia   The condition of having fat in the blood.

lipidemia   Abnormally high concentration of fat in the blood.

lipids   Fats and fatlike substances in the body.

Lipitor   Brand name for atorvastatin; used to counteract high levels of lipids in the blood.

lipoma   A fatty tumor; adipoma.

lipopenia   A deficiency of lipids (fat) in the body.

lipuria   Fat in the urine; adiposuria.

lithium   A generic agent that is effective in the treatment of psychoses.

Lithotabs   Brand name for lithium; used to treat psychoses; a major tranquilizer.

lithotripsy   The operation of crushing a stone.

Loniten   Brand name for minoxidil; used to dilate blood vessels.

lumbar   Pertaining to the lower back region; the loin region.

lumbosacral plexus   A network of nerves in the loin region.

Luminal   Brand name for phenobarbital; used to prevent or relieve convulsions.

luteinizing hormone   A hormone that causes ovulation; stimulates progesterone (in females) and testosterone (in males).

lymph   A colorless liquid made up of fluid from the spaces between cells plus various salts, sugar, water, and waste products.

lymph(o)   A combining form indicating lymph or the lymphatic glands or vessels.

lymphadenitis   Inflammation of the lymph glands.

lymphangioma   A tumor rich in blood vessels.

lymphedema   Swelling of subcutaneous tissue due to excessive lymph fluid.

lymphocyte   A white cell that is formed in the lymph glands.

lymphocytopenia   Reduction in the number of lymphocytes in the blood.

lymphopathy   Any disease of the lymphatic system.

lymphopenia   Deficiency of lymph cells.

lymphopoiesis   Making or developing lymph.

lymphostasis   Stoppage of lymph flow.

M

malleus   The bone shaped like a hammer, located in the middle ear, that transmits vibrations to the cochlea.

mammaplasty   Mastoplasty; plastic surgery of the breast.

mammary   Pertaining to the breast.

mammogram   A roentgenography of the breast.

mandible   The lower jawbone.

-mania or -manic   Suffixes denoting an abnormal love for or compulsion.

masochistic type   A personality disorder in which the person seems to derive pleasure from physical or psychological pain inflicted on oneself either by the self or by others.

masseter muscle   A muscle located at the side of the mandible; used for chewing and for closing the jaw.

mast(o)   A combining form denoting relationship to the breast or mammary gland.

mastectomy   Excision of all or part of a breast.

mastication   The act or process of chewing.

mastitis   Inflammation of the breast.

mastoid   Resembling a nipple or breast.

mastopexy   Surgical reattachment of a breast.

mastoplasty   Plastic surgery of the breast; mammaplasty.

maxilla   The upper jawbone.

Maxipime   Brand name for cefepime; used to kill infectious agents or prevent them from spreading.

meatus   An opening; an orifice.

Mectizan   Brand name for ivermectin; used to destroy parasites.

medullary hormones   Epinephrine and norepinephrine.

megalomania   Delusions of grandeur; unreasonable conviction of one's own greatness.

melanin   Pigment granules in the skin that determine color.

melanocyte-stimulating hormone   A hormone that stimulates skin pigmentation; MSH.

melanuria   Black or dark discoloration of the urine.

melatonin   A hormone related to day/night cycle; levels increase before sleep.

melena   Dark, black feces containing blood.

menarche   The beginning of the menstrual function.

meningeal   Pertaining to the meninges.

meninges   The membranes that cover the brain and the spinal cord; singular spelling is *meninx*.

meningioma   Any swelling or tumor of the meninges.

meningitis   Inflammation of the meninges.

meningocele   Herniation of the meninges.

meningomyelitis   Inflammation of the meninges and the spinal cord.

meningopathy   Any disease of the meninges.

meningorrhagia   Excessive bleeding of the meninges.

menopause   Cessation of the menses.

menorrhagia   Excessive bleeding during the menses.

menorrhea   Normal discharge of the menses.

menses   The monthly flow of blood from the genital tract of women.

menstrual   Pertaining to the menses.

metacarpals   Hand bones that extend from the wrist.

Metamucil   Brand name for psyllium; used to promote peristalsis and bowel evacuation.

metatarsals   Foot bones that extend from the ankle.

metr(o), metr(a)   Combining forms denoting the uterus.

metritis   Inflammation of the uterus.

metrocolpocele   Hernia of the uterus and vagina.

metropathy   Any uterine disease; hysteropathy.

metroptosis   Prolapse of the uterus; hysteroptosis.

metrorrhagia   Abnormal bleeding from the uterus.

metrorrhea   Uterine bleeding.

metrostenosis   Narrowing of the uterus.

Mevacor   Brand name for lovastatin; used to counteract high levels of lipids in the blood.

microglia   A type of neuroglial cells that respond to infections.

millivolt   One one-thousandth (1/1000) of a volt.

Monistat   Brand name for miconazole; used to destroy fungus or suppress its growth.

monochromatic   Having only one color.

monorchism   Having only one testicle in the scrotum.

morphine   Generic agent used to relieve pain.

mucolytics   Agents that destroy or dissolve mucus.

Mucomyst   Brand name for acetylcystein; used to destroy or dissolve mucus.

Mucosil   Brand name for acetylcystein; used to destroy or dissolve mucus.

multicellular   Composed of many cells.

muscle relaxant   Agent that reduces muscle tension.

muscular   Pertaining to muscles.

my(o)   A combining form denoting muscle.

myalgia   Muscle pain.

Mycostatin   Brand name for nystatin; used to destroy fungus or suppress its growth.

mydriatics   Agents used to dilate the pupils.

myel, myel(o)   Combining forms that denote the spinal cord or bone marrow.

myelin   A sheath surrounding some nerve cells; functions as an electrical insulator.

myelitis   Inflammation of the spinal cord.

myelogram   Roentgenogram of the spinal cord.

myeloneuritis   Inflammation of the spinal cord and peripheral nerves.

myelopathy   Any disease of the spinal cord.

myocardial   Pertaining to the muscular tissue of the heart.

myocarditis   Inflammation of the myocardium.

myocardium   The heart muscle.

myocele   Muscle herniation.

myopathy   Any disease of the muscles.

myorrhaphy   Suturing of a muscle.

myotomy   The cutting or dissection of a muscle.

myringectomy   Excision of the tympanic membrane, or eardrum.

myringitis   Inflammation of the tympanic membrane, or eardrum.

myringomycosis   Fungal condition of the tympanic membrane, or eardrum.

myx(o)   A combining form denoting mucus or mucous membrane.

myxadenitis   Inflammation of a mucous gland.

myxadenoma   A tumor with the structure of the mucous gland.

myxorrhea   A flow of mucus.

N

naproxen sodium   An agent that counteracts or suppresses inflammation.

narcissistic type   A personality disorder in which interpersonal problems arise because of an inflated sense of self-worth.

narcolepsy   Recurrent uncontrollable brief episodes of sleep.

narcoleptic   Pertaining to narcolepsy.

nares   The external orifice of the nose; nostrils; singular spelling *naris*.

naris   One of the openings of the nose; one nostril; plural spelling *nares*.

nas(o)   A combining form denoting the nose.

nasal   Pertaining to the nares; pertaining to the nose.

nasal bone   The bone that forms the bridge of the nose.

nasogastric   Pertaining to the nose and the stomach.

nasopharyngeal   Pertaining to the nasopharynx.

nasopharynx   The part of the pharynx above the level of the soft palate.

nasoscope   An instrument for visual examination of the nose.

nasoseptal   Pertaining to the nasal septum.

Nembutal   Brand name for phenobarbital; used for short-term treatment of insomnia.

neonatal   Pertaining to the first four weeks after birth.

neoplasm   Any new or abnormal growth.

nephr(o)   A combining form denoting relationship to the kidney.

nephrectomy   Excision of a kidney.

nephritis   Inflammation of the kidney.

nephrohydrosis   An accumulation of water or fluid in the kidneys.

nephrolithiasis   Condition of having kidney stones.

nephrologist   A specialist in the diagnosis and treatment of kidney disorders and diseases.

nephrology   The study of the science of the kidneys.

nephropathy   Any kidney disease.

nephropexy   Surgical reattachment of a kidney.

nephroptosis   Downward displacement of the kidney.

neur(o)   A combining form denoting the nerves or nervous system.

neural   Pertaining to the nerves.

neuralgia   Nerve pain.

neuritis   Inflammation of the nerves.

neuroglia   Supporting structure of nervous tissue; literally "nerve glue."

neurohypophysis   Posterior lobe of the pituitary gland; also called the neurohypophysis cerebri.

neurohypophysis cerebri   Posterior lobe of the pituitary gland.

neurologist   A specialist in the disorders of the nervous system caused by organic disease or injury.

neurology   The study of the science of the nervous system.

neuropathy   Any disease of the nervous system.

neuroplasty   Plastic surgery of the nerves.

neuroplexus   A network of nerves.

neurosis   An emotional (nervous) disorder characterized by anxiety.

neurosurgeon (neurosurgery)   A specialist in the diagnosis and mainly surgical treatment of diseases and disorders of the central nervous system (brain and spinal cord).

Nexium   Brand name for omeprazole; used to neutralize acidity in the stomach.

nightmare disorder   Repeated awakenings from sleep caused by extremely frightening dreams.

Nitro-Bid (ointment)   Brand name for nitroglycerin; used to alleviate angina pectoris.

Nitrocine (transdermal)   Brand name for nitroglycerin; used to alleviate angina pectoris.

Nitrogard (buccal tablets)   Brand name for nitroglycerin; used to alleviate angina pectoris.

nitroglycerin   Generic agent used to alleviate angina pectoris; also used to dilate blood vessels.

Nitrolingual (spray)   Brand name for nitroglycerin; used to alleviate angina pectoris.

noctiphobia   Irrational fear of night and darkness.

nocturia   Excessive urination at night.

nonopiod analgesics   Agents that provide an analgesic, anesthetic effect on the urinary tract; also eliminate urinary spasms.

nonspecific   Not due to any single known cause, as to a pathogen.

nonviable   Not capable of living.

norepinephrine   A hormone that raises blood pressure, constricts vessels.

Novocain   Brand name for procaine; used to reduce or eliminate the perception of sensation.

nuclear medicine   The branch of medicine concerned with the use of radionuclides in the diagnosis and treatment of disease.

nymphomania   Abnormal, excessive sexual desire in the female.

Nytol   Brand name for diphenhydramine; used for short-term treatment of insomnia.

O

obsessive-compulsive disorders   Disorders marked by recurrent compulsions (repetitive behaviors) and obsessions (persistent ideas, thoughts, and impulses). Compulsions may involve repetitive washing of hands, checking constantly to see if a door is locked, etc. Obsessions may involve repeated thoughts such as becoming contaminated by shaking hands.

obsessive-compulsive type   A personality disorder characterized by a preoccupation with orderliness, perfection, and control.

obstetrician (obstetrics)   A specialist in pregnancy, prenatal care, and childbirth and its aftermath.

occipital bone   The bone at the back of the skull forming the base.

occlusion   The natural closure and fitting together of the upper and lower teeth.

ocular   Pertaining to the eye; ophthalmic.

oculi   Plural spelling for eyes.

oculus   Singular spelling for the eye.

odontalgia   Toothache.

oligemia   Deficiency in the volume of blood.

oligodendroglia   A type of neuroglial cells that aid in the development of myelin.

oliguria   Diminished secretion of urine.

oncology (oncologist)   The branch of medicine that deals with tumors, primarily cancer.

onych(o)   A combining form denoting the nails.

onychogenic   Producing nail substance.

onychoma   A tumor of the nail or nail bed.

onychomalacia   Abnormally soft nail.

onychomycosis   A fungus condition of the nails.

onychophagia   Habitual biting of the nails.

onychoptosis   Falling off of the nail.

onychorrhexis   Splitting or rupture of the nails.

onychosis   Abnormal condition of the nails.

oophor(o)   A combining form denoting the ovaries.

oophorectomy   Excision of an ovary; an ovariectomy.

oophoritis   Inflammation of an ovary; ovaritis.

oophoroma   Tumor of the ovary.

oophoroplasty   Plastic surgery on the ovary.

oophororrhagia   Hemorrhage or bleeding from an ovary.

oophorostomy   The making of an opening into an ovarian cyst to provide drainage.

ophthalm(o)   A combining form denoting the eye.

ophthalmic   Pertaining to the eye; ocular.

ophthalmologist   A physician who deals with all areas involving the eye.

ophthalmomycosis   A fungal condition of the eye.

ophthalmopathy   Any disease of the eye.

ophthalmoscope   An instrument to examine the eye.

ophthalmology   The study or science of the eye and its structure.

optical   Pertaining to vision.

optometer   An instrument used to measure ocular refraction.

Ora-Jel   Brand name for benzocaine; used on the skin to abolish the sensation of pain.

oral   Pertaining to the mouth.

orchiditis   Inflammation of a testis; orchitis.

orchidoplasty   Plastic surgery of a testis.

orchiopathy   Any disease of the testes.

orchiopexy   Surgical fixation in the scrotum of an undescended testis.

orchitis   Inflammation of a testis; orchiditis.

organ of Corti   Small nerve endings in the cochlea that transmit impulses to the brain via the auditory nerve; also called the hairs of Corti.

orolingual   Pertaining to the mouth and tongue.

oropharynx   The division of the pharynx between the soft palate and the upper edge of the epiglottis.

Ortho-Novum   Brand name for estrogen and progestin; used to prevent conception or impregnation.

orthopedic surgeon (orthopedist) (orthopedic surgery)   A surgeon who deals with the diagnosis and mainly surgical treatment of the musculoskeletal system.

orthopnea   Inability to breathe unless one is in an upright position.

oscheal   Pertaining to the scrotum.

oscheitis   Inflammation of the scrotum.

oscheoma   Tumor of the scrotum.

oscheoplasty   Plastic surgery of the scrotum.

ossification   Formation of bone.

oste(o)   A combining form denoting the bones.

osteitis   Inflammation of a bone.

osteoclasis   Breaking or fracturing a bone.

osteolysis   Breaking down bone.

osteomalacia   Softening of the bones.

osteomyelitis   Inflammation of bone marrow.

osteoporosis   Increased porousness of bones.

ot(o)   A combining form indicating the ear.

otalgia   Earache—pain in the ear.

otics   Agents used to treat ear disorders.

otitis   Inflammation of the ear.

otolaryngologist (otolaryngology)   A specialist in the diagnosis and treatment of diseases of the ear, nose, and throat.

otomycosis   Abnormal condition of fungus in the ear.

otoscope   An instrument used for viewing the ear.

ova   Plural spelling of *ovum*.

ovari(o)   A combining form denoting relationship to the ovary.

ovariectomy   Excision or removal of an ovary; an oophorectomy.

ovariocele   Herniation of an ovary.

ovariocentesis   Surgical puncture of an ovary.

ovariopathy   Ovarian disease.

ovariopexy   Surgically reattaching an ovary to the abdominal wall.

ovariorrhaphy   Rupture of an ovary.

ovariorrhexis   Rupture of an ovary.

ovaritis   Inflammation of an ovary; oophoritis.

ovary (ovaries)   Endocrine glands that secrete estrogen and progesterone, and produce the female gametes.

oviducts   Tubes that connect the ovaries to the uterus; fallopian tubes; uterine tubes.

oviform   Egg-shaped.

ovocyte   A developing egg cell; an oocyte.

ovogenesis   The process of formation of the female gametes (ova); oogenesis.

ovum   The female sex cell.

oximeter   Photoelectric device used for determining the oxygen saturation in the blood.

oxycodone   Generic agent used to relieve pain.

oxytocin   Hormonal agent that promotes uterine contractions and promotes labor.

oxytocins   Agents that promote uterine contractions and promote labor.

P

pain disorder   A somatoform disorder characterized by pain, for which there is no physical finding, in one or more parts of the body; causes distress or impairs work or social functioning.

palate   The roof of the mouth.

pancreas   A gland located behind the stomach that produces insulin and glucagon.

pancreat(o)   A combining form denoting relationship to the pancreas.

pancreatectomy   Surgical removal of the pancreas.

pancreatic   Pertaining to the pancreas.

pancreatitis   Inflammation of the pancreas.

pancreatolith   A stone or calculus in the pancreas.

pancreatolithectomy   Excision of pancreatic stones.

pancreatopathy   A disease of the pancreas.

pancreolysis   The breaking down of the pancreas.

panhysterectomy   Total removal of the uterus and cervix (total hysterectomy).

panic attack   A period of intense fear or discomfort, with fears of dying or losing control. Some physical symptoms include smothering sensations and trembling.

para   A word denoting a woman who has produced a viable offspring, regardless of whether the child was living a birth.

paranoid type   A personality disorder characterized by a pattern of distrust and suspiciousness of others without reason.

paraplegia   Paralysis in the legs and the lower part of the body.

paraplegic   Pertaining to paraplegia.

parasiticides   Agents that destroy parasites.

parasomnias   A category of sleep disorders in which abnormal events occur during sleep.

parasympathetic nerves   The part of the autonomic nervous system that restore the body's systems to normal; it lowers blood pressure and decreases heart rate.

parathormone   Another name for PTH, parathyroid hormone.

parathyroid hormone (PTH)   A hormone that regulates the metabolism of calcium and phosphorous.

parathyroidal   Pertaining to the parathyroid gland.

parathyroidectomy   Excision of a parathyroid gland.

parathyroidoma   A tumor of the parathyroid gland.

parathyroids   Four glands located beside the thyroid gland that produce PTH (parathyroid hormone).

parathyropathy   Any disease of the parathyroid glands.

parietal bone   The bone on the side of the skull behind the frontal bone.

parturition   The act or process of giving birth to a child.

passive-aggressive type   A personality disorder marked by aggressive behavior manifested in a passive way, such as pouting, procrastination, or stubbornness.

patella   Kneecap.

pathological gambling   Morbid preoccupation with gambling; a need to gamble.

pathologist   A specialist dealing primarily with the diagnosis of disease.

pathology   The study of diseases.

Paxil   Brand name for paroxetine; used to prevent or relieve depression.

pectoralis major   A chest muscle that flexes and rotates the arm medially.

pectoralis minor   A chest muscle that draws the shoulder downward.

pediatrician (pediatrics)   A specialist in the diagnosis and treatment of diseases of children.

pelvic   Pertaining to the pelvis.

Penetrex   Brand name for enoxacin; used to kill infectious agents or prevent them from spreading.

penicillin   The generic name for various brand names such as V-cillin K, Ledercillin VK, and PenVee K, used to treat infections.

pentad   Any group of five (5).

Pentothal   Brand name for thiopental sodium; used to reduce or eliminate the perception of sensation.

Pepcid   Brand name for famotidine; used to neutralize acidity in the stomach and to counteract diarrhea.

Pepto-Bismol   Brand name for bismuth subsalicylate; used to neutralize acidity in the stomach.

pericarditis   Inflammation of the pericardium.

pericardium   The fibroserous sac surrounding the heart.

perineum   The area in females between the base of the vulva and anus; in males, the area between the base of the scrotum and anus.

periosteum   Connective tissue surrounding bones.

peripheral nervous system   The brain stem, cerebrum, and cerebellum.

personality disorders   Mental disorders characterized by an inflexible and poorly adaptive personality. These traits result in definite impairment in social functioning. Because of these impairments, the patient's actions may have a generally adverse effect on society.

phacocele   Herniation of a lens of the eye.

phacomalacia   A soft cataract.

phakitis   Inflammation of a lens of the eye.

phalanx, phalanges (pl.)   Finger and toe bones; also called dactyls or digits.

pharmacologist   One who specializes in the study of the action of drugs.

pharyng(o)   A combining form denoting the pharynx.

pharyngeal   Pertaining to the pharynx.

pharyngectomy   Excision of all or part of the throat.

pharyngitis   Inflammation of the pharynx.

pharyngomycosis   Any fungal infection of the throat.

pharyngonasal   Pertaining to the nose and pharynx.

pharyngoplegia   Paralysis of the muscles of the throat.

pharyngoscope   An instrument used for viewing the throat.

pharyngostenosis   Narrowing of the throat.

pharynx   The musculo-membranous passage between the mouth and posterior nares and the larynx and the esophagus; the throat.

Phenergan   Brand name for promethazine; used to prevent or alleviate nausea and vomiting.

Phenergan with codeine   Brand name for promethazine hydrochloride; used to alleviate or prevent coughs.

phenobarbital   A generic agent that prevents or relieves convulsions; also used for short-term treatment of insomnia.

phenylephrine   A generic agent used to counteract low blood pressure by causing contraction of blood vessels.

-phil(ia)   A suffix denoting love or attraction to.

phleb(o)   A combining form denoting a vein or the veins.

phlebitis   Inflammation of a vein.

phleborrhagia   Excessive bleeding from a vein.

phlebosclerosis   Hardening of the walls of the veins.

phlebostenosis   Narrowing or constricting of a vein.

phlebotomy   Incision into a vein.

physiatrist   A specialist in the diagnosis and treatment of disease with the aid of physical agents such as heat, light, water, or mechanical apparatus.

physical medicine and rehabilitation   The diagnosis and treatment of disease with the aid of physical agents such as heat, light, water, or mechanical apparatus.

pia mater   The inner layer of the meninges; contains blood vessels.

pineal gland   The pinecone shaped gland in the brain that secretes serotonin and melatonin; also called the pineal body.

pinealectomy   Excision of the pineal gland.

pinealopathy   Any disease of the pineal gland.

Pitocin   Brand name for oxytocin; used to promote uterine contractions and promote labor.

pituitary gland   A gland located in the brain that produces hormones that direct the functions of the other endocrine glands; also called the hypophysis cerebri.

placenta   An organ characteristic of true mammals during pregnancy, joining mother and offspring; provides nutrients for the developing fetus.

plastic surgeon (plastic surgery)   A specialist in the restoration or repair of defects of the human body.

platelets   Thrombocytes; clotting cells.

pleocytosis   The presence of a greater number of cells than normal.

pleur(o)   A combining form indicating the pleura (the membrane lining the chest cavity and covering the lungs).

pleura, pleurae (pl)   The serous membrane surrounding the lungs.

pleural   Of or relating to the pleura.

pleuralgia   Pain in the pleural region.

pleurectomy   Excision of the pleura.

pleurisy   Inflammation of the pleura; pleuritis.

pleuritis   Inflammation of the pleura; pleurisy.

pleurocele   Herniation of lung tissue or of the pleura.

pleurocentesis   Surgical puncture or tap of the pleura.

pleurotomy   Incision into the pleura.

plexus   A network.

-pnea   A word ending denoting breathing or air or gas.

pneum(a),pneum(o),pneum(ato),pneumon(o)   Combining forms denoting the lungs, respiration, air, or gas.

pneumocentesis   Surgical puncture for aspiration of the lung.

pneumoconiosis   A disease caused by dust or other particulates in the lungs.

pneumodynamics   The dynamics of the respiratory system.

pneumoencephalography   Radiographic films of the brain utilizing injections of air or gas.

pneumomelanosis   The blackening of the lungs as from coal dust.

pneumonitis   Inflammation of the lung.

pneumonography   X-ray of the lung.

pneumothorax   Accumulation of air in the chest cavity.

poliomyelitis   Inflammation of the gray matter of the spinal cord.

polycythemia   An increase in the number of red blood cells in the blood.

polydipsia   Excessive thirst, symptomatic of diabetes.

polyphagia   Excessive eating or overeating (bulimia).

polyuria   Excessive production of urine.

postmortem   Occurring or performed after death.

postnasal   Situated or occurring behind the nose.

postoperative   Occurring after an operation.

postpartum   Occurring after labor and childbirth.

post-traumatic stress disorder (PTSD)   Psychological symptoms occurring after a traumatic event, such as military combat, flood, fire, or automobile accident.

prednisone   An adrenal cortex steroid used to alleviate or to decrease inflammation; also for immunosuppression or allergies

premenstrual   Before the onset of the menses.

prenatal   Before childbirth.

preoperative   Occuring before an operation.

prepartal   Occurring before labor.

presbycusis   Loss of hearing due to old age.

presbyopia   Loss of vision due to old age; hardening of the lens due to aging.

preventive medicine   The branch of study and practice of medicine that aims at the prevention of disease.

primipara   A woman who has had one viable offspring.

Prinivil   Brand name for lisinopril; used to counteract high blood pressure.

Procardia   Brand name for nifedipine; used to counteract high blood pressure.

proct(o)   A combining form denoting the rectum or anus.

proctatresia   Anal atresia, the absence of a proper rectal opening.

proctocele   Hernial protrusion of the rectum.

proctologist (proctology)   A specialist in the diagnosis and treatment of diseases and disorders of the rectum and sigmoid colon.

proctopexy   Surgical fixing or fastening of the rectum.

proctoptosis   Prolapse or falling of the rectum.

proctorrhea   Flow from the rectum or anus.

proctoscopy   Examination of the rectum by the use of a proctoscope.

progesterone   A hormone that increases the development of female sexual characteristics; involved in female reproduction.

prolactin   A hormone that stimulates the development of the breast and the production of milk during pregnancy.

prostate   A gland in the male that surrounds the neck of the urinary bladder and the urethra; contributes fluid to seminal fluid to protect sperm.

prostatectomy   Excision of the prostate gland.

prostatic   Pertaining to the prostate gland.

prostatitis   Inflammation of the prostate gland.

prostatotomy Incision into the prostate gland.

prosthesis The replacement of part of the body by an artificial part such as a denture.

protoplasia The primary formation of tissue.

Proventil Brand name for albuterol; used to expand the air passages in the lungs.

Prozac Brand name for fluoxetine; used to prevent or relieve depression.

psych(o), psych Combining forms denoting the mind or the mental faculties.

psychiatrist (psychiatrics) A specialist in the functional disorders of the mind.

psychogenic Originating or developing in the mind.

psychology The branch of medicine that studies the mind.

psychoneurosis A mental or behavioral disorder that presents symptoms of functional nervous disease.

psychoses A group of severe mental disorders marked by gross impairment in reality testing, typically shown by delusions, hallucinations, incoherent speech, or disorganized or agitated behavior.

psychosexual gender identity disorders Disorders involving a repeated desire to be of the opposite sex or a belief that one was born the wrong sex.

psychosomatic Pertaining to the mind–body relationship.

psychotherapy Treatment of emotional, behavioral, and mental disorders.

pubis One of two bones that connect at the midline of the base of the pelvis.

pulmonary Pertaining to the lungs.

pulmonary disease The branch of medicine that diagnoses and treats diseases of the chest or thorax.

pulmonectomy Excision of all or part of a lung.

pulmonic Pertaining to the lungs.

pulmonitis Inflammation of the lung; pneumonitis.

pulmonologist A lung specialist.

pupil The perforation in the center of the iris.

pupillary Pertaining to a pupil of the eye.

pyel(o) A combining form denoting the pelvis of the kidney.

pyelectasis Dilatation (dilation) of the kidney pelvis.

pyelitis Inflammation of the pelvis of the kidney.

pyelography Roentgenographic study of the kidney and renal collecting system.

pyelolithotomy The operation of removing a renal calculus (kidney stone) from the pelvis of the kidney.

pyelonephritis Inflammation of the pelvis of the kidney.

pyeloscopy Examination or observation of the kidney pelvis via a fluoroscope.

pyosis Abnormal condition of containing pus.

pyromania A morbid compulsion to set fires. Deliberate and purposeful fire-setting that brings a sense of gratification. Not to be confused with arson, which is usually done for a profit motive.

pyuria Presence of pus in the urine.

Q

quadriplegia Paralysis in all four limbs.

quadruped Four-footed, such as many animals.

R

rachialgia Pain in the spine.

rachitis Inflammation of the spine; rickets.

radial keratotomy Incisions made in the cornea from its outer edge toward its center in spokelike fashion; flattens the cornea and corrects myopia.

radiologist (radiology) A specialist in the diagnostic and therapeutic use of radiant energy.

radius The forearm bone connected to the thumb side; the shorter of the two forearm bones.

rectal Pertaining to the rectum.

rectosigmoidectomy Excision of the rectum and the sigmoid.

rectum Distal portion of the large intestine.

rectus abdominus Straight abdominal muscle; supports the abdomen, flexes the lumbar vertebrae.

rectus femoris muscle Straight muscle from the iliac spine to the patella; flexes the thigh.

regurgitate To flow backward; to vomit.

renal Pertaining to a kidney.

renal cortex The outer covering of the kidney.

reniform Kidney shaped.

renocortical Pertaining to the cortex of a kidney.

retina A membrane inside the eye that connects to the optic nerve and transmits light impulses to the brain.

Retin-A Brand name for tretinoin; used to soften the horny layer of the epidermis.

retinal Pertaining to the retina of the eye.

retinitis Inflammation of the retina.

retinopathy Any disease of the retina.

retinoscopy   Visual examination of the retina to look for refractive errors.

retractor   An instrument to draw back and hold the edges of a wound.

retroflexed   Bent backward.

rheumatologist (rheumatology)   A specialist in the diagnosis and treatment of rheumatism, a variety of disorders involving connective tissues (joints and related structures).

rhin(o)   A combining form denoting the nose.

rhinesthesia   Pertaining to the sense of smell.

rhinitis   Inflammation of the mucous membrane of the nose.

rhinocheiloplasty   Plastic surgery on the lip and nose.

rhinodynia   Pain in the nose or nasal area.

rhinolith   A stone or concretion of the nose.

rhinomycosis   Abnormal condition of having fungus in the nose.

rhinoplasty   Plastic surgery of the nose.

rhinorrhagia   Abnormal bleeding from the nose; abnormal nasal hemorrhage.

ribs   Pairs of bones attached to each side of the twelve thoracic vertebrae.

Robitussin   Brand name for guaifenesin; used to alleviate or prevent coughs and to promote the ejection of mucus from the lower respiratory tract.

rods/cones   Photoreceptor cells in the retina of the eye.

Rolaids   Brand name for calcium carbonate; used to neutralize acidity in the stomach.

rubeosis   Redness of an area.

S

sacral   Pertaining to the sacrum.

sacrum   Five fused vertebrae superior to the tailbone.

salping(o)   A combining form denoting the uterine (fallopian) tube or auditory (eustachian) tube.

salpingitis   Inflammation of a uterine tube; inflammation of the eustachian tube.

salpingocele   Hernial protrusion of a uterine tube.

salpingography   Roentgenogram or X-ray picture of the uterine tube.

salpingo-oophorectomy   Excision of the ovary and the uterine tube.

salpingopexy   Surgical fixing or fastening of a uterine tube.

salpingorrhagia   Hemorrhage from a fallopian tube.

salpingorrhaphy   Suture or surgical repair of the uterine tube.

salpingoscopy   Visual examination of the eustachian tube or of the uterine tube.

salpingotomy   Surgical incision into the uterine tube.

sarc(o)   A combining form denoting flesh or connective tissue.

sarcoblast   A primitive or immature cell that develops into connective tissue.

sarcogenic   Forming flesh.

sarcoid   Resembling flesh.

sarcolysis   Destruction or dissolution of flesh.

sarcoma   A tumor of fleshy or connective tissue.

sarcopoietic   Producing flesh or muscle.

sarcosis   Abnormal increase in flesh.

sartorius muscle   The muscle located at the side of the proximal end of the tibia that flexes the thigh and leg; also called the tailor's muscle.

satyriasis   Abnormal, excessive sexual desire in the male.

scapula   Shoulderblade.

schizoid type   A personality disorder in which there is withdrawal from affectional and social contacts.

schizophrenia   A group of major mental disorders characterized by distortion in thinking, bizarre delusions, and hallucinations.

schizotypal type   A personality disorder that appears to be a form of schizoid personality. Individuals with this disorder manifest oddities of thinking, perception, communication, and behavior.

sclera   The white portion of the eyeball.

sebaceous glands   Oil-producing glands in the skin.

Seconal   Brand name for secobarbital; used for short-term treatment of insomnia.

sedatives (hypnotics)   Agents that allay activity and excitement; used for short-term treatment of insomnia.

semicircular canals   Canals located in the inner ear that function to maintain equilibrium during movement.

semicoma   A stupor from which the patient may be aroused.

semilunar   Resembling a crescent or half-moon.

seminal   Pertaining to semen.

seminal vesicles Two membranous pouches that unite with the excretory ducts of the testes; they provide most of the fluid component of semen.

seminiferous Conveying semen.

seminiferous tubules Small coiled tubes inside the testis in which sperm are produced.

seminology The scientific study of semen and spermatozoa.

seminoma Malignant neoplasm of the testis.

septic Pertaining to the presence of pathogenic organisms; toxic.

septicemia Systemic disease associated with the presence and persistence of microorganisms and toxins in the blood.

Serevent Brand name for salmeterol; used to expand the air passages in the lungs.

serotonin A hormone whose function is unclear; a precursor to melatonin; inhibits gastric secretion, serves as a central neurotransmitter.

Sertan Brand name for primidone; used to prevent or relieve convulsions.

sexual deviations Abnormal sexual inclinations or behaviors (paraphilias).

sexual masochism A paraphilia in which sexual gratification is derived from being humiliated or hurt by another.

sexual sadism A paraphilia in which sexual gratification is derived from humiliating or hurting another.

sigmoid A word denoting the S-shaped portion of the colon.

sigmoidectomy Excision of the sigmoid.

sigmoiditis Inflammation of the sigmoid.

sigmoidoscope Illuminated endoscope for examination of the sigmoid.

sinistral Pertaining to the left.

sinistrocardia Location of the heart in the left side of the thorax.

sleep terror disorder Parasomnia marked by panic and confusion when abruptly awakening from sleep.

sleepwalking Recurrent episodes of arising from bed during sleep and walking about.

social phobia Anxiety provoked by exposure to types of social or performance situations. Example: performing in front of others.

Solarcaine Brand name for lidocaine topical; used on the skin to abolish the sensation of pain.

soleus muscle A muscle extending from the fibula, fascia at the back of the knee, to the tibia; flexes the ankle joint.

Solfoton Brand name for phenobarbital; used to prevent or relieve convulsions.

somatic nervous system The part of the peripheral nervous system responsible for voluntary activities.

somatization disorder A disorder marked by multiple physical complaints not fully explained by any known medical condition.

somatoform disorders A group of disorders with symptoms suggesting physical ailments but *without* organic findings evident.

somatotropin Growth hormone.

Sominex 2 Brand name for diphenhydramine; used for short-term treatment of insomnia.

specific phobia Intense fear caused by a specific object or situation. Examples: *claustrophobia*—fear of closed places; *acrophobia*—fear of heights; *ailurophobia*—fear of cats; *xenophobia*—fear of strangers.

sperm Semen; testicular secretion.

sperm(a), sperm(i), sperm(o), spermat(o) Combining forms denoting a seed, usually the male generative element (semen).

spermatic Pertaining to semen.

spermatism Promoting secretion of semen.

spermatocyte A sperm cell.

spermatogenesis The process of producing spermatozoa.

spermatogenic Producing semen or spermatozoa.

spermatolysis Destruction of spermatozoa.

spermatopoietic Pertaining to a condition in which semen is produced or discharged.

spermatorrhea An involuntary discharge of semen without orgasm.

spermicide An agent that is destructive to spermatozoa.

sphenoid bone The winglike structure wedged in the front portion of the cranium.

sphincter A ringlike band of muscle fibers that constricts a passage or closes a natural orifice.

sphygm(o) A combining form denoting the pulse or blood pressure.

sphygmic Pertaining to a pulse.

sphygmoid Resembling the pulse.

sphygmology The study or science of the pulse.

sphygmomanometer An instrument for measuring blood pressure.

sphygmopalpation Palpating or feeling the pulse.

sphygmoscopy Examination of the pulse.

splen(o) A combining form denoting the spleen.

splenatrophy Atrophy or wasting away of the spleen.

splenectomy Excision or removal of the spleen.

splenic Pertaining to the spleen.

splenocele Herniation or swelling of the spleen.

splenohepatomegaly Enlargement of the spleen and liver.

splenomegaly Abnormally large spleen.

splenophrenic Pertaining to the spleen and diaphragm.

splenorrhagia Bleeding or hemorrhage from the spleen.

spondyl(o) A combining form indicating the vertebrae or spinal column.

spondylitis Inflammation of a vertebra.

spondylosis Degenerative disease of the vertebrae.

Sporanox Brand name for itraconazole; used to destroy fungus or suppress its growth.

stapes The bone shaped like a stirrup, located in the middle ear, that transmits vibrations to the cochlea.

steatorrhea An excessive amount of fats in the feces; usually results from malabsorption syndrome.

sternocleidomastoid muscle The muscle that connects the sternum to the clavicle and the mastoid process; pulls the head laterally and toward chest, and raises breastbone.

sternum The breastbone, located in the front midline of the chest.

stomatalgia Pain in the mouth.

stomatic Pertaining to the mouth.

stomatitis Inflammation of the oral mucosa.

stomatology The study of the science of the mouth.

stomatopathy Any disease of the mouth.

stomatoplasty Plastic surgery of the mouth.

stomatoscope An instrument for visual examination of the mouth.

streptokinase A generic agent used to dissolve blood clots or to thin the blood.

subcutaneous Located beneath the cutis; the innermost layer of skin tissue.

sublingual Under the tongue.

sudoriferous glands Sweat-producing glands in the skin.

superior A directional term meaning located above something.

suprarenal Above the kidney; adrenal gland.

supratympanic Situated above the tympanum.

surgeon A specialist in treating pathologic or traumatic conditions by operative procedures.

surgery The branch of medicine that treats pathologic or traumatic conditions by operative procedures.

symbiotic psychosis A condition found in 2- to 4-year-old children with an abnormal relationship to a mothering figure, marked by autism and regression.

sympathetic nerves The part of the autonomic nervous system that prepare the body for stress and action; slows digestion and increases heart rate.

syndesm(o) A combining form denoting ligaments.

syndesmectomy Excision or resection of a ligament.

syndesmopexy Surgical reattachment of a ligament.

syphilis A sexually transmitted disease caused by the bacterium *Treponema pallidum*.

systole The active phase of contraction of the heart.

systolic pressure The pressure of the active phase of contraction of the heart; the higher of the two blood pressures.

T

tachycardia Excessive rapidity in the action of the heart, usually in the pulse rate.

tachypnea Abnormally fast rate of breathing.

Tagamet Brand name for cimetidine; used to neutralize acidity in the stomach.

tarsals Ankle bones.

temporal bone The bone connected to the parietal bone and the base of the skull.

ten(o), **tend(o)** Combining forms denoting a tendon.

tenalgia Pain in a tendon.

tendinitis Inflammation of a tendon.

tendon Connective tissue within muscle that attaches to the periosteum of the bone.

tertian Recurring every third day.

Tessalon Perles Brand name for benzonatate; used to alleviate or prevent coughs and to promote the ejection of mucus from the lower respiratory tract.

testicular Pertaining to the testis.

testis Male gonad; endocrine gland that produces testosterone.

testitis Inflammation of the testis; orchitis.

testosterone A hormone that promotes the development of male sexual characteristics; affects reproduction.

tetradactyly The condition of having four digits on the hands or feet.

thorac(o) A combining form denoting the chest or thorax.

thoracentesis Surgical puncture of the chest wall for aspiration of fluids; thoracocentesis.

thoracic Pertaining to the chest.

thoracic surgeon (thoracic surgery) A specialist in the diagnosis and treatment (mainly surgical) of disorders of the organs of the thoracic cavity, generally the heart and lungs.

thoracocentesis Surgical puncture of the chest wall for aspiration of fluids; thoracentesis.

thoracotomy Incision into the chest.

Thorazine Brand name for chlorpromazine; used to treat psychoses; a major tranquilizer.

thromb(o) A combining form indicating a blood clot, or thrombus.

thrombectomy Excision of a blood clot or thrombus.

thrombin A generic agent used to arrest the flow of blood.

thromboarteritis Inflammation of an artery with a clot present.

thromboclasis Breaking down a blood clot.

thrombocytes Clotting cells; platelets.

thrombolytic An agent that dissolves or splits a blood clot.

thrombopathy Disease involving the clotting cells.

thrombophlebitis Inflammation of a vein in which a clot is present.

thrombopoiesis The formation of clotting cells.

thrombosis The formation of clots or thrombi.

thymectomy Excision of the thymus gland.

thymic Pertaining to the thymus gland.

thymitis Inflammation of the thymus gland.

thymopathy Any disease of the thymus gland.

thymosin A hormone that regulates immune response.

thymus An endocrine gland located in the area between the lungs and behind the sternum; secretes the hormone thymosin

thyr(o) A combining form denoting the thyroid gland.

thyrocele A thyroid tumor; goiter.

thyroid gland The largest endocrine gland, located in the neck below the larynx; produces thyronine, triiodothyronine, and calcitonin.

thyroidectomy Excision of the thyroid gland.

thyroidotomy Incision into the thyroid gland.

thyroid-stimulating hormone Stimulates thyroid secretion; TSH.

thyropathy Any disease of the thyroid gland.

thyrotoxic Pertaining to toxic levels of thyroid hormones.

thyrotoxicosis Overproduction of thyroid hormones.

thyroxin (T4) Tetraiodothyronine; a hormone that regulates metabolism.

tibia Shinbone.

topical anesthetics Agents used on the skin to abolish the sensation of pain.

trache(o) A combining form indicating the trachea or windpipe.

tracheitis Inflammation of the trachea.

tracheopathy Any disease of the trachea.

tracheoplasty Plastic surgery on the trachea.

tracheorrhaphy Surgical repair or suture of the trachea.

tracheostenosis Narrowing of the trachea.

tracheostomy Surgical creation of an opening into the trachea.

tracheotomy Incision into the trachea.

transabdominal Through the abdominal wall.

transdermal Through the skin.

transfusion Transfer of blood components from a donor to a receptor.

transvestism "Cross-dressing"; the practice of wearing articles of clothing commonly worn by the opposite sex.

trapezius muscle A muscle located in the back shoulder region that raises the shoulder and arm.

Trasylol Brand name for aprotinin; used to arrest the flow of blood.

triceps muscle The three-headed muscle at the side and middle of the forearm; extends the forearm, extends the arm.

trich, trich(o)   Combining forms indicating the hair or capillary (hairlike) vessels.

trichalgia   Pain when the hair is touched.

trichogenous   Promoting growth of hair.

trichoglossia   A hairy condition of the tongue.

trichology   The study of the hair.

trichomonas   A sexually transmitted disease caused by the bacterium *Trichomonas vaginalis*.

trichomycosis   A fungus infection of the hair.

trichopathy   A disease of the hair.

trichoschisis   Splitting of the hair.

tricuspid valve   A heart valve with three leaflets.

triiodothyronine (T3)   A hormone that regulates metabolism.

Tri-Norinyl   Brand name for estrogen and progestin; used to prevent conception or impregnation.

triorchidism   The condition of having three testes.

Tums   Brand name for calcium carbonate; used to neutralize acidity in the stomach.

Tylenol   Brand name for acetaminophen; used to relieve pain.

tympanic   Pertaining to the tympanic membrane or the eardrum.

tympanic cavity   The middle ear.

tympanic membrane   The eardrum.

tympanotomy   Incision into the tympanic membrane, or eardrum.

U

ulna   The longer of the two forearm bones.

ultrasonic   Having a frequency above sound.

unilateral   Pertaining to or affecting only one side.

ureter   The tube that connects the kidney to the urinary bladder.

ureteral   Pertaining to the ureter.

ureteralgia   Pain in the ureter.

ureterectasis   Distension of the ureter.

ureterectomy   Excision of a ureter.

ureterolith   A stone/calculus in the ureter.

ureterolithiasis   Formation of stones/calculi in the ureter.

ureteropathy   Any disease of the ureter.

ureteroplasty   Plastic surgery of the ureter.

urethra   The tube that connects the urinary bladder to the outside of the body.

urethral   Pertaining to the urethra.

urethrectomy   Excision of all or part of the urethra.

urethritis   Inflammation of the urethra.

urethrophraxis   Obstruction of the urethra.

urethroplasty   Plastic surgery of the urethra.

urethrorrhagia   Excessive bleeding from the urethra.

urethrorrhaphy   Suturing of the urethra.

urethrospasm   Spasm of the urethra.

-uria   A suffix denoting urine or urination.

uricosurics   Agents that promote the excretion of uric acid in the urine; used in the treatment of gout.

Urogesic   Brand name for phenazopyridine; used to eliminate urinary spasms.

urologist (urology)   A specialist in the diagnosis and treatment of disorders and diseases of the urinary system in both sexes and the genital system in the male.

uterocervical   Relating to the cervix of the uterus.

uterogenic   Formed in the uterus.

uteroplasty   Plastic surgery of the uterus.

uterus   A pear-shaped organ designed to hold and to nourish a developing fetus.

V

vaginal   Pertaining to the vagina.

vaginitis   Inflammation of the vagina; colpitis.

vaginopathy   Any disease of the vagina.

vaginoscopy   Visual examination of the vagina.

Valium   Brand name for diazepam; used to reduce or eliminate anxiety; a minor tranquilizer; also used to prevent or relieve convulsions.

vas(o)   A combining form denoting a vessel or duct.

vascular   Pertaining to blood vessels or indicating a copious blood supply.

vasculitis   Inflammation of vessels, especially blood vessels.

vasculopathy   Any disease of blood vessels.

vasectomy   Surgical removal of all or part of the ductus (vas) deferens.

vasodilator   An agent that causes dilation of a blood vessel.

vasodilators   Agents that dilate blood vessels.

vasography   X-ray picture, or roentgenography, of the blood vessels.

vasorrhaphy   Suture of the ductus (vas) deferens.

vasospasm   Contraction of a vessel.

vasotomy   An incision into the ductus (vas) deferens.

veins   Blood vessels that return blood to the heart.

vena, venae   Singular and plural terms referring to a vein or veins.

venipuncture   Surgical puncture of a vein.

venous   Pertaining to a vein.

ventricles   The two heart chambers that pump the blood.

Versed   Brand name for midazolam; used to reduce or eliminate the perception of sensation.

vertebral   Pertaining to the vertebrae.

vertebrocostal   Pertaining to the vertebrae and the ribs.

vesiculectomy   Excision of a vesicle, especially a seminal vesicle.

vesiculitis   Inflammation of a vesicle, especially a seminal vesicle.

vesiculotomy   Incision into a vessel, especially a seminal vesicle.

Viagra   Brand name for sildenafil; used to enhance erectile function of the penis.

Vicodin   Brand name for hydrocodone; used to relieve pain.

vitreous humor   A gelatinous fluid in the posterior (vitreous chamber) cavity of the eye that works with the aqueous humor and the lens to refract light.

voluntary muscles   Skeletal muscles that you can move at will.

voyeurism   A disorder marked by recurrent sexual urges to watch unsuspecting people who are naked, disrobing, or engaging in sexual activities; "peeping Tom".

vulva   The external female genitalia; the mons pubis, the labia, Bartholin's glands, and the clitoris.

W

warfarin   A generic agent used to dissolve blood clots or to thin the blood.

X

Xanax   Brand name for alprazolam; used to reduce or eliminate anxiety; a minor tranquilizer.

xanthochromic   Denoting a yellow discoloration of the skin or spinal fluid.

xanthoderma   Any yellow discoloration of the skin.

Xylocaine   Brand name for lidocaine topical; used on the skin to abolish the sensation of pain.

Z

Zantac   Brand name for ranitidine; used to neutralize acidity in the stomach.

Zestril   Brand name for lisinopril; used to counteract high blood pressure.

Zithromax   Brand name for azithromycin; used to kill infectious agents or prevent them from spreading.

Zocor   Brand name for simvastatin; used to counteract high levels of lipids in the blood.

Zoloft   Brand name for sertaline; used to prevent or relieve depression.

zoophilia   A disorder involving sexual activity with animals.

zoophobia   Abnormal fear or dread of animals.

zygomatic bone   Cheekbone.

Zyloprim   Brand name for allopurinol; used in the treatment of gout.

Zyrtec   Brand name for cetirizine; used to treat allergies.

Index

sarcolysis, 89
sarcoma, 89
sarcopoietic, 89
sarcosis, 90
sartorius, 406, 407
satyriasis, 485
scapula, 390, 395
-schesis, 515
-schisis, 515
schizoid type, 474
schizophrenia, 481
schizotypal type, 474
sciatic nerve, 335
-scirrhus, 515
sclera, 422, 423
sclero-, 510
-sclerosis, 515
-scope, 4, 515
-scopy, 7, 515
scrotum, 268, 269–270
sebaceous gland, 80, 81
secretory glands, 140
-sect(ion), 515
sedatives
    nervous system, 343
    psychiatric conditions, 491
semen, 281
semi-, 510
semicircular canals, 422, 433
semicoma, 61
semilunar, 58
seminal, 281
seminal vesicle, 268, 269, 277–278
seminiferous, 281
seminiferous tubules, 268
seminology, 281
seminoma, 281
sensory neurons, 326
-sepsis, 515
septic, 5
septicemia, 211
serotonin, 372
serum albumin, 208
serum globulin, 208
sexual deviation, 485
sexual identity disorders, 485
sexually transmitted diseases
    female reproductive system,
        296, 511
    male reproductive system and,
        268, 511
sexual masochism, 485
sexual sadism, 485
sigmoid, 154
sigmoid colon, 140, 153
sigmoidectomy, 154
sigmoiditis, 154
sigmoidoscope, 154
sinistral, 38
sinistro-, 38, 510
sinistrocardia, 38
skeletal muscles, 388
skeletal system. See
    musculoskeletal system
skin, 80, 81–82
skull bones, 389, 390–391
sleep disorders, 486
sleep terror disorder, 486
sleepwalking, 486
small intestine, 140, 141,
    147–150
smooth muscles, 388
social phobia, 477
sodium, 367–368
soft palate, 109, 142

soleus, 405, 406, 407
somat-, 510
somatic nervous system, 326
somatization disorder, 478
somatoform disorders, 477
somatotropin, 371
-spasm, 515
specific phobia, 477
sperm, 268, 281
sperm(a), 281
spermatic, 281
spermat(o), 281
spermatocyte, 281
spermatogenesis, 281
spermatolysis, 281
spermatopoietic, 281
spermatorrhea, 281
sperm(i), 281
spermicide, 281
sphenoid, 391
sphenoid bone, 389
sphincter muscles, 148
sphincters, 140
sphygmic, 194
sphygm(o), 193–194
sphygmoid, 193
sphygmology, 193
sphygmomanometer, 176,
    193, 194
sphygmopalpation, 194
sphygmoscopy, 194
spinal cord, 326, 327,
    331–332
spine, 399–400
spleen, 208, 219–220
splenatrophy, 220
splenectomy, 220
splenic, 220
splen(o), 220
splenocele, 220
splenohepatomegaly, 220
splenomegaly, 14
splenophrenic, 220
splenorrhagia, 220
spondylitis, 400
spondyl(o), 400
spondylosis, 400
stapes, 422, 433
-stasis, 515
-stat, 515
steat(o), 93
steatorrhea, 93
steno-, 510
-stenosis, 19, 515
sternocleidomastoid, 405, 406
sternum, 390, 391
steroid hormones, 372
-sthenia, 515
stomach, 140, 141, 147–150, 219
stomatalgia, 142
stomatic, 142
stomatitis, 142
stomat(o), 142
stomatopathy, 142
stomatoplasty, 7, 142
stomatoscope, 142
-stomy, 515
sub-, 510
subcutaneous layer, 80, 81
sublingual, 61, 143
suffixes, 3–4
    diagnosis, symptoms and
        procedures, 7–8
    dilation, constriction, narrowing
        and deficiencies, 17–18

diseases and abnormal
    conditions, 13–14
superior vena cava, 177
supra-, 32, 511
suprarenal, 32, 241
supratympanic, 32, 61
surgeon, 459
surgery, 459
suspensory ligaments, 423
sweat, 93–94
symbiotic psychosis, 482
sympathetic nerves, 326
symphysis pubis, 269, 297
syn-, 511
syndesmopexy, 8
systemic circulation, 185
systole, 194
systolic, 194
systolic pressure, 176

tachy-, 511
tachycardia, 180
tachypnea, 123
tarsals, 390, 396
tear gland, 429–430
tear sac, 430
tele-, 511
temporal, 391
temporal bone, 389
tenalgia, 408
tendinitis, 408
tendons, 388, 405–408
ter-, 511
tertian, 61
testes, 268, 269–270, 354,
    355, 373
testicular, 270
testis, 270
testitis, 270
testosterone, 268, 373
tetra-, 511
tetradactyly, 57
-therapy, 515
thoracic, 5, 123, 391
thoracic bones, 391
thoracic curvature, 399
thoracic surgeon, 459
thoracic surgery, 459
thoracic vertebrae, 399
thorac(o), 123
thoracocentesis, 123
thoracotomy, 7, 123
thorax, 108
throat, 113–114,
    141–143
thrombectomy, 8, 216
thromb(o), 216
thromboclasis, 22
thrombocyte, 208, 215, 216
thrombolytic, 216
thrombolytics
    cardiovascular
        system, 197
thrombopathy, 216
thrombophlebitis, 216
thrombopoiesis, 216
thrombosis, 216
thymectomy, 363
thymic, 363
thymitis, 363
thym(o), 363
thymopathy, 363
thymosin, 372

thymus, 208, 219, 354, 355, 363–
    364, 372
thyr(o), 359
thyrocele, 14, 359
thyroidectomy, 359
thyroid gland, 219, 354, 355,
    359–360, 372
thyroid hormone
    endocrine system, 377
thyroidotomy, 359
thyroid-stimulating
    hormone, 371
thyropathy, 359
thyrotoxic, 359
thyroxine, 372
tibia, 388, 390, 396
-tomy, 7, 515
tongue, 109, 141–143
tonsils, 208
topical anesthetics
    integumentary system, 97
-toxic(in), 515
trachea, 108, 109, 117–118,
    122, 219
tracheitis, 117
tracheopathy, 117
tracheoplasty, 117
tracheorrhaphy, 117
tracheostenosis, 117
tracheostomy, 117
tracheotomy, 7, 117
trach(o), 117
-tractor, 515
tranquilizers, major
    nervous system, 343
    psychiatric conditions, 491
tranquilizers, minor
    nervous system, 343
    psychiatric conditions, 491
trans-, 33, 38, 511
transabdominal, 38
transdermal, 38
transfusion, 5
transverse colon, 140, 153
transvestism, 485
trapezius, 406
tri-, 33, 42, 511
triceps, 407
triceps brachii, 406
trich, 85
trichalgia, 85
trich(o), 85
trichogenous, 85
trichoglossia, 85
trichology, 85
trichomycosis, 85
trichopathy, 85
trichoschisis, 85
triiodothyronine, 372
triorchidism, 42, 57
-tripsy, 5, 515
-trophy, 515
tympanic, 437
tympanic cavity, 422, 433
tympanic membrane,
    422, 433
tympan(o), 437
tympanotomy, 437

ulna, 390, 395
ulnar nerve, 335
ultra-, 511
ultrasonic, 62